Mood Disorders

Mood Disorders

Brain Imaging and Therapeutic Implications

Edited by

Sudhakar Selvaraj
McGovern Medical School at UTHealth, Houston, TX

Paolo Brambilla
University of Milan, Italy

Jair C. Soares
McGovern Medical School at UTHealth, Houston, TX

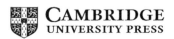

CAMBRIDGE
UNIVERSITY PRESS

CAMBRIDGE
UNIVERSITY PRESS

University Printing House, Cambridge CB2 8BS, United Kingdom

One Liberty Plaza, 20th Floor, New York, NY 10006, USA

477 Williamstown Road, Port Melbourne, VIC 3207, Australia

314–321, 3rd Floor, Plot 3, Splendor Forum, Jasola District Centre,
New Delhi – 110025, India

79 Anson Road, #06–04/06, Singapore 079906

Cambridge University Press is part of the University of Cambridge.

It furthers the University's mission by disseminating knowledge in the pursuit
of education, learning, and research at the highest international levels of excellence.

www.cambridge.org
Information on this title: www.cambridge.org/9781108427128
DOI: 10.1017/9781108623018

© Cambridge University Press 2021

First published 2021

Printed in the United Kingdom by TJ Books Limited, Padstow Cornwall

A catalogue record for this publication is available from the British Library.

Library of Congress Cataloging-in-Publication Data
Names: Selvaraj, Sudhakar, editor. | Brambilla, Paolo, editor. | Soares, Jair C., editor.
Title: Mood disorders : brain imaging and therapeutic implications /
edited by Sudhakar Selvaraj, Paolo Brambilla, Jair Soares.
Description: Cambridge, United Kingdom ; New York, NY : Cambridge University Press, 2020. |
Includes bibliographical references and index.
Identifiers: LCCN 2020022964 (print) | LCCN 2020022965 (ebook) | ISBN 9781108427128 (hardback) |
ISBN 9781108623018 (ebook)
Subjects: LCSH: Affective disorders – Imaging. | Affective disorders – Treatment. | Brain – Imaging.
Classification: LCC RC537 .M6635 2020 (print) | LCC RC537 (ebook) | DDC 616.85/2707548–dc23
LC record available at https://lccn.loc.gov/2020022964
LC ebook record available at https://lccn.loc.gov/2020022965

ISBN 978-1-108-42712-8 Hardback

....

Every effort has been made in preparing this book to provide accurate and up-to-date information that is in accord with accepted standards and practice at the time of publication. Although case histories are drawn from actual cases, every effort has been made to disguise the identities of the individuals involved. Nevertheless, the authors, editors, and publishers can make no warranties that the information contained herein is totally free from error, not least because clinical standards are constantly changing through research and regulation. The authors, editors, and publishers therefore disclaim all liability for direct or consequential damages resulting from the use of material contained in this book. Readers are strongly advised to pay careful attention to information provided by the manufacturer of any drugs or equipment that they plan to use.

Contents

Section 5 Therapeutic Applications of Neuroimaging in Mood Disorders

Colour plates can be found between pages 148 and 149

Contributors

Amit Anand
Center for Behavioral Health Cleveland Clinic
and Lerner School of Medicine of Case Western
Reserve University, Ohio, USA

Danilo Arnone
Department of Psychiatry and Behavioral Science,
College of Medicine and Health Sciences,
United Arab Emirates University, Al Ain, UAE and
Centre for Affective Disorders, Psychological
Medicine, Institute of Psychiatry, Psychology and
Neuroscience, King's College London,
London, UK

Isabelle E. Bauer
Louis A. Faillace, MD Department of Psychiatry
and Behavioral Sciences, McGovern Medical School
University of Texas Health Science Center at
Houston, Texas, USA

Francesco Benedetti
Vita-Salute San Raffaele University, Milan, Italy

Paolo Brambilla
University of Milan, Milan, Italy, Psychiatric
Clinic at Fondazione IRCCS Ca' Granda Ospedale
Maggiore Policlinico, Milan, Italy, USA

Jungwon Cha
Center for Behavioral Health Cleveland Clinic
and Lerner School of Medicine of Case Western
Reserve University, Ohio, USA

Ziqi Chen
Huaxi MR Research Center (HMRRC),
Department of Radiology, West China Hospital of
Sichuan University, Chengdu, PR China

Raymond Y. Cho
Baylor College of Medicine, Department of
Psychiatry and Behavioral Sciences
Houston, TX, USA

Philip J. Cowen
Psychopharmacology Research Unit (PPRU),
University Department of Psychiatry, University
of Oxford, UK

Beata R. Godlewska
Psychopharmacology Research Unit (PPRU),
University Department of Psychiatry, University
of Oxford, UK

Qiyong Gong
Huaxi MR Research Center (HMRRC),
Department of Radiology, West China Hospital of
Sichuan University, Chengdu, PR China

Sameer Jauhar
Department of Psychological Medicine, Institute
of Psychiatry, Psychology and Neuroscience,
King's College, London, UK

Su Hyun Jeong
McGovern Medical School, The University of
Texas Health Science Center at Houston,
Houston, TX, USA

Yueyi Jiang
Laboratory for Affective and Translational
Neuroscience; McLean Hospital/Harvard Medical
School, Massachusetts, USA

Vivian Kafantaris
Donald and Barbara Zucker School of Medicine at
Hofstra/Northwell, Department of Psychiatry,
Hempstead, NY, USA; Northwell Health System –
The Zucker Hillside Hospital, Department of
Psychiatry, Glen Oaks, NY, USA; Feinstein
Institute for Medical Research, Manhasset,
NY, USA

Jasmine Kaur
Donald and Barbara Zucker School of Medicine at
Hofstra/Northwell, Department of Psychiatry,

Hempstead, NY, USA; Northwell Health System –
The Zucker Hillside Hospital, Department of
Psychiatry, Glen Oaks, NYPark Center, Inc.,
Psychiatric Medical Services, Fort Wayne,
Indiana, USA

Brent M. Kiou
Department of Psychiatry, University of Utah,
Salt Lake City, USA

Poornima Kumar
Laboratory for Affective and Translational
Neuroscience, McLean Hospital/Harvard Medical
School, Massachusetts, USA

David E.J. Linden
Department of Psychiatry and Neuropsychology,
School for Mental Health and Neuroscience,
Maastricht University Medical Centre,
Maastricht, NL

Rodrigo Machado-Vieira
Experimental Therapeutics and Molecular
Pathophysiology Program, Louis A. Faillace, MD
Department of Psychiatry and Behavioral
Sciences, McGovern Medical School
University of Texas Health Science Center at
Houston, Texas, USA

Koji Matsuo
Department of Psychiatry, Saitama Medical
University, Moroyama, Iruma, Saitama, Japan

Toshio Matsubara
Division of Neuropsychiatry, Department of
Neuroscience, Yamaguchi University Graduate
School of Medicine, Ube, Yamaguchi, Japan
Health Service Center, Yamaguchi University
Organization for University Education,
Yamaguchi, Yamaguchi, Japan

Elena Mazza
Vita-Salute San Raffaele University, Milan, Italy

Colm McDonald
Centre for Neuroimaging & Cognitive Genomics
(NICOG), Clinical Neuroimaging Laboratory,
NCBES Galway Neuroscience Centre, National
University of Ireland, Galway, Ireland

Jeffrey H. Meyer
Brain Imaging Health Centre, Family Mental
Health Imaging Centre, CAMH Department of
Psychiatry, University of Toronto, Toronto,

Ontario, Canada Department of Pharmacology
and Toxicology, University of Toronto, Toronto,
Ontario, Canada

Thomas D. Meyer
Louis A. Faillace, MD Department of Psychiatry
and Behavioral Sciences, McGovern Medical
School University of Texas Health Science Center
at Houston, Texas, USA

Nicholas Murphy
Baylor College of Medicine, Department of
Psychiatry and Behavioral Sciences
Houston, TX, USA

Benson Mwangi
Louis A. Faillace, MD Department of Psychiatry
and Behavioral Sciences, McGovern Medical
School University of Texas Health Science Center
at Houston, Texas, USA

Allison C Nugent
Magnetoencephalography Core Facility, National
Institute of Mental Health, National Institutes of
Health, Bethesda, Maryland, NIMH, NIH, MD,
USA

Maria Concepcion Garcia Otaduy
University of Sao Paulo, School of Medicine

Mary Melissa Packer
Stanford University, Department of Psychiatry
and Behavioral Sciences, Stanford, CA, USA

James J. Peters
VA Medical Center, Mental Health Patient Care
Center and Mental Illness Research Education
Clinical Center (MIRECC), Bronx, NY, USA

Sara Poletti
Vita-Salute San Raffaele University, Milan, Italy

Nithya Ramakrishnan
Baylor College of Medicine, Department of
Psychiatry and Behavioral Sciences
Houston, TX, USA

Perry F. Renshaw
Diagnostic Neuroimaging, Department of
Psychiatry, University of Utah, Salt Lake City,
USA

Estêvão Scotti-Muzzi
Faculty of Medicine, University of Sao Paulo, Sao
Paulo, Brazil

Sudhakar Selvaraj
Depression Research Program, Louis A. Faillace, MD Department of Psychiatry and Behavioral Sciences, McGovern Medical School University of Texas Health Science Center at Houston, Texas, USA

Manpreet K. Singh
Stanford University, Department of Psychiatry and Behavioral Sciences, Stanford, CA, USA

Leon Skottnik
Department of Psychiatry and Neuropsychology, School for Mental Health and Neuroscience, Maastricht University Medical Centre, Maastricht, NL

Jair C. Soares
Professor and Chairman, Pat R. Rutherford Chair in Psychiatry, Louis A. Faillace, MD Department of Psychiatry and Behavioral Sciences; Executive Director, UT Harris County Psychiatric Center; Director, UT Center of Excellence on Mood Disorders, UTHealth School of Medicine, Houston, TX, USA

Márcio Gerhardt Soeiro-de-Souza
University of Sao Paulo, School of Medicine, Sao Paulo, Brazil

Philip R. Szeszko
Icahn School of Medicine at Mount Sinai, Department of Psychiatry, New York, NY; James J. Peters VA Medical Center, Mental Health Patient Care Center and Mental Illness Research Education Clinical Center (MIRECC), Bronx, NY, USA

Whitney Tang
Stanford University, Department of Psychiatry and Behavioral Sciences, Stanford, CA, USA

Natasha Topolski
McGovern Medical School, The University of Texas Health Science Center at Houston, Houston, TX, USA

Giulia Tronchin
Centre for Neuroimaging & Cognitive Genomics (NICOG), Clinical Neuroimaging Laboratory, NCBES Galway Neuroscience Centre, National University of Ireland Galway, H91TK33 Galway, Ireland

Benedetta Vai
Vita-Salute San Raffaele University, Milan, Italy

Alexis E. Whitton
The Black Dog Institute and The University of New South Wales, Sydney, Australia

Preface

Over the past four decades, advances in in vivo brain imaging have transformed our understanding of brain mechanisms involved in mental health processes and psychiatric illnesses. The methods for in vivo brain imaging investigations have become more sophisticated with higher spatial and temporal resolution to study anatomical and functional processes in the in vivo human brain.

Mood disorders are one of the most common mental illnesses that pose a substantial burden to patients, their families, and society in general. Despite the enormous importance of these major health problems and significant progress made in the research, the exact biological causative mechanisms are still elusive. The application of brain imaging methods to study mood disorders has expanded over the years to study different aspects of brain structure and function to understand the underlying biological mechanisms involved in these disorders and the mechanisms of action of available treatments. As the causation of these major psychiatric disorders remains largely unknown, there is considerable hope that these studies will substantially contribute to major advances linked to developments in the fields of genetics, pharmacology, and neurosciences.

Anatomical studies in mood disorders initially involved anatomical computerized tomography (CT) and magnetic resonance image (MRI) studies, but the evolution of high-resolution diffusion-weighted imaging (DTI) based techniques now allows us to map the cortical tracts involved in mood disorders. Functional molecular imaging applications such as single-photon emission computed tomography (SPECT) and positron emission tomography (PET) have started to examine possible abnormalities in biological pathways in addition to studying brain blood flow and metabolism. Functional magnetic resonance imaging (fMRI) has contributed to higher resolution studies of brain networks possibly involved in the pathophysiology of these disorders and potential applications

as biomarkers as well as in treatment. Magnetoencephalography (MEG) imaging technique offers a very direct measurement of neural electrical activity and provides high temporal resolution complementing fMRI. Developments in magnetic resonance spectroscopy (MRS), along with SPECT and PET radiotracer studies as well, have allowed unprecedented in vivo neurochemical investigations of the human brain. Receptor-ligand PET imaging has become an integral component in the central nervous system drug discovery and is routinely employed in antidepressant target validation and therapeutic dosing. The emerging findings from available studies suggest anatomical, functional, and chemical abnormalities in cortical and subcortical brain regions, and in related neuroanatomic circuits possibly involved in mood regulation. This important new area of investigation in neuropsychiatry has been growing rapidly over the past few years.

In conclusion, the application of newly available methods from brain imaging to the study of mood disorders holds substantial promise to elucidate the brain mechanisms implicated in these illnesses. The latest advances in this important research have not yet been reviewed in a comprehensive and authoritative textbook that would provide complete and easily accessible information on the recent developments. This textbook will include chapters from leading authorities in this field and will therefore fill an important gap in the neuropsychiatric literature. It should be an invaluable resource for practitioners in the fields of psychiatry, neurology, primary care medicine, and related mental health professions, as well as researchers, graduate and postgraduate trainees, and students, as a source of the most updated information on new developments in brain imaging applied to the study of brain mechanisms involved in causation of mood disorders and the mechanisms of action of available treatments.

Chapter 1

Brain Imaging Methods in Mood Disorders

Sudhakar Selvaraj, Paolo Brambilla, and Jair C. Soares

1.1 Introduction

Mood disorders are the most common mental illnesses with a lifetime prevalence of up to 20% worldwide (1). Major depressive disorder (MDD) and bipolar disorder (BD) are significant health problems in the United States and worldwide (2). In the United States alone, the lifetime prevalence of MDD is up to 17%, and that of BD about 2.1% (2) that can go up to 4% of individuals with mood episodes not meeting episodic criteria included. Both are chronic illnesses characterized by recurrent episodes of depression and mania and depression in MDD and BD, respectively. Severe and disabling forms of BD and MDD are associated with increased risk of suicide, decline of physical health, and reduced productivity, and both conditions are associated with high rates of completed suicide of up to 8% (3). Furthermore, MDD and BD are associated with substantial economic burden of over $200 billion (4) and $45.2 billion each year (5), respectively, in USA alone that are primarily related to lost productivity (6).

1.2 Clinical Features

Typically the depression symptoms are similar in both conditions and characterized by symptoms such as depressed or irritable mood, tiredness, lack of interest in pleasurable activities, poor sleep and appetite, low self-esteem, cognitive difficulties, and suicidal thoughts. BD is characterized by recurrent periods of elevated and depressed mood and energy levels with marked deficits in cognitive function interspersed with periods of euthymia. Mania and depression episodes are also associated with impairment in reward processing with excessive pleasure-seeking behavior (7). The diagnoses of MDD and BD are primarily clinical and are currently made by the use of clinical interview, or by using reliable diagnostic interviews such as the Diagnostic and Statistical Manual of Mental Disorders, or DSM, and the International Classification of Diseases (ICD). The precise boundary between major depression and BD is a matter of current active research, but patients who suffer from milder forms of mania (hypomania) are now classified as bipolar II disorder. Whether the presence of lesser degrees of mood elevation in patients with major depression should lead to a diagnosis of bipolar spectrum disorder is still uncertain, and more research is required (8, 9). DSM-5 also contains a new illness specifier for "mixed episode" when mania and depression symptoms overlap and thus illustrate the diagnostic complexities when based on clinical signs and symptoms alone.

Furthermore, cognitive deficits, long duration of illness, persistent depression symptoms, and level of education have been associated with employment among people with BD (10, 11) and contribute to poor clinical outcomes in patients. Cognitive deficits (verbal learning, memory, sustained attention, and executive functioning) (12, 13) are present as early in the first manic episode even after clinical remission (14); are unaffected by medication status (15); and are shown to be strongly predictive of subsequent occupational recovery (16).

Current treatments are usually selected on a trial-and-error basis, uninformed by illness- or treatment-specific biomarker (17, 18), with nearly 50% of depressed patients unfortunately not adequately responding to treatment (24, 26). In BD, conventional antidepressants are either not effective (19) or may increase the risk of a switch into mania (20) and thus associated with treatment resistance and substantial morbidity (17). Accordingly, personalizing treatment by developing noninvasive and clinically useful biomarkers of antidepressant response is a critical priority.

1.3 Etiology and Pathophysiology of Mood Disorders

The etiology of mood disorders is multifactorial and is conceived as an illness with a polygenic basis and environmental interactions contributing to the etiology and pathogenesis of the illness. MDD runs in families, and twin and adoption studies have shown that this can be accounted for in some measure by genetic factors (21, 22), although heritability estimates (37%) are substantially less than those for BP (85%) and schizophrenia (83%) (23). Progress in identifying specific genes predisposing to mood disorders through association and linkage studies is still ongoing. Genetic similarities with bipolar I disorder and schizophrenia are high, and so is the correlation of bipolar II disorder with MDD. Genome-wide linkage studies in BP found involvement of biological pathways that include glutamate signaling calcium channels, second messenger systems, and hormonal regulation (24).

The biochemical pathophysiology of depression and BP is not well known. Astute clinical observations and serendipitous discoveries of psychotropic medications led to the neurotransmitter-based theories that dominated the biological research over the last five decades. Monoamine hypothesis suggests that depression is caused by either a functional deficiency of noradrenaline (25–27) or serotonin function, or both, in the central nervous system (28–30). Similarly, dopaminergic models of the mania symptoms are well researched. Pathophysiology of BD is mostly unknown, but disrupted energy metabolism (31) and mitochondrial dysfunction have been proposed as pathophysiology of BD (32–35). Lithium's neurotrophic and neuroprotective effect is thought to be related to the treatment response in BD and changes in glutamate excitatory and inhibitory GABA mechanisms that underlie antiepileptic drugs are also relevant in the treatment of the BD.

1.4 Neuroimaging Techniques

Neuroimaging has played remarkably in the progress of clinical neurological practice and has been widely used in the diagnosis, prognosis, treatment, and monitoring of many neurological conditions. X-rays of the skull were the first neuroimaging tool but now are mostly replaced by the use of newer technologies such as computed tomography (CT scans) and magnetic resonance imaging (MRI). Functional brain activity can be studied using magnetic resonance spectroscopy (MRS), positron emission tomography (PET), and functional magnetic resonance imaging and spectroscopy (fMRI and fMRS). MRI has become a powerful tool in medical practice and research due to its noninvasive approach and the unmatched anatomical detail that it captures. MRI combined with new methods of processing and analysis has transformed the field of structural and functional brain imaging. With the advent of higher-resolution scanners, MRI allows the study of changes in brain volume or size in greater detail than previous imaging techniques such as CT scans. MRI-based fiber tract studies use advanced techniques such as diffusion tensor imaging and magnetization transfer to study white matter integrity and fiber tracts involved in functional integration between anatomically separate cortical regions. Positron emission tomography is a three-dimensional imaging technique based on nuclear medicine principles to study biological, pharmacological, and physiological functions in vivo. Positron emission tomography, when combined with a suitable radiotracer, can be a potent tool to study a protein target such as receptors, transporters, enzymes, or similar biological targets. The uptake of (18 F) Fludeoxyglucose (18 F-FDG) by tissues has been widely used in clinical medicine as a marker for the tissue glucose uptake correlating with metabolism. Magnetoencephalography (MEG) and Electroencephalogram (EEG) are combined with other imaging modalities and used to study electrical brain signals and for mapping brain activity. Now, neurological diagnostic examination often involves neuroimaging to investigate brain tumors, degeneration, vascular and other lesions, and functional changes.

1.5 Clinical Applications of Neuroimaging

Multiple sclerosis (MS) is a good case example of the clinical application of neuroimaging. Multiple sclerosis is a chronic, progressive, relapsing, and remitting neurological disease characterized by damage to myelin and axons of the central nervous system causing several motor, sensory, and cognitive consequences, and also highly comorbid with mood disorders. MRI has remarkably transformed the clinical diagnosis, treatment, and prognosis. It helped to establish the evidence of structural and functional lesions in MS and thus is widely used as a disease biomarker (36, 37). Until the 1980s, the diagnosis of MS was mainly made using clinical features but now it is primarily MRI based using McDonald's criteria (38).

Our understanding of putative neural substrates and pathophysiology of MDD and BD is increasingly advanced by imaging technology. Studies utilizing these techniques continue to provide growing insight into the pathophysiology of BD. MRI brain anatomical studies show widespread cortical and subcortical brain volume changes and increased rates of deep white matter hyperintensities in BD. Although several brain regions have been implicated as abnormal using MRI in BD, the prefrontal cortex (PFC) is of particular interest, and several studies have uncovered structural pathology in the PFC among patients with BD. These volume changes are consistent with postmortem studies that found reductions in neuronal size and neuropil volume in the hippocampus and reductions in glial cell numbers in PFC (39) and brain volume in BD patients (40). Functional MRI studies consistently found alterations in cortico-limbic-striatal responses to emotional stimuli in mood disorders in frontal, amygdalar, and striatal regions in response to negative stimuli when compared to positive stimuli (41). Deficits in cognitive control, memory, and attention are consistently observed in adults and children with BD and their family members, which indicates that dysfunctions in fronto-limbic and temporal circuitry and cognitive impairment are endophenotypic markers for BD (42). Mania and depression episodes are also associated with excessive pleasure-seeking behavior and reduced hedonic capacity, respectively, which suggests alterations in neural processing and regulation of reward function (7, 43). These findings support the hypothesis of a shared, interactive brain network for cognition and mood. Emerging neuropsychological and functional brain imaging studies suggest abnormalities in reward processing in patients with BD even during euthymic periods (7). Thus neuroimaging uncovers several areas of brain function abnormalities and may help develop a more comprehensive and evidence-based assessment of mood disorder symptoms.

1.6 Conclusion

Mood disorders, both MDD and BD, are devastating illnesses with deleterious functional and social consequences for both the affected individuals and their families. Multiple lines of evidence suggest anatomical alternations and impairment of neurocircuitry in the critical mood and cognitive circuits. Advances in neuroimaging have made phenomenal changes in the practice of neurology. Similar changes in the clinical practice of psychiatry are long overdue. The application of newly available methods from brain imaging to the study of mood disorders holds substantial promise to elucidate the brain mechanisms implicated in these illnesses. Neuroimaging combined with other developments in the field of clinical neuroscience can leapfrog the current deficits in our understanding of mood disorders and help develop biological markers and evidence-based treatments.

References

1. Kessler RC, Angermeyer M, Anthony JC, et al. Lifetime prevalence and age-of-onset distributions of mental disorders in the world health organization's world mental health survey initiative. *World Psychiatry*. 2007; **6**(3): 168–176.

2. Merikangas KR, Akiskal HS, Angst J, et al. Lifetime and 12-month prevalence of bipolar spectrum disorder in the national comorbidity survey replication. *Arch Gen Psychiatry*. 2007; **64**(5): 543–552.

3. Nordentoft M, Mortensen PB, Pedersen CB. Absolute risk of suicide after first hospital contact in mental disorder. *Arch Gen Psychiatry*. 2011; **68**(10): 1058–1064.

4. Greenberg PE, Fournier AA, Sisitsky T, Pike CT, Kessler RC. The economic burden of adults with major depressive disorder in the United States (2005 and 2010). *J Clin Psychiatry*. 2015; **76**(2): 155–162.

5. Cloutier M, Greene M, Guerin A, Touya M, Wu E. The economic burden of bipolar I disorder in the United States in 2015. *Journal of affective disorders*. 2018; **226**: 45–51.

6. Wyatt RJ, Henter I. An economic evaluation of manic-depressive illness–1991. *Soc Psychiatry Psychiatr Epidemiol*. 1995; **30**(5): 213–219.

7. Pizzagalli DA, Goetz E, Ostacher M, Iosifescu DV, Perlis RH. Euthymic patients with bipolar disorder show decreased reward learning in a probabilistic reward task. *Biol Psychiatry*. 2008; **64**(2): 162–168.

8. Angst J. The emerging epidemiology of hypomania and bipolar II disorder. *J Affect Disord*. 1998; **50**(2–3): 143–151.

9. Akiskal HS, Bourgeois ML, Angst J, et al. Re-evaluating the prevalence of and diagnostic composition within the broad clinical spectrum of bipolar disorders. *J Affect Disord*. 2000; **59** Suppl 1: S5–S30.

10. Gilbert E, Marwaha S. Predictors of employment in bipolar disorder: A systematic review. *Journal of affective disorders*. 2013; **145**(2): 156–164.

11. Tse S, Chan S, Ng KL, Yatham LN. Meta-analysis of predictors of favorable employment outcomes among individuals with bipolar disorder. *Bipolar disorders*. 2014; **16**(3): 217–229.

12. Quraishi S, Frangou S. Neuropsychology of bipolar disorder: A review. *Journal of Affective Disorders*. 2002; **72**(3): 209–226.

13. Robinson LJ, Thompson JM, Gallagher P, et al. A meta-analysis of cognitive deficits in euthymic patients with bipolar disorder. *Journal of Affective Disorders*. 2006; **93**(1–3): 105–115.

14. Torres IJ, Defreitas VG, Defreitas CM, et al. Neurocognitive functioning in patients with bipolar I disorder recently recovered from a first manic episode. *J Clin Psychiatry*. 2010 September; **71**(9):1234–1242.

15. Pavuluri MN, Schenkel LS, Aryal S, et al. Neurocognitive function in unmedicated manic and medicated euthymic pediatric bipolar patients. *Am J Psychiatry*. 2006; **163**(2): 286–293.

16. Bearden CE, Shih VH, Green MF, et al. The impact of neurocognitive impairment on occupational recovery of clinically stable patients with bipolar disorder: A prospective study. *Bipolar Disorders*. 2011; **13**(4): 323–333.

17. Phillips ML, Kupfer DJ. Bipolar disorder diagnosis: Challenges and future directions. *Lancet*. 2013; **381**(9878):1663–1671.

18. Teixeira AL, Colpo GD, Fries GR, Bauer IE, Selvaraj S. Biomarkers for bipolar disorder: Current status and challenges ahead. *Expert Rev Neurother*. 2019; **19**(1): 67–81.

19. Sachs GS, Nierenberg AA, Calabrese JR, et al. Effectiveness of adjunctive antidepressant treatment for bipolar depression. *N Engl J Med*. 2007; **356**(17): 1711–1722.

20. Post RM, Altshuler LL, Leverich GS, et al. Mood switch in bipolar depression: Comparison of adjunctive venlafaxine, bupropion and sertraline. *Br J Psychiatry*. 2006; **189**: 124–131.

21. Kendler KS, Gatz M, Gardner CO, Pedersen NL. A Swedish national twin study of lifetime major depression. *Am J Psychiatry*. 2006; **163**(1): 109–114.

22. Kendler KS, Prescott CA. A population-based twin study of lifetime major depression in men and women. *Arch Gen Psychiatry*. 1999; **56**(1): 39–44.

23. Bienvenu OJ, Davydow DS, Kendler KS. Psychiatric "diseases" versus behavioral disorders and degree of genetic influence. *Psychol Med*. 2011; **41**(1): 33–40.

24. Craddock N, Sklar P. Genetics of bipolar disorder. *Lancet*. 2013; **381**(9878): 1654–1662.

25. Bunney WE, Jr., Davis JM. Norepinephrine in depressive reactions. A review. *Arch Gen Psychiatry*. 1965; **13**(6): 483–494.

26. Schildkraut JJ. The catecholamine hypothesis of affective disorders: A review of supporting evidence. *Am J Psychiatry*. 1965; **122**(5): 509–522.

27. Schildkraut JJ, Kety SS. Biogenic amines and emotion. *Science*. 1967; **156**(771): 21–37.

28. Coppen A, Shaw DM, Malleson A, Eccleston E, Gundy G. Tryptamine metabolism in depression. *Br J Psychiatry*. 1965; **111**(479): 993–998.

29. Lapin IP, Oxenkrug GF. Intensification of the central serotoninergic processes as a possible determinant of the thymoleptic effect. *Lancet*. 1969; **1**(7586): 132–136.

30. Coppen AJ. Biochemical aspects of depression. *Int Psychiatry Clin*. 1969; **6**(2): 53–81.

31. Jun C, Choi Y, Lim SM, et al. Disturbance of the glutamatergic system in mood disorders. *Exp Neurobiol*. 2014; **23**(1): 28–35.

32. Manji H, Kato T, Di Prospero NA, et al. Impaired mitochondrial function in psychiatric disorders. *Nat Rev Neurosci*. 2012; **13**(5): 293–307.

33. Kato T. Mitochondrial dysfunction as the molecular basis of bipolar disorder: Therapeutic implications. *CNS Drugs*. 2007; **21**(1): 1–11.

34. Stork C, Renshaw PF. Mitochondrial dysfunction in bipolar disorder: Evidence from magnetic resonance spectroscopy research. *Mol Psychiatry*. 2005; **10**(10): 900–919.

35. Konradi C, Sillivan SE, Clay HB. Mitochondria, oligodendrocytes and inflammation in bipolar disorder: Evidence from transcriptome studies points to intriguing parallels with multiple sclerosis. *Neurobiol Dis*. 2012; **45**(1): 37–47.

36. Filippi M, Rocca MA. MR imaging of multiple sclerosis. *Radiology*. 2011; **259**(3): 659–681.

37. Filippi M. Multiple sclerosis in 2010: Advances in monitoring and treatment of multiple sclerosis. *Nat Rev Neurol*. 2011; **7**(2): 74–75.

38. Polman CH, Reingold SC, Banwell B, et al. Diagnostic criteria for multiple sclerosis: 2010 revisions to the McDonald criteria. *Ann Neurol.* 2011; **69**(2): 292–302.

39. Miller AH, Maletic V, Raison CL. Inflammation and its discontents: The role of cytokines in the pathophysiology of major depression. *Biol Psychiatry.* 2009; **65**(9): 732–741.

40. Wise T, Radua J, Via E, et al. Common and distinct patterns of grey-matter volume alteration in major depression and bipolar disorder: Evidence from voxel-based meta-analysis. *Mol Psychiatry.* 2017; **22**(10): 1455–1463.

41. Bertocci M, Bebko G, Mullin B, et al. Abnormal anterior cingulate cortical activity during emotional n-back task performance distinguishes bipolar from unipolar depressed females. *Psychological Medicine.* 2012; **42**(7): 1417.

42. Glahn DC, Bearden CE, Niendam TA, Escamilla MA. The feasibility of neuropsychological endophenotypes in the search for genes associated with bipolar affective disorder. *Bipolar Disorders.* 2004; **6**(3): 171–182.

43. Di Nicola M, De Risio L, Battaglia C, et al. Reduced hedonic capacity in euthymic bipolar subjects: A trait-like feature? *Journal of Affective Disorders.* 2013; **147**(1–3): 446–450.

2 Neuroanatomical Findings in Unipolar Depression and the Role of the Hippocampus

Danilo Arnone

2.1 Introduction

Depressive disorders are common conditions with a life prevalence of 15% in high-income countries (1) and significant economic implications for individuals and society. Major depressive disorders have negative repercussions on the overall quality of life of the people affected with an excess number of years lived with a disability (2). Although effective treatment is available, up to 65% of individuals do not fully respond or continue to experience residual symptoms, which contribute to significant disease burden (3). It is essential to improve our understanding of the neuroanatomy of depressive disorders and the functional implications to develop new targets for more efficacious treatments.

This chapter reviews the current neuroanatomical evidence for abnormalities identified in major depression by focusing on selected research findings emerging from structural neuroimaging and postmortem studies. It also gives a perspective on the role played by the hippocampus in view of the described effects of stress on this region (4).

2.2 Structural Magnetic Resonance Imaging in Major Depressive Disorders

Since the introduction of magnetic resonance imaging (MRI) in the 1990s, several hundred cross-sectional studies have investigated structural changes in depressive disorders mostly in comparison with healthy controls by adopting a region of interest (ROI) approach (which involves delineation of anatomical boundaries of selected ROIs) or by using voxel-based morphometry (VBM) (which is based on measurements of anatomical differences of volume at voxel level across the whole brain). According to structural

MRI and differently from bipolar disorder, major depression is characterized not by global brain volumetric reduction but by regional morphometric changes in a number of brain regions implicated in mood regulation (5–7). A number of meta-analyses of MRI studies have reported consistent volumetric reductions in prefrontal areas, more extensively in the orbitofrontal and anterior cingulate cortices and limbic regions such as the amygdala and hippocampus. Other areas in the prefrontal cortex also commonly described include the dorsomedial and ventromedial prefrontal cortices (5, 6, 8). Recent work reporting data from twenty cohorts of patients worldwide indicated that these regions are also characterized by cortical thinning, and aside from the orbitofrontal cortex and anterior cingulate cortex, other regions include the posterior cingulate cortex, temporal lobes, and insula (9). Volumetric reduction in the temporal regions, including the insula, has also been reported in an independent study (10). Their involvement is hardly surprising considering that the temporal lobes and the insula are known to be involved in automatic responses, including multisensory recognition and participation in the processing of emotions (11, 12).

The role of subcortical regions in the neuroanatomy of depression has been of great interest in view of the role of the limbic system in the processing of emotions. Several studies have evaluated structural changes in the hippocampus complex, the most investigated limbic region in major depression (5), whereas the amygdala is the second brain region most extensively researched in this type of studies in depressive disorders (6). Findings in the literature tend to vary from no volumetric difference at all to increase or decrease in volume in comparison with healthy volunteers (13). This variability can be explained by the significant heterogeneity in the patients included, the methods applied to measure differences, and the presence of comorbidities (6, 13). Bora and others, for instance, found evidence of amygdala morphometric reduction in depression when comorbid anxiety was present (8). Overall, the most consistent evidence suggests a volumetric reduction in this region (5, 10, 14). Other regions involved in depression include the basal ganglia (ventral striatum), thalamus, pituitary region, corpus callosum, and cerebellum (5, 10, 14)).

Studies that have used diffusion tensor imaging techniques in major depression have identified white matter disconnectiviy in several areas associated with decreased fractional anisotropy. These have included bilateral frontal white matter, right fusiform gyrus, right occipital lobe and the right inferior longitudinal fasciculus, the right inferior fronto-occipital fasciculus, the right posterior thalamic radiation, and interhemispheric fibers crossing the genu and the body of the corpus callosum (15). Consistent with earlier MRI studies in affective disorders (5, 16), a recent systematic analysis of diffusion tensor imaging studies carried out by using a conservative approach indicated that the most reliable finding of decreased functional connectivity is located in the genu of the corpus callosum, crucially important in interhemispheric prefrontal connectivity relevant to affective regulation (14).

In summary, current evidence suggests that in the absence of global gray matter loss in major depression, several regions have been implicated in the neuroanatomy of this disorder. Involved brain areas include the prefrontal brain, temporal regions, and the insula. White matter disconnectivity in the genu of the corpus callosum is the most reliable finding identified by using diffusion tensor imaging. Within the limbic system the amygdala and the hippocampus are the most investigated regions. Hippocampal volumetric reduction is considered the most consistent finding.

2.3 Postmortem Studies in Depression

Posthumous evidence in major depression is based on a relatively small number of studies. Direct neuropathological abnormalities have been observed in groups of individuals with mood disorders compared with healthy controls and in some instances in relation to other conditions like schizophrenia. A reduction in glial cell number and/or density in major depression, especially in individuals with positive family history for mood disorders, has been described in the subgenual prefrontal cortex (17), supracallosal areas (18, 19), and dorsolateral and orbitofrontal regions (18, 20). In these brain areas, other abnormalities have included neurons with smaller cell body size versus larger body size found in cortical layers II, V, and VI of the prefrontal cortex, which may account for volumetric reduction in depression (18, 20, 21).

In the hippocampus complex, an increase in glial cell density with no changes in the size of glial nuclei has been associated with a decrease in the size of the soma of pyramidal and granule cells (22). Further evidence supports neuronal loss in advancing age, independent from neurocognitive degeneration and cerebrovascular pathology (23). A reduction in glial cell density has also been reported in the amygdala (24), and reduced hypothalamic volume has been described in the literature (25). The ventrolateral component of the dorsal raphe nucleus has also been demonstrated to be reduced in volume in patients with mood disorders with a smaller number of triangular neurons in this region (26). There is also indirect evidence emerging from markers of neuronal activity. For example, lower density of Immune reactive calretinin, a marker of GABAergic activity in neurons and glia, has been described in layer I of the dorsolateral prefrontal cortex (27). Further evidence of disruption in the glutamatergic function includes abnormalities in glutamate signaling genes SLC1A2, SLC1A3, and GLUL found in the locus coeruleus (28). Other abnormalities involve growth factor genes FGFR3 and TrkB, and other genes expressed in the astrocytes (28). Some of the limitations of this literature are the possible contamination of the sample with other conditions, the small sample size and the retrospective nature of diagnoses and cause of death, limited clinical and treatment history, and the possibility that tissue changes might have occurred prior to cellular analysis.

In summary, there is evidence of neuropathological abnormalities in depressive disorders affecting primarily prefrontal areas and limbic regions and including both neurons and glial cells, pointing toward a reduction in brain volume.

2.4 Evidence of Structural Changes in Depression Following Prolonged Stress, and the Role of the Hippocampus and Hypothalamic–Pituitary–Adrenal Axis

One of the etiological models of depression central to the pathophysiology of the disorder proposes that prolonged stress mediates over-activation of the hypothalamic–pituitary–adrenal (HPA) axis (29). Stress and glucocorticoids, the end product of HPA axis hyperactivity, generate a cascade of intracellular events known to downregulate brain neurotrophic factors (e.g., nerve growth factor), brain-derived neurotrophic factor (BDNF), and neurotrophin-3 (30). BDNF is essential for survival, differentiation, and functioning of neurons in the brain (31). Downregulation of BDNF demonstrated in rodents exposed to prolonged stress is believed to reduce cellular resilience and to lower the threshold for hippocampal cellular damage in animal models of depression (32). Stress and high levels of circulating corticosteroids may be responsible for the volumetric reduction, which is measured in a number of regions, including the hippocampus (33, 34), and could be the result of intracellular mechanisms leading to homeostatic modification and cellular damage (32, 35). Cellular alteration is likely to be mediated by postsynaptic mechanisms in response to receptors' activation. Animal studies suggest that BDNF-mediated long-term synaptic potentiation could act via N-methyl D-aspartate (NMDA) receptors (36). NMDA receptors' stimulation appears key to hippocampal toxicity and cellular stress and includes NMDA receptors' direct interaction with the neurotransmitter glutamate facilitated by elevated glucocorticoid levels (32, 37). Increased expression of BDNF and its receptor TrkB in the dentate gyrus and the CA3 region of the hippocampus following sustained administration of antidepressant treatment in animal studies (38) might be key to treatment response in humans. This effect appears mediated by cyclic adenosine monophosphate (cAMP) dependent phosphorylation in postmortem studies (39). cAMP-response element-binding (CREB) protein mRNA levels in the CA1, CA3, and dentate gyrus regions of the hippocampus (35, 40) have been shown to be associated with hippocampal neuronal sprouting and neurogenesis and could explain recovery following treatment (35). Supporting evidence suggests low circulating levels of BDNF in unmedicated currently depressed patients correlating with hippocampal volume (41) normalization following administration of an antidepressant and clinical remission (42). Indirect evidence from MRI longitudinal studies also supports greater hippocampal volumes in medicated depressed patients that appear to be associated with remission at one year follow-up (43). Although findings in the literature are not always consistent, discrepancies could be expression of depression heterogeneity, inclusion/exclusion of comorbidities, sample size, length of pharmacological treatment, and methodological differences. Lai and others, for instance, did not find that six-week treatment with duloxetine affected gray matter in the hippocampus in a sample of depressed patients with comorbid panic disorder (44). Evidence from cross-sectional studies overall supports greater hippocampal volumes following response to treatment and remission and greater hippocampal volumes in responders to pharmacological treatment in comparison with nonresponders (45). Furthermore, lower hippocampal volume at baseline has been shown to predict non-remission to antidepressant treatment in a study in older adults (46) and first presenters (47). Other postsynaptic mechanisms linked with neurotrophic effects related to efficacious treatments of mood episodes include lithium-mediated gene expression, resulting in the induction of protein bcl-2, as shown in the frontal cortex and hippocampus (and also cerebellar granule cells and striatum) of rodents and in human neuroblastoma cells (48–50), and the modulation of protein kinase C (PKC) alpha and epsilon, as shown in rodent frontal cortex and hippocampus following administration of lithium and sodium valproate (51). Finally, lithium and antidepressants modulate adenylate cyclase systems by reducing receptor/G protein coupling (52).

In summary, a range of animal and human studies support the notion that stress can induce neuroendocrine changes occurring in depressive disorders and that a cascade of postsynaptic events is likely to increase the susceptibility of hippocampal structures to cellular damage. Although the molecular nature of volumetric loss detectable with MRI in depression is not clearly established, pharmacological treatment could be implicated in volumetric normalization associated with treatment response. Conventional pharmacological compounds associated with treatment response are believed to act on intracellular mechanisms and neurotrophic pathways.

2.5 Hippocampal Abnormalities: State versus Trait Marker for a Depressive Episode

Volumetric reduction in the hippocampus is the most replicated finding in major depression, consistent with the involvement of this region in the processing of emotions (11). Evidence from meta-analyses suggests that the effect is larger with increasing proportion of patients currently depressed (5). This notion is supported by experimental data indicating a reduction in the gray matter of the hippocampus in currently depressed subjects in comparison with healthy controls (53–60), also in unmedicated patients (44, 61–64), and not in individuals with remitted depression (64). The association between remission and full volumetric recovery is complicated by several factors impacting on the overall measured effect, such as illness duration (65, 66) or age of onset (e.g., proxy of illness duration) (67), number of episodes (68), severity of symptoms (45), the presence of treatment resistance, or a chronic illness course (which could be expression of a different biological subtype of depression, not necessarily representative of the disorder) (43). There may also be some biological characteristics intrinsic to remission including scar effects. Salvadore and others, for example, compared unmedicated remitted patients with a chronic course of illness versus currently depressed and healthy controls and reported prefrontal gray matter changes only in currently depressed patients in comparison with both the other groups (69). Another factor is the possibility that bipolar disorder can present as unipolar depression at disease onset, which could dilute morphometric differences, and greater hippocampal reduction has been associated with major depression in comparison with bipolar disorder (13, 70). Some research studies include participants with positive family history for major depressive disorders, and often no sufficient attention is given to the presence of early developmental adversity. Increasing evidence suggests that these are very important contributors to hippocampal integrity. There is in fact evidence of reduced hippocampal volume in subjects with parental history of depression prior to developing major depression (71, 72), whereas a known independent interaction exists between hippocampal volume, early developmental adversity, and risk of developing depressive symptoms in the future (71, 73). The increased risk of developing depression in the presence of early life stressors has been shown to be attributable to the excess of BDNF Val66Met variant (the BDNF transcript with the amino acid valine in position 66 instead of methionine) resulting in decreased secretion of BDNF and volumetric reduction in the hippocampus in individuals who experienced traumatic events. Another mechanism of action has been attributed to the predominance of the short allele variant of the serotonin transporter, resulting in less effective serotonergic neurotransmission and vulnerability to stress (74). In this context, volumetric reduction in the hippocampus could be the result of neurotoxicity induced by stress-related glucocorticoids release and decrease in neurotrophic factors, with evidence of reduction in the size of the soma of hippocampal pyramidal and granule glial cells (22) and decreased density of dendrites and spines in the hippocampal subregion CA3 detected in subjects with higher anxiety and depression scores (75), potentially in combination with a stress-prone less-efficient serotonergic neurotransmission.

In summary, there is compelling evidence suggesting hippocampal volumetric reduction in symptomatic individuals. The resolution of symptoms suggests a degree of amelioration supportive of a "state effect." Moderating factors of morphometric normalization include the number of episodes, age of onset/duration of illness, severity of the disorder, family history, the experience of traumatic events, especially at young age, and cumulative effects of pharmacological and psychological treatment.

2.6 Neuroanatomical Circuitry Involved in Major Depression

Several brain regions have been implicated in major depression, which are part of circuits involved in instinctual behaviors, homeostatic mechanisms, and covert processing of emotional information mostly located in subcortical regions including the hippocampus, amygdala, hypothalamus, thalamus, with brain regions located in the forebrain, inner temporal lobes (insula), and the cingulate area (76). The overtone of emotional regulation is the result of the interaction between subcortical regions and neocortical associative areas where information regarding the "state" of the body is integrated, resulting in a range of cognitive and executive functions filtered through socially relevant norms (77). This is consistent with animal and lesion studies that suggest that pivotal brain areas participating in mood regulation are located in the prefrontal cortex and that important pathways connect the orbitofrontal cortex with the thalamus and hypothalamus/brain stem. These studies also suggest that the ventromedial prefrontal cortex is involved in appraisal of behavioral consequences in humans. Lesions in this region abolish the normal automatic visceral response to emotive stimuli, and affected individuals become unaware of long-term consequences of their behaviors (78, 79).

Brain regions where morphometric changes, often in the direction of a reduction, have been reported in major depression include the ventromedial prefrontal cortex, orbitofrontal cortex, anterior cingulate cortex, posterior cingulate cortex, temporal areas, basal nuclei, and the limbic system.

From the medial prefrontal cortex, projections reach the superior temporal gyrus, anterior cingulate cortex, entorhinal cortex, parahippocampal gyrus (80), and the limbic system (hypothalamus, periaqueductal gray matter, and amygdala) to exercise control over visceral functions in relation to mood state (81). Direct somatotopic reciprocal cortico-thalamic connections are described to originate from medial and lateral prefrontal cortices with an indirect thalamic pathway via striato-pallido intermediate stations. In these networks, medial components of the prefrontal cortex (orbito-medial and orbitofrontal) project to the ventromedial part of the striatum, including caudate nucleus and putamen, and to the paraventricular thalamic nucleus (which also exchange connections with the ventromedial striatum) (81). The paraventricular thalamic nucleus is important in circuits of mood regulation because it is involved in autonomic responses and stress regulation. Such responses require interactions with limbic regions including amygdala, hypothalamus, and periaqueductal gray matter (81, 82).

Mayberg described the coexistence of two virtual anatomically related systems (83, 84): a system that primarily processes cognitive information in response to emotional stimuli and an interoceptive system that mediates covert responses (83, 84). In this model, subcortical areas, which include thalamus and ventral striatum, are implicated in the implicit processing of novel emotional and nonemotional information together with limbic regions such as the amygdala and the hippocampus complex (83, 84). Prefrontal regions, particularly medial cortical areas, exercise cognitive control and appraisal of emotional states (85).

In summary, the effective processing of emotional information is the result of a synergy between subcortical regions integrating information with cortical areas. Whereas subcortical regions host more automated functions, cortical areas are essential associative areas coordinating emotional information with the environmental milieu of the individual. The frontal brain, particularly the orbito-medial prefrontal areas, coordinates emotional responses with executive functions so to guide the provision of coherent behavioral responses.

References

1. Bromet E, Andrade LH, Hwang I, et al. Cross-national epidemiology of DSM-IV major depressive episode. *BMC Med.* 2011 July; **26**(9): 90.

2. WHO. *World Health: Reducing Risks, Promoting Health Life.* WHO, Geneva, Switzerland; 2002.

3. Cleare A, Pariante CM, Young AH, et al. Evidence-based guidelines for treating depressive disorders with antidepressants: a revision of the 2008 British Association for Psychopharmacology guidelines. *J Psychopharmacol Oxf Engl.* 2015 May; **29**(5): 459–525.

4. Lee AL, Ogle WO, Sapolsky RM. Stress and depression: possible links to neuron death in the hippocampus. *Bipolar Disord.* 2002 April; **4**(2): 117–128.

5. Arnone D, McIntosh AM, Ebmeier KP, Munafò MR, Anderson IM. Magnetic resonance imaging studies in unipolar depression: systematic review and meta-regression analyses. *Eur Neuropsychopharmacol J Eur Coll Neuropsychopharmacol.* 2012 January; **22**(1): 1–16.

6. Koolschijn PCMP, van Haren NEM, Lensvelt-Mulders GJLM, Hulshoff Pol HE, Kahn RS. Brain volume abnormalities in major depressive disorder: a meta-analysis of magnetic resonance imaging studies. *Hum Brain Mapp.* 2009 November; **30**(11): 3719–3735.

7. Arnone D, Cavanagh J, Gerber D, et al. Magnetic resonance imaging studies in bipolar disorder and schizophrenia: meta-analysis. *Br J Psychiatry J Ment Sci.* 2009 September; **195**(3): 194–201.

8. Bora E, Fornito A, Pantelis C, Yücel M. Gray matter abnormalities in major depressive disorder: a meta-analysis of voxel based morphometry studies. *J Affect Disord.* 2012 April; **138**(1–2): 9–18.

9. Schmaal L, Hibar DP, Sämann PG, et al. Cortical abnormalities in adults and adolescents with major depression based on brain scans from 20 cohorts worldwide in the ENIGMA major depressive disorder working group. *Mol Psychiatry.* 2017; **22**(6): 900–909.

10. Arnone D, Job D, Selvaraj S, et al. Computational meta-analysis of statistical parametric maps in major depression. *Hum Brain Mapp.* 2016 April; **37**(4): 1393–1404.

11. Adolphs R. Neural systems for recognizing emotion. *Curr Opin Neurobiol.* 2002 April; **12**(2): 169–177.

12. Phillips ML, Ladouceur CD, Drevets WC. A neural model of voluntary and automatic emotion regulation: implications for understanding the pathophysiology and neurodevelopment of bipolar disorder. *Mol Psychiatry.* 2008 September; **13**(9): 829, 833–857.

13. Kempton MJ, Salvador Z, Munafò MR, et al. Structural neuroimaging studies in major depressive disorder: meta-analysis and comparison with bipolar disorder. *Arch Gen Psychiatry.* 2011 July; **68**(7): 675–690.

14. Wise T, Radua J, Nortje G, et al. Voxel-based meta-analytical evidence of structural disconnectivity in major depression and bipolar disorder. *Biol Psychiatry.* 2016 February 15; **79**(4): 293–302.

15. Liao Y, Huang X, Wu Q, et al. Is depression a disconnection syndrome? Meta-analysis of diffusion tensor imaging studies in patients with MDD. *J Psychiatry Neurosci JPN.* 2013 January; **38**(1): 49–56.

16. Arnone D, McIntosh AM, Chandra P, Ebmeier KP. Meta-analysis of magnetic resonance imaging studies of the corpus callosum in bipolar disorder. *Acta Psychiatr Scand.* 2008 November; **118**(5): 357–362.

17. Ongür D, Drevets WC, Price JL. Glial reduction in the subgenual prefrontal cortex in mood disorders. *Proc Natl Acad Sci U S A.* 1998 October 27; **95**(22): 13290–13295.

18. Cotter D, Mackay D, Chana G, et al. Reduced neuronal size and glial cell density in area 9 of the dorsolateral prefrontal cortex in subjects with major depressive disorder. *Cereb Cortex N Y N 1991.* 2002 April; **12**(4): 386–394.

19. Uranova NA, Vostrikov VM, Orlovskaya DD, Rachmanova VI. Oligodendroglial density in the prefrontal cortex in schizophrenia and mood disorders: a study from the Stanley Neuropathology Consortium. *Schizophr Res.* 2004 April 1; **67**(2–3): 269–275.

20. Rajkowska G, Miguel-Hidalgo JJ, Wei J, et al. Morphometric evidence for neuronal and glial prefrontal cell pathology in major depression. *Biol Psychiatry.* 1999 May 1; **45**(9): 1085–1098.

21. Cotter D, Mackay D, Landau S, Kerwin R, Everall I. Reduced glial cell density and neuronal size in the anterior cingulate cortex in major depressive disorder. *Arch Gen Psychiatry.* 2001 June; **58**(6): 545–553.

22. Stockmeier CA, Mahajan GJ, Konick LC, et al. Cellular changes in the postmortem hippocampus in major depression. *Biol Psychiatry.* 2004 November 1; **56**(9): 640–650.

23. Tsopelas C, Stewart R, Savva GM, et al. Neuropathological correlates of late-life depression in older people. *Br J Psychiatry J Ment Sci.* 2011 February; **198**(2): 109–114.

24. Bowley MP, Drevets WC, Ongür D, Price JL. Low glial numbers in the amygdala in major depressive disorder. *Biol Psychiatry.* 2002 September 1; **52**(5): 404–412.

25. Bielau H, Brisch R, Gos T, et al. Volumetric analysis of the hypothalamus, amygdala and hippocampus in non-suicidal and suicidal mood disorder patients–a post-mortem study. *CNS Neurol Disord Drug Targets.* 2013 November; **12**(7): 914–920.

26. Baumann B, Bielau H, Krell D, et al. Circumscribed numerical deficit of dorsal raphe neurons in mood disorders. *Psychol Med.* 2002 January; **32**(1): 93–103.

27. Oh DH, Son H, Hwang S, Kim SH. Neuropathological abnormalities of astrocytes, GABAergic neurons, and pyramidal neurons in the dorsolateral prefrontal cortices of patients with major depressive disorder. *Eur Neuropsychopharmacol J Eur Coll Neuropsychopharmacol.* 2012 May; **22**(5): 330–338.

28. Bernard R, Kerman IA, Thompson RC, et al. Altered expression of glutamate signaling, growth factor, and glia genes in the locus coeruleus of patients with major depression. *Mol Psychiatry.* 2011 June; **16**(6): 634–646.

29. Cowen PJ. Not fade away: the HPA axis and depression. *Psychol Med.* 2010 January; **40**(1): 1–4.

30. Duman RS, Monteggia LM. A neurotrophic model for stress-related mood disorders. *Biol Psychiatry*. 2006 June 15; **59**(12): 1116–1127.

31. Lanfumey L, Mongeau R, Cohen-Salmon C, Hamon M. Corticosteroid-serotonin interactions in the neurobiological mechanisms of stress-related disorders. *Neurosci Biobehav Rev*. 2008 August; **32**(6): 1174–1184.

32. Manji HK, Drevets WC, Charney DS. The cellular neurobiology of depression. *Nat Med*. 2001 May; **7**(5): 541–547.

33. Sapolsky RM. Glucocorticoids and hippocampal atrophy in neuropsychiatric disorders. *Arch Gen Psychiatry*. 2000 October; **57**(10): 925–935.

34. Young LT, Bakish D, Beaulieu S. The neurobiology of treatment response to antidepressants and mood stabilizing medications. *J Psychiatry Neurosci JPN*. 2002 July; **27**(4): 260–265.

35. Campbell S, Macqueen G. The role of the hippocampus in the pathophysiology of major depression. *J Psychiatry Neurosci JPN*. 2004 November; **29**(6): 417–426.

36. Leal G, Comprido D, de Luca P, et al. The RNA-binding protein hnRNP K mediates the effect of BDNF on dendritic mRNA metabolism and regulates synaptic NMDA receptors in hippocampal neurons. *eNeuro*. 2017 December 12; **4**(6): ENEURO.0268–17.2017.

37. Arnone D, Mumuni AN, Jauhar S, Condon B, Cavanagh J. Indirect evidence of selective glial involvement in glutamate-based mechanisms of mood regulation in depression: meta-analysis of absolute prefrontal neuro-metabolic concentrations. *Eur Neuropsychopharmacol J Eur Coll Neuropsychopharmacol*. 2015 August; **25**(8): 1109–1117.

38. MacQueen GM, Campbell S, McEwen BS, et al. Course of illness, hippocampal function, and hippocampal volume in major depression. *Proc Natl Acad Sci U S A*. 2003 February 4; **100**(3): 1387–1392.

39. Stewart RJ, Chen B, Dowlatshahi D, MacQueen GM, Young LT. Abnormalities in the cAMP signaling pathway in post-mortem brain tissue from the Stanley Neuropathology Consortium. *Brain Res Bull*. 2001 July 15; **55**(5): 625–629.

40. Dowlatshahi D, MacQueen GM, Wang JF, Young LT. Increased temporal cortex CREB concentrations and antidepressant treatment in major depression. *Lancet Lond Engl*. 1998 November 28; **352**(9142): 1754–1755.

41. Eker C, Kitis O, Taneli F, et al. Correlation of serum BDNF levels with hippocampal volumes in first episode, medication-free depressed patients. *Eur Arch Psychiatry Clin Neurosci*. 2010 October; **260**(7): 527–533.

42. Aydemir O, Deveci A, Taneli F. The effect of chronic antidepressant treatment on serum brain-derived neurotrophic factor levels in depressed patients: a preliminary study. *Prog Neuropsychopharmacol Biol Psychiatry*. 2005 February; **29**(2): 261–265.

43. Frodl T, Meisenzahl EM, Zill P, et al. Reduced hippocampal volumes associated with the long variant of the serotonin transporter polymorphism in major depression. *Arch Gen Psychiatry*. 2004 February; **61**(2): 177–183.

44. Lai C-H, Hsu Y-Y. A subtle grey-matter increase in first-episode, drug-naive major depressive disorder with panic disorder after 6 weeks' duloxetine therapy. *Int J Neuropsychopharmacol*. 2011 March; **14**(2): 225–235.

45. Vakili K, Pillay SS, Lafer B, et al. Hippocampal volume in primary unipolar major depression: a magnetic resonance imaging study. *Biol Psychiatry*. 2000 June 15; **47**(12): 1087–1090.

46. Hsieh M-H, McQuoid DR, Levy RM, et al. Hippocampal volume and antidepressant response in geriatric depression. *Int J Geriatr Psychiatry*. 2002 June; **17**(6): 519–525.

47. MacQueen GM, Yucel K, Taylor VH, Macdonald K, Joffe R. Posterior hippocampal volumes are associated with remission rates in patients with major depressive disorder. *Biol Psychiatry*. 2008 November 15; **64**(10): 880–883.

48. Chen RW, Chuang DM. Long term lithium treatment suppresses p53 and Bax expression but increases Bcl-2 expression. A prominent role in neuroprotection against excitotoxicity. *J Biol Chem*. 1999 March 5; **274**(10): 6039–6042.

49. Manji HK, Moore GJ, Chen G. Lithium at 50: have the neuroprotective effects of this unique cation been overlooked? *Biol Psychiatry*. 1999 October 1; **46**(7): 929–940.

50. Goodwin GM, Haddad PM, Ferrier IN, et al. Evidence-based guidelines for treating bipolar disorder: revised third edition recommendations from the British Association for Psychopharmacology. *J Psychopharmacol Oxf Engl*. 2016; **30**(6): 495–553.

51. Manji HK, Bebchuk JM, Moore GJ, et al. Modulation of CNS signal transduction pathways and gene expression by mood-stabilizing agents: therapeutic implications. *J Clin Psychiatry*. 1999; **60**(Suppl. 2): 27–39;discussion 40–41, 113–116.

52. Chen G, Hasanat KA, Bebchuk JM, et al. Regulation of signal transduction pathways and gene expression by mood stabilizers and

antidepressants. *Psychosom Med*. 1999 October; **61**(5): 599–617.

53. Abe O, Yamasue H, Kasai K, et al. Voxel-based analyses of gray/white matter volume and diffusion tensor data in major depression. *Psychiatry Res*. 2010 January 30; **181**(1): 64–70.

54. Bell-McGinty S, Butters MA, Meltzer CC, et al. Brain morphometric abnormalities in geriatric depression: long-term neurobiological effects of illness duration. *Am J Psychiatry*. 2002 August; **159**(8): 1424–1427.

55. Bergouignan L, Chupin M, Czechowska Y, Kinkingnéhun S, Lemogne C, Le Bastard G, et al. Can voxel based morphometry, manual segmentation and automated segmentation equally detect hippocampal volume differences in acute depression? *NeuroImage*. 2009 March 1; **45**(1): 29–37.

56. Kim MJ, Hamilton JP, Gotlib IH. Reduced caudate gray matter volume in women with major depressive disorder. *Psychiatry Res*. 2008 November 30; **164**(2): 114–122.

57. Mak AKY, Wong MMC, Han S-H, Lee TMC. Gray matter reduction associated with emotion regulation in female outpatients with major depressive disorder: A voxel-based morphometry study. *Prog Neuropsychopharmacol Biol Psychiatry*. 2009 October 1; **33**(7): 1184–1190.

58. Peng J, Liu J, Nie B, et al. Cerebral and cerebellar gray matter reduction in first-episode patients with major depressive disorder: A voxel-based morphometry study. *Eur J Radiol*. 2011 November; **80**(2): 395–399.

59. Shah PJ, Ebmeier KP, Glabus MF, Goodwin GM. Cortical grey matter reductions associated with treatment-resistant chronic unipolar depression. Controlled magnetic resonance imaging study. *Br J Psychiatry J Ment Sci*. 1998 June; **172**: 527–532.

60. Wagner G, Koch K, Schachtzabel C, et al. Structural brain alterations in patients with major depressive disorder and high risk for suicide: Evidence for a distinct neurobiological entity? *NeuroImage*. 2011 January 15; **54**(2): 1607–1614.

61. Cheng Y-Q, Xu J, Chai P, et al. Brain volume alteration and the correlations with the clinical characteristics in drug-naïve first-episode MDD patients: A voxel-based morphometry study. *Neurosci Lett*. 2010 August 9; **480**(1): 30–34.

62. Lai C-H, Hsu Y-Y, Wu Y-T. First episode drug-naïve major depressive disorder with panic disorder: Gray matter deficits in limbic and default network structures. *Eur Neuropsychopharmacol J Eur Coll Neuropsychopharmacol*. 2010 October; **20**(10): 676–682.

63. Zou K, Deng W, Li T, et al. Changes of brain morphometry in first-episode, drug-naïve, non-late-life adult patients with major depression: An optimized voxel-based morphometry study. *Biol Psychiatry*. 2010 January 15; **67**(2): 186–188.

64. Arnone D, et al. State-dependent changes in hippocampal grey matter in depression. 2013; Available from: http://doi.org/10.1038/mp.2012.150

65. McKinnon MC, Yucel K, Nazarov A, MacQueen GM. A meta-analysis examining clinical predictors of hippocampal volume in patients with major depressive disorder. *J Psychiatry Neurosci JPN*. 2009 January; **34**(1): 41–54.

66. Gerritsen L, Comijs HC, van der Graaf Y, et al. Depression, hypothalamic pituitary adrenal axis, and hippocampal and entorhinal cortex volumes–the SMART Medea study. *Biol Psychiatry*. 2011 August 15; **70**(4): 373–380.

67. Hickie I, Naismith S, Ward PB, et al. Reduced hippocampal volumes and memory loss in patients with early- and late-onset depression. *Br J Psychiatry J Ment Sci*. 2005 March; **186**: 197–202.

68. Videbech P, Ravnkilde B. Hippocampal volume and depression: A meta-analysis of MRI studies. *Am J Psychiatry*. 2004 November; **161**(11): 1957–1966.

69. Salvadore G, Nugent AC, Lemaitre H, et al. Prefrontal cortical abnormalities in currently depressed versus currently remitted patients with major depressive disorder. *NeuroImage*. 2011 February 14; **54**(4): 2643–2651.

70. Wise T, Radua J, Via E, et al. Common and distinct patterns of grey-matter volume alteration in major depression and bipolar disorder: Evidence from voxel-based meta-analysis. *Mol Psychiatry*. 2017 October; **22**(10): 1455–1463.

71. Rao U, Chen L-A, Bidesi AS, et al. Hippocampal changes associated with early-life adversity and vulnerability to depression. *Biol Psychiatry*. 2010 February 15; **67**(4): 357–364.

72. Amico F, Meisenzahl E, Koutsouleris N, et al. Structural MRI correlates for vulnerability and resilience to major depressive disorder. *J Psychiatry Neurosci JPN*. 2011 January; **36**(1): 15–22.

73. Vythilingam M, Vermetten E, Anderson GM, et al. Hippocampal volume, memory, and cortisol status in major depressive disorder: Effects of treatment. *Biol Psychiatry*. 2004 July 15; **56**(2): 101–112.

74. Kaufman J, Yang B-Z, Douglas-Palumberi H, et al. Brain-derived neurotrophic factor-5-HTTLPR gene interactions and environmental modifiers of

depression in children. *Biol Psychiatry*. 2006 April 15; **59**(8): 673–680.

75. Soetanto A, Wilson RS, Talbot K, et al. Association of anxiety and depression with microtubule-associated protein 2- and synaptopodin-immunolabeled dendrite and spine densities in hippocampal CA3 of older humans. *Arch Gen Psychiatry*. 2010 May; **67**(5): 448–457.

76. Wise T, Cleare AJ, Herane A, Young AH, Arnone D. Diagnostic and therapeutic utility of neuroimaging in depression: An overview. *Neuropsychiatr Dis Treat*. 2014; **10**: 1509–1522.

77. Antonio Damasio. *Descartes' Error: Emotion, Reason and the Human Brain*. Random House; 2008.

78. Damasio AR, Tranel D, Damasio H. Individuals with sociopathic behavior caused by frontal damage fail to respond autonomically to social stimuli. *Behav Brain Res*. 1990 December 14; **41**(2): 81–94.

79. Bechara A, Damasio H, Damasio AR. Emotion, decision making and the orbitofrontal cortex. *Cereb Cortex N Y N 1991*. 2000 March; **10**(3): 295–307.

80. Saleem KS, Kondo H, Price JL. Complementary circuits connecting the orbital and medial prefrontal networks with the temporal, insular, and opercular cortex in the macaque monkey. *J Comp Neurol*. 2008 February 1; **506**(4): 659–693.

81. Price JL, Drevets WC. Neurocircuitry of mood disorders. *Neuropsychopharmacol Off Publ Am Coll Neuropsychopharmacol*. 2010 January; **35**(1): 192–216.

82. Spencer SJ, Fox JC, Day TA. Thalamic paraventricular nucleus lesions facilitate central amygdala neuronal responses to acute psychological stress. *Brain Res*. 2004 February 6; **997**(2): 234–237.

83. Mayberg HS. Limbic-cortical dysregulation: A proposed model of depression. *J Neuropsychiatry Clin Neurosci*. 1997; **9**(3): 471–481.

84. Mayberg HS. Targeted electrode-based modulation of neural circuits for depression. *J Clin Invest*. 2009 April; **119**(4): 717–725.

85. Adolphs R. Neural systems for recognizing emotion. *Curr Opin Neurobiol*. 2002 April; **12**(2): 169–177.

Chapter 3

Neuroanatomical Findings in Bipolar Disorder

Giulia Tronchin and Colm McDonald

3.1 Introduction

Over the past three decades, numerous cross-sectional neuroimaging studies have reported neuroanatomical abnormalities in patients with bipolar disorder compared with healthy volunteers. These studies have highlighted those anatomical regions likely to harbor pathophysiological abnormalities underpinning the disorder. However, there are inconsistencies in several of the findings reported, and the precise etiology of structural brain abnormalities remains unclear – for example, the extent to which neuroanatomical abnormalities are driving illness development as distinct from consequential to its treatment. Between-study clinical and methodological heterogeneity, as well as low sample size, doubtless contributes to the inconsistent results in the literature. Systematic reviews and recent combinations of datasets through meta- and mega-analyses have sought to resolve individual study variation by maximizing statistical power and exploring sources of heterogeneity in large samples. Whereas meta-analyses combine metrics from previously analyzed studies, mega-analysis refers to a technique whereby individual level neuroimaging data, along with associated demographic and clinical variables, are gathered from multiple participating research groups for combined analyses. In this chapter, we will first review the main regional macroscopic neuroanatomical deviations derived from case-control MRI studies of bipolar disorder to date, with an emphasis on those findings that have emerged from large-scale studies employing meta- and mega-analyses. We will then review how the neuroanatomical deviations of bipolar disorder contrast with the related disorders of schizophrenia and major depressive disorder and discuss the likely sources of heterogeneity in neuroanatomical variation, including the impact of sociodemographic, clinical, and pharmacotherapy variables.

3.2 Case-Control Studies

Structural magnetic resonance imaging (MRI) enables high-resolution anatomical imaging in vivo to investigate global and regional variation in gray/white matter and cerebrospinal fluid. Manual, semiautomated, and fully automated techniques have been developed to extract structural information from MRI datasets. Manual segmentation techniques are labor intensive, and automated approaches, such as voxel-based morphometry, have often been employed to derive global and regional estimates of gray and white matter volume in bipolar disorder studies. Subcortical gray matter structures can be assessed by their regional volume or shape. Cortical gray matter can be assessed using measures of volume, surface area, and thickness. Cortical thickness is a measure of neuron numbers within a cortical layer, and surface area represents a measure of cortical column layer number. Given that cortical surface area and thickness are driven by cellular mechanisms, which are separable and highly heritable (1), several studies focus on these metrics rather than regional cortical volume.

3.2.1 Lateral Ventricles

Patients with manic depressive illness were first reported to display increased ventricular area compared with controls in a computerized axial tomography study in 1985 (2). Since then, there has been consistent evidence from numerous MRI studies that enlarged volume of the lateral ventricles characterizes bipolar disorder, emphatically confirmed by systematic reviews and by combining datasets through meta- and mega-analyses (3–8). In contrast to schizophrenia (9), there is evidence for more prominent ventriculomegaly on the right side (4, 5, 7), the reason for which is unclear, but it echoes reports of cortical and subcortical right hemisphere pathologies being more frequently associated with bipolar disorder (10).

3.2.2 Subcortical Structures

Many imaging studies of bipolar disorder have focused on subcortical structures, especially anterior limbic system structures, given their key role in emotional regulation. Recent meta- and mega-analyses have highlighted the markedly heterogeneous nature of studies into volume deviation of the hippocampus and amygdala, reported variously in individual studies as being increased, decreased, or unchanging in volume compared with controls, with no overall change when these studies were combined (4, 7, 11). There is also evidence from meta-analytical studies for increased striatal volumes in bipolar disorder, including right putamen (7), left putamen (12), and globus pallidus (6). As well as clinical heterogeneity, methodological heterogeneity may be contributing to the mixed results for small gray matter structures such as the hippocampus, which are difficult to segment precisely using fully automated techniques (13).

The largest international collaborative meta-analytic combination of such data to date is through the Bipolar Disorder Working Group of ENIGMA (Enhancing Neuroimaging Genetics Through Meta-analysis) by Hibar et al. (8), which incorporated MRI data from 1,710 bipolar disorder patients and 2,594 healthy controls and a consistent image segmentation process. This study identified a small but significant volume reduction of the hippocampus, amygdala, and thalamus in bipolar disorder. This small bilateral hippocampal volume reduction is consistent with the most recent systematic review of twenty-one published studies, which reported that the deficit was more pronounced in early-onset cases (14). The weight of this current evidence toward medial temporal lobe and thalamic deficits in bipolar disorder is in keeping with the functional neuroanatomy of these limbic structures and their role in the neurocircuitry of emotional processing and declarative memory, which are characteristically impaired in the illness.

3.2.3 Cortical Regions

Whereas global cerebral volume is generally preserved in bipolar disorder in most – although not all (11) – meta-analyses (4, 5, 7), there is evidence of regional gray matter deficit in the frontal cortex (6). Several meta-analyses of whole brain voxel-based morphometry studies in bipolar disorder compared with controls using differing methodologies have now been conducted. These have reported further gray matter deficits in the bilateral insula and anterior cingulate (15), the fronto-insular cortex (16, 17), bilateral ventrolateral and right dorsolateral prefrontal gray matter (18), right-sided frontotemporal gray matter incorporating prefrontal cortex, anterior temporal cortex, claustrum, and insula (19), and in the left medial frontal gyrus and right inferior/precentral gyri incorporating the insula (12).

Other large-scale studies have focused on regional parcellated cortical volume and estimates of cortical thickness and surface area. A systematic review of seventeen studies of cortical thickness in bipolar disorder identified illness-related decreased cortical thickness in bilateral prefrontal regions, left anterior cingulate, paracingulate, and superior temporal gyrus (20). The ENIGMA consortium completed a highly powered analysis of individual-level data on a cohort of 1,837 participants with bipolar disorder and 2,582 healthy controls, conducted with a harmonized software processing pipeline (21). Bipolar patients displayed a widespread pattern of bilaterally reduced thickness in frontal, temporal, and parietal regions, with the largest effect in the left pars opercularis, left fusiform gyrus, and left rostral middle frontal cortex. Cortical surface area differences were not found between adult patients with bipolar disorder and healthy controls (21), indicating that the cortical volume loss associated with bipolar disorder is consequential to the reduced thickness and preserved surface area. Taken together, these cortical studies identify illness-related gray matter deficits in paralimbic, frontotemporal, and prefrontal cortex anatomical regions subserving emotional processing, attentional, and executive functions known to be abnormal in bipolar disorder.

3.2.4 White Matter

With the advent of MRI technology in the early 1990s, studies began reporting the excessive presence of qualitatively assessed white matter hyperintensities in bipolar disorder (22, 23). Subsequent meta-analyses demonstrated that bipolar disorder was associated with a threefold increase in the rates of deep white matter hyperintensities compared with controls (5, 24), more marked in the right hemisphere and frontoparietal regions (5), and suggestive of white matter damage disrupting brain connectivity in bipolar illness.

Meta-analyses have reported that bipolar disorder is associated with a reduced area of the corpus callosum, the largest white matter inter-hemispheric pathway responsible for the integration of inter-hemispherical information (5, 11). A recent international multicenter study indicated that callosal area reductions in bipolar disorder are most prominent in the posterior sections of the corpus callosum (25).

As with gray matter volume, meta-analyses indicate that global white matter volume appears to be preserved in bipolar disorder (4–6), but there is evidence for regional white matter deficit. A meta-analysis of voxel-based morphometry studies (12) reported a reduction in white matter density in the left corona radiata, inferior longitudinal fasciculus, and posterior cingulum. A recent meta-analysis of voxel-based studies using seed-based mapping analysis of white matter (26), including 765 patients with bipolar disorder and 1,055 healthy controls, reported a large region of decreased white matter volume in the posterior corpus callosum and posterior cingulate gyrus in bipolar disorder.

3.2.5 Diffusion Tensor Imaging

Diffusion tensor imaging (DTI) can be used as an indirect measure of white matter microstructural organization by measuring directional constraint of the diffusivity of water molecules due to the local cellular environment (27). The most commonly employed metric to quantify white matter organization is fractional anisotropy (FA), which represents the level of regional organization within fiber bundles (28). Studies in bipolar disorder have repeatedly identified reduced regional FA in patients compared with healthy volunteers. The first meta-analysis conducted by Vederine and colleagues (29) of ten whole brain DTI studies, employing an activation likelihood estimation technique, demonstrated two significant clusters of decreased FA in the right hemisphere in bipolar disorder. One of these regions, close to the para-hippocampal gyrus, has a role in subprocesses associated with automatic emotion regulation (30), and

the other, close to the right anterior cingulate cortex and subgenual cortex, is important in the identification of emotionally salient stimuli and automatic emotion regulation (30, 31). A further systematic review and meta-analysis using effect size-signed differential mapping of fifteen whole brain DTI studies reported widespread FA reductions in bipolar disorder across commissural, association, and projection tracts, with the meta-analysis identifying FA reductions in the right parieto-occipital, left mid-posterior cingulate, and left anterior cingulate white matter (32). The specific white matter tracts involved in these regions of FA deficit include the long association tracts of the inferior longitudinal fasciculus and inferior frontal-occipital fasciculus, as well as anterior limbic system tracts, and indicate that white matter microstructural abnormalities might underpin the cognitive deficits as well as affective deficits linked to bipolar disorder (32). A further meta-analysis of voxel-based DTI studies, employing anisotropic effect size-signed differential mapping and including eighteen studies, identified FA deficits in bipolar patients that incorporated the left cingulum, right anterior superior longitudinal fasciculus, and genu, extending to the frontolimbic tracts, including the uncinate fasciculus (33).

DTI studies also confirm abnormal white matter integrity in all divisions of the corpus callosum in patients with bipolar disorder compared to healthy controls (29, 32–36), extending callosal area studies to further implicate disrupted inter-hemispheric communication in the illness. Taken together, these DTI studies indicate that bipolar disorder is associated with widespread microstructural disorganization of white matter tracts consistent with structural dysconnectivity in anatomical regions underpinning the emotional dysregulation and cognitive dysfunction associated with the disorder (37, 38).

3.2.6 Structural Network Findings

The abnormalities described thus far in gray and white matter regions are focal; however, the brain functions via a series of interconnected neuroanatomical networks. The "dysconnectivity" theory postulates that major psychotic illnesses can be explained by impaired integration between brain regions, rather than specific focal brain abnormalities (39). Through graph theory, it is now possible to investigate topology within the brain's global structural connectivity network in vivo using data derived from structural MRI to define cortical and subcortical gray matter regions ("nodes") and from diffusion MRI to define the white matter tracts interconnecting these regions ("edges")(40). Such structural connectivity investigations comparing patients with bipolar disorder and controls report evidence of impaired integration (34, 41–43) and segregation (34, 42–44) in bipolar disorder. Specific brain networks found to have abnormal anatomical connectivity include those incorporating left orbitofrontal cortex, left hippocampus, bilateral isthmus cingulate (34), left cuneus, right cerebellum, inferior frontal gyrus, right calcarine gyrus (43), superior and middle frontal gyri (42, 44), and superior and middle occipital gyri (42). Furthermore, there is evidence from these network analyses of impaired inter-hemispheric integration in bipolar disorder (34, 41, 45, 46), with interhemispheric dysconnectivity especially prominent in the frontal lobes (34). Rich club connectivity, which plays an important role in integrating information across functionally specialized neural circuits (47), is also reported to be reduced in bipolar disorder (42, 43), although there is conflicting evidence for this (41). Taken together, these findings provide network-level evidence for altered anatomical brain connectivity in BD that disrupts global integration and local segregation and extends across anterior, posterior, and interhemispheric regional networks.

3.3 Bipolar Disorder Compared with Schizophrenia and Major Depressive Disorder

There are blurred clinical and etiological boundaries between bipolar disorder and the other major psychotic/mood disorder diagnoses of schizophrenia and major depressive disorder. The extent to which these disorders may share or differ in their neuroanatomical substrate has been a source of research interest. The ENIGMA consortium has published meta-analyses of MRI studies on schizophrenia and major depressive disorder as well as bipolar disorder. These demonstrate that all three disorders are associated with significant reduction of the hippocampus when compared with healthy controls (8, 48, 49), with the effect size greatest for schizophrenia, less so for bipolar disorder and smallest for major depressive disorder, where it was largely driven by patients with the recurrent illness. Similarly enlargement of the lateral ventricles and reduced volume of other subcortical structures such as amygdala and thalamus are more prominent in schizophrenia than in bipolar disorder (6, 8, 48). Moreover, schizophrenia is associated with more widespread subcortical neuroanatomical deficits, with a volume reduction of the nucleus accumbens and enlargement of globus pallidus that are not found in bipolar disorder (48).

Cortical gray matter thinning is also more prominent in schizophrenia (especially frontotemporal) than in bipolar disorder, and schizophrenia, in contrast, does display reduced cortical surface area (21, 50). Cortical thinning in major depressive disorder is heterogeneous and potentially dynamic, depending on the age of onset and recurrence of illness, but like bipolar disorder is prominent in regions linked to the limbic system such as orbitofrontal cortex, cingulate, and insula (51). As with bipolar disorder, the cortical surface area is preserved in adult patients with major depressive disorder (51).

More prominent and widespread gray matter deficits associated with schizophrenia in comparison with bipolar disorder are also supported by a meta-analysis of voxel-based morphometry studies (15). This analysis reported that schizophrenia was characterized by regional gray matter deficits in frontal, temporal, cingulate, insula, and thalamus, and increased gray matter in the basal ganglia; whereas bipolar disorder was associated with overlapping gray matter deficit in the insula, but distinctive gray matter deficit in the anterior cingulate (15). In a large direct comparison of the two disorders using voxel-based morphometry (52), more severe and widespread gray matter deficits were reported in schizophrenia, which was shared in frontotemporal regions with bipolar disorder. There was a more prominent volume reduction of the thalamus and insula in schizophrenia, but anterior cingulate gray matter reduction was more specific for bipolar disorder (52). Major depressive disorder and bipolar disorder are reported by a meta-analysis of voxel-based morphometry studies to share gray matter deficits across the medial prefrontal cortex, anterior cingulate, and insula (53), with specific gray matter deficit in major depressive disorder in the right dorsolateral prefrontal cortex and left hippocampus.

Bipolar disorder is more commonly associated with white matter hyperintensities and reduced corpus callosum area compared to major depressive disorder (54). However, both schizophrenia and bipolar disorder are characterized by white matter abnormalities as evidenced by widespread fractional anisotropy reductions, especially in frontal and callosal regions (55–58). Emerging studies from complex network analyses also implicate white matter dysconnectivity, especially in frontal areas, in both schizophrenia and bipolar disorder (59).

Taken together, it appears from the current literature that schizophrenia displays more prominent gray matter abnormalities than bipolar disorder, which could be related to the neuroprogressive trajectory that characterizes the former (60), and that both bipolar disorder and major depressive disorder share specific gray matter deficits in the anterior cingulate and insula that are likely to underpin mood dysregulation. Widespread white matter abnormalities characterize both schizophrenia and bipolar disorder, suggesting that structural dysconnectivity is a phenotype that characterizes the broad spectrum of psychosis.

3.4 Sources of Heterogeneity

The vast majority of structural neuroimaging studies of bipolar disorder have been conducted cross-sectionally. While the recent large studies and meta- or mega-analyses have provided considerable statistical power to detect the subtle mean regional neuroanatomical changes that characterize the disorder in case-control studies, there is substantial variability in these measures among patients. In the absence of longitudinal studies to track neuroimaging changes over time in individual patients, sources of the evident heterogeneity in case-control studies have been explored using post hoc statistical analyses such as through correlations, subdividing patient samples, assessing interactions, and metaregression analyses.

3.4.1 Psychotropic Medication

Considerable attention has been given to the effect of medication use on brain structure in bipolar disorder. The effect of lithium, in particular, has been investigated extensively in post hoc analyses, in part because of the preclinical evidence that lithium activates neurotrophic and neuroprotective pathways and associated signaling mechanisms (61), which may be detectable macroscopically using MRI. An early meta-analysis by Kempton et al. (5) included a meta-regression which demonstrated that those studies with a higher proportion of patients taking lithium reported higher cerebral gray matter for patients. Hallahan and colleagues' mega-analysis (7) confirmed an increase of global cerebral volume in bipolar patients taking lithium at the time of scanning. Besides, they demonstrated that such patients had larger bilateral hippocampal and amygdala volume than controls, whereas patients not taking lithium had volume deficit of these structures. Another recent meta-analysis (62) based on fifteen studies reported that global gray matter was significantly larger in patients treated with lithium compared with patients who were not treated with lithium. A large case-control study based on 266 patients and 171 healthy volunteers reported that patients on lithium had a significantly larger total brain, thalamus, putamen, pallidum, hippocampus, and accumbens volumes compared to lithium-free patients (63). The ENIGMA meta-analyses reported larger thalamic volume in patients treated with lithium compared with patients not taking lithium (8), as well as significantly increased cortical thickness in patients taking lithium, most prominently in the left paracentral gyrus and left and right superior parietal gyrus, and increased surface area of the left paracentral lobule (21). The small number of longitudinal studies performed in bipolar disorder also indicate that treatment with lithium is associated with volume increases in gray matter, prefrontal gray matter, and hippocampal volume (64–66).

In contrast, the ENIGMA meta-analyses reported reduced hippocampal volume (8) and reduced cortical thickness in the left and right lateral occipital gyrus and right paracentral gyrus (21) in patients taking antiepileptic mood stabilizers compared with patients not taking antiepileptic medications. However, other individual studies report no differences or even gray matter increases in the prefrontal cortex and anterior cingulate in bipolar patients treated with antiepileptic mood stabilizers [67, 68]. Studies report antipsychotic medication use is associated with reduced gray matter volume in schizophrenia (69, 70). Similarly, there is evidence for reduced cortical surface area with atypical antipsychotic treatment in bipolar patients, compared with those patients not taking atypical antipsychotics, in the right rostral middle frontal gyrus and right superior frontal gyrus in the ENIGMA meta-analysis (21). Arnone and colleagues (6) reported a significant association between antipsychotic use in bipolar disorder and reduced volume of gray matter and right amygdala. A reduction of volume in the right amygdala was also associated with antidepressant exposure in this meta-analysis (6).

The effect of psychotropic medications on white matter metrics has been less widely investigated than gray matter structures. In the largest single-site DTI study to date of patients with bipolar disorder and healthy volunteers that explored the impact of pharmacotherapy, Abramovic and colleagues (71) reported that patients off lithium showed a significant lower fractional anisotropy values than patients on lithium in the corpus callosum, fornix, and the major and minor forceps. Although evidence is mixed to date, some other individual DTI studies have also reported a normalizing effect of lithium on fractional anisotropy reductions in bipolar disorder (68). No differences have been reported in network-level connectivity measures between patients on and off lithium (41, 42), nor in patients exposed or not exposed to antipsychotic medications (41).

Overall, evidence from both large-scale cross-sectional and longitudinal structural neuroimaging studies in bipolar disorder are that medication use is a significant source of heterogeneity, and that treatment with lithium has an ameliorating effect on gray matter and subcortical structures, possibly through the neuroprotective properties of this medication, and might also attenuate white matter aberrations. Whereas it is difficult to separate medication use from clinical course characteristics in observational cross-sectional studies (e.g., patients with more severe or persistent symptoms may be more likely to be prescribed antipsychotic medications long term and also have more cortical thinning), the evidence to date from neuroimaging studies indicates that antiepileptic mood stabilizers have a less ameliorating effect than lithium, and that antipsychotic medications are associated with gray matter deficits.

3.4.2 Demographic and Clinical Variables

Increasing age has been linked in the ENIGMA meta-analyses to proportionately greater hippo-campal volume deficits in bipolar disorder (8) and reduced cortical thickness more prominently in the left rostral middle frontal gyrus (21). These effects are subtle, however, and indicate that the accelerated aging of the brain reported in schizophrenia is not mirrored in bipolar disorder (72, 73). An association with gender was also identified for subcortical structures, with increased thalamic volume in female patients with bipolar disorder (8). However, there was no impact of gender on cortical volume or thickness (17, 21). This is in contrast to schizophrenia where male dominated samples with poorer prognosis, and more neurodevelopmental compromise may be partially driving the more substantial gray matter deficits in this syndrome than a bipolar disorder (17). Analyses of white matter metrics, such as through volume or network analyses, have mostly not reported links with age or gender (26, 34, 41, 46). However, there are individual studies that do report associations between increasing age and reduced fractional anisotropy in frontal tracts (74).

Age of onset and duration of illness are often assessed as sources of variation when analyzing changes in cortical and subcortical regions in patients with bipolar disorder. Hallahan et al.'s mega-analysis (7) reported a significant association between earlier age of onset in patients with bipolar disorder and reduced cerebral volume and left thalamic volume, as well as increased left amygdala volume. There was no association between age of onset and subcortical volume in the ENIGMA meta-analysis (8); however, reduced cortical thickness was associated with longer illness duration, with the strongest effect present bilaterally in the pericalcarine gyrus, left rostral anterior cingulate gyrus, and right cuneus, while a significant association with increased thickness was found in the right entorhinal gyrus (21). Longer duration of illness has been associated with more cerebral gray matter volume loss (6), but with increased gray matter in limbic system structures such as the amygdala, thalamus, and anterior cingulate (6,16). Of course, other variables correlated with duration of illness (such as the amount of time on lithium or other mood stabilizers) may be driving the associations reported between increased duration of illness and increased volume of anterior limbic system structures. Pezzoli et al.'s meta-analysis (26) reported no significant association between age of onset or duration of illness and regional white matter volume, and individual DTI studies largely do not report such associations either (35, 42).

Although some individual studies report bipolar subtype differences, the largest and most statistically powerful studies failed to detect any significant difference in volume, cortical thickness, surface area, or white matter regional volume when comparing bipolar I disorder and bipolar II disorder (5, 6, 8, 21, 26) A large multicenter DTI study reported greater microstructural impairment of the corpus callosum body (36) in bipolar patients with a history of psychotic symptoms than in those patients without psychotic features.

Ultimately cross-sectional studies assessing the impact of demographics or clinical variables on brain structure in bipolar disorder are limited by their methodology, given the nonlinear trajectory of brain development, and that illness of varying severity can emerge across the age range. For example, studies on clinical subgroups suggest that childhood onset bipolar disorder is associated with more prominent and progressive gray matter deficits in emotional regulation regions and that late-onset bipolar disorder is more likely to be associated with white matter abnormalities (75). The interaction between risk factors (and ameliorative factors such as psychotropic medication) and neuroanatomy in the context of dynamic processes underpinning brain development are difficult to decipher post hoc, even with large-scale observational studies. Longitudinal neuroimaging studies with rich phenotyping are required to dissect the likely complex interplay between the progression of illness with age and with other modulating factors such as medication use, age of onset, bipolar subtype, genotypic variation, and environmental risk factors.

3.4.3 Longitudinal

A review of twenty longitudinal structural neuroimaging studies (76), which included juvenile onset and first-episode psychosis samples, reported some consistency for progressive loss of gray matter volume in prefrontal cortex, anterior cingulate cortex, and sub-genual region in bipolar disorder, with relative preservation of temporal, ventricular, and subcortical structures – in contrast to longitudinal studies of schizophrenia,

which also identify progression in these regions. Gray matter loss was more extensive and progressive in young-onset bipolar disorder patients (76). There is also evidence that patients experiencing repeated mood exacerbations do display greater frontal and temporal gray matter loss than those with more stable illness course (77, 78). Longitudinal studies examining medication impact, which are largely shorter scale in follow-up, are consistent in demonstrating that lithium treatment is associated with increased cerebral gray matter in bipolar disorder (68).

3.5 Conclusions

Large neuroimaging studies and collaborative initiatives combining data in order to maximize statistical power have now emphatically demonstrated that the diagnostic category of bipolar disorder is associated with small subtle deviations in neuroanatomy (summarized in Table 3.1). These include lateral ventricular enlargement and gray matter deficits in thalamus, hippocampus, amygdala, insula, anterior cingulate, and prefrontal cortex. The illness is associated with decreased white matter in the posterior corpus callosum and posterior cingulate gyrus and disrupted white matter microstructural integrity incorporating diverse transverse and longitudinal tracts, indicating that structural dysconnectivity also characterizes the disorder. Reflecting the clinical and course variation of the illness itself, neuroanatomical deviations are heterogenous. Sources of heterogeneity clearly include lithium treatment, which is associated with attenuated or reversed subcortical volume deficit and apparent reversal of cortical thinning. Indices of severity such as longer duration of illness and repeated episodes of mood exacerbation are associated with progressive gray matter deficits. At this stage, further structural neuroimaging studies of small unselected samples are unlikely to be informative. Future research to elucidate the factors impacting on regional neuroanatomy in bipolar disorder will include large-scale longitudinal studies with repeated scanning and rich phenotyping, tracking clinically homogenous subgroups, incorporating multimodal imaging (to include physiological or molecular level metrics to better understand the functional consequences of deviant neuroanatomy),

Table 3.1 Summary of neuroanatomical deviations associated with bipolar disorder

	Structure	△Compared with healthy volunteers	Sources of heterogeneity	References
Global measures				
	Global cerebral volume	↔	Age of onset ↓	(4,5,7)
	Global gray matter volume	↔	Lithium ↑ Antipsychotic ↓ Longer duration of illness ↑	(5,6,62,63)
	Global white matter volume	↔		(4–6)
Gray matter subcortical structures				
	Lateral ventricles	↑⁺⁺⁺	Lithium ↑	3–7)
	Hippocampus	↓⁺⁺	Lithium ↑ Antiepileptic ↓ Older age ↓	(7,8,14,63)
	Thalamus	↓⁺⁺	Lithium ↑ Female gender ↑ Earlier age of onset ↓ Longer duration of illness ↑	(6–8,16,63)
	Amygdala	↓⁺⁺	Lithium ↑ Antidepressant ↓ Antipsychotic ↓ Earlier age of onset ↑ Longer duration of illness ↑	(6–8,16)
	Putamen	↑⁺⁺	Lithium ↑	(7,12,63)
	Globus pallidus	↑⁺	Lithium ↑	(6,63)
	Nucleus accumbens	↔	Lithium ↑	(63)
Volume cortical regions				
	Prefrontal	↓	Lithium ↑ Antiepileptic ↑ Longitudinal ↓	(18,66,67,68,76)
	Frontal	↓⁺⁺⁺		(6,12,16–18)
	Insular cortex	↓⁺⁺⁺		(12,15,16,18)
	Temporal	↓		(18)
	Anterior cingulate	↓⁺	Longitudinal ↓ Antiepileptic ↑ Longer duration of illness ↑	(6,15,16,67,68,76)
Thickness cortical regions				
	Prefrontal regions	↓⁺		(20,21)
	Frontal regions	↓	Lithium ↑ Antiepileptic ↓ Older age ↓	(21,71)

Table 3.1 (cont.)

	Structure	△Compared with healthy volunteers	Sources of heterogeneity	References
	Temporal regions	↓+		(20,21)
	Parietal regions	↓	Lithium ↑	(21)
White matter				
	Deep white matter hyperintensities	↑+		(5,24)
	Corpus callosum	↓++	History of psychotic features↑	(6,11,25,26)
	Association tracts	↓FA+		(29,32)
	Projection tracts	↓FA+		(29,32)
	Inter-hemispheric tracts	↓FA+	Lithium FA↑	(29,32,71)
Network connectivity				
	Integration	↓+++		(37,41–43,45)
	Segregation	↓++		(37,42–44)
	Centrality	Altered		(37,43)

+ strength of evidence, ↑ increase, ↓ decrease, ↔ preserved; FA fractional anisotropy; Integration: global and inter-regional communication across the network. Segregation: local communication between neighboring regions. Centrality: importance of brain regions within the network.

linking genotypic variation with neuroimaging metrics, and including neuroimaging assessments as a potential biomarker in clinical trials.

References

1. Panizzon MS, Fennema-Notestine C, Eyler LT, et al. Distinct genetic influences on cortical surface area and cortical thickness. *Cereb Cortex*. 2009; **19**(11): 2728–2735.

2. Pearlson GD, Garbacz DJ, Moberg PJ, et al. Symptomatic, familial, perinatal, and social correlates of computerized axial tomography (CAT) changes in schizophrenics and bipolars. *Journal of Nervous and Mental Disease*. 1985; **173**: 42–50.

3. Strakowski SM, DelBello MP, Adler CM. The functional neuroanatomy of bipolar disorder: a review of neuroimaging findings. *Mol Psychiatry*. 2005; **10**(1): 105–116.

4. McDonald C, Zanelli J, Rabe-Hesketh S, et al. Meta-analysis of magnetic resonance imaging brain morphometry studies in bipolar disorder. *Biol Psychiatry*. 2004; **56**(6): 411–417.

5. Kempton MJ, Geddes JR, Ettinger U, et al. Meta-analysis, database, and meta-regression of 98 structural imaging studies in bipolar disorder. *Arch Gen Psychiatry*. 2008; **65**(9): 1017–1032.

6. Arnone D, Cavanagh J, Gerber D, et al. Magnetic resonance imaging studies in bipolar disorder and schizophrenia: meta-analysis. *Br J Psychiatry*. 2009; **195**(3): 194–201.

7. Hallahan B, Newell J, Soares JC, et al. Structural magnetic resonance imaging in bipolar disorder: an international collaborative mega-analysis of individual adult patient data. *Biol Psychiatry*. 2011; **69**(4): 326–335.

8. Hibar DP, Westlye LT, Van Erp TGM, et al. Subcortical volumetric abnormalities in bipolar disorder. *Mol Psychiatry*. 2016; **21**(12): 1710–1716.

9. Wright IC, Rabe-Hesketh S, Woodruff PWR, et al. Meta – analysis of regional brain volumes in schizophrenia. *American Journal of Psychiatry*. 2000 January; **157**(1): 16–25.

10. Starkstein SE, Fedoroff P, Berthier ML, et al. Manic-depressive and pure manic states after brain lesions. *Biol Psychiatry*. 1991; **29**(2): 149–158.

11. Arnone D, McIntosh AM, Chandra P, et al. Meta-analysis of magnetic resonance imaging studies of

the corpus callosum in bipolar disorder. *Acta Psychiatr Scand.* 2008; **118**(5): 357–362.

12. Ganzola R, Duchesne S. Voxel-based morphometry meta-analysis of gray and white matter finds significant areas of differences in bipolar patients from healthy controls. *Bipolar Disord.* 2017; **19**(2): 74–83.

13. Akudjedu TN, Nabulsi L, Makelyte M, et al. A comparative study of segmentation techniques for the quantification of brain subcortical volume. *Brain Imaging Behav.* 2018 December; **12**(6): 1678–1695.

14. Otten M, Meeter M. Hippocampal structure and function in individuals with bipolar disorder: a systematic review. *J Affect Disord.* 2015; **174**: 113–125.

15. Ellison-Wright I, Bullmore E. Anatomy of bipolar disorder and schizophrenia: a meta-analysis. *Schizophr Res.* 2010; **117**(1): 1–12.

16. Bora E, Fornito A, Yücel M, et al. Voxelwise meta-analysis of gray matter abnormalities in bipolar disorder. *Biol Psychiatry.* 2010; **67**(11): 1097–1105.

17. Bora E, Fornito A, Yücel M, et al. The effects of gender on grey matter abnormalities in major psychoses: a comparative voxelwise meta-analysis of schizophrenia and bipolar disorder. *Psychol Med.* 2012; **42**(2): 295–307.

18. Houenou J, Frommberger J, Carde S, et al. Neuroimaging-based markers of bipolar disorder: evidence from two meta-analyses. *J Affect Disord.* 2011; **132**(3): 344–355.

19. Selvaraj S, Arnone D, Job D, et al. Grey matter differences in bipolar disorder: a meta-analysis of voxel-based morphometry studies. *Bipolar Disord.* 2012; **14**(2): 135–145.

20. Hanford LC, Nazarov A, Hall GB, et al. Cortical thickness in bipolar disorder: a systematic review. *Bipolar Disord.* 2016; **18**(1): 4–18.

21. Hibar DP, Westlye LT, Doan NT, et al. Cortical abnormalities in bipolar disorder: an MRI analysis of 6503 individuals from the ENIGMA Bipolar Disorder Working Group. *Mol Psychiatry.* 2018; **23**(4): 932–942.

22. Altshuler LL, Curran J, Hauser P, et al. T2 hyperintensities in bipolar disorder: magnetic resonance imaging comparison and literature meta-analysis. *Am J Psychiatry.* 1995; **152**: 1139–1144.

23. Swayze VW, Andreasen NC, Alliger RJ, et al. Structural brain abnormalities in bipolar affective disorder: ventricular enlargement and focal signal hyperintensities. *Arch Gen Psychiatry.* 1990; **47**(11): 1054–1059.

24. Beyer JL, Young R, Kuchibhatla M, et al. Hyperintense MRI lesions in bipolar disorder: a meta-analysis and review. *Int Rev Psychiatry.* 2009; **21**(4): 394–409.

25. Sarrazin S, d'Albis MA, McDonald C, et al. Corpus callosum area in patients with bipolar disorder with and without psychotic features: an international multicentre study. *J Psychiatry Neurosci.* 2015; **40**(5): 352–359.

26. Pezzoli S, Emsell L, Yip SW, et al. Meta-analysis of regional white matter volume in bipolar disorder with replication in an independent sample using coordinates, T-maps, and individual MRI data. *Neurosci Biobehav Rev.* 2018; **84**: 162–170.

27. Le Bihan D, Mangin J-F, Poupon C, et al. Diffusion tensor imaging: concepts and applications. *J Magn Reson Imaging.* 2001; **13**(4): 534–546.

28. Jones DK. Challenges and limitations of quantifying brain connectivity *in vivo* with diffusion MRI. *Imaging Med.* 2010; **2**(3): 341–355.

29. Vederine FE, Wessa M, Leboyer M, et al. A meta-analysis of whole-brain diffusion tensor imaging studies in bipolar disorder. *Prog Neuro-Psychopharmacology Biol Psychiatry.* 2011; **35**(8): 1820–1826.

30. Phillips ML, Ladouceur CD, Drevets WC. A neural model of voluntary and automatic emotion regulation: implications for understanding the pathophysiology and neurodevelopment of bipolar disorder. *Mol Psychiatry.* 2008; **13**(9): 833–857.

31. Phillips ML, Drevets WC, Rauch SL, et al. Neurobiology of emotion perception II: implications for major psychiatric disorders. *Biol Psychiatry.* 2003; **54**(5): 515–528.

32. Nortje G, Stein DJ, Radua J, et al. Systematic review and voxel-based meta-analysis of diffusion tensor imaging studies in bipolar disorder. *J Affect Disord.* 2013; **150**(2): 192–200.

33. Wise T, Radua J, Nortje G, et al. Voxel-based meta-analytical evidence of structural disconnectivity in major depression and bipolar disorder. *Biol Psychiatry.* 2016; **79**(4): 293–302.

34. Leow A, Ajilore O, Zhan L, et al. Impaired inter-hemispheric integration in bipolar disorder revealed with brain network analyses. *Biol Psychiatry.* 2013; **73**(2): 183–193.

35. Emsell L, Leemans A, Langan C, et al. Limbic and callosal white matter changes in euthymic bipolar I disorder: an advanced diffusion magnetic resonance imaging tractography study. Biol Psychiatry. 2013; **73**(2): 194–201.

36. Sarrazin S, Poupon C, Linke J, et al. A multicenter tractography study of deep white matter tracts in bipolar I disorder: psychotic features and interhemispheric disconnectivity. *JAMA Psychiatry*. 2014; **71**(4): 388–396.

37. Emsell L, McDonald C. The structural neuroimaging of bipolar disorder. *Int Rev Psychiatry*. 2009; **21**(4): 297–313.

38. Mahon K, Burdick KE, Szeszko PR. A role for white matter abnormalities in the pathophysiology of bipolar disorder. *Neurosci Biobehav Rev*. 2010; **34**(4): 533–554.

39. Stephan KE, Friston KJ, Frith CD. Dysconnection in schizophrenia: from abnormal synaptic plasticity to failures of self-monitoring. *Schizophr Bull*. 2009; **35**(3): 509–527.

40. O'Donoghue S, Cannon DM, Perlini C, et al. Applying neuroimaging to detect neuroanatomical dysconnectivity in psychosis. *Epidemiol Psychiatr Sci*. 2015; **24**(4): 298–302.

41. Collin G, van den Heuvel MP, Abramovic L, et al. Brain network analysis reveals affected connectome structure in bipolar I disorder. *Hum Brain Mapp*. 2016; **37**(1): 122–134.

42. O'Donoghue S, Kilmartin L, O'Hora D, et al. Anatomical integration and rich-club connectivity in euthymic bipolar disorder. *Psychol Med*. 2017; **47**(9): 1609–1623.

43. Wang Y, Deng F, Jia Y, et al. Disrupted rich club organization and structural brain connectome in unmedicated bipolar disorder. 2019 February; 49(3): 510–518.

44. Forde NJ, O'Donoghue S, Scanlon C, et al. Structural brain network analysis in families multiply affected with bipolar I disorder. *Psychiatry Res – Neuroimaging*. 2015; **234**(1): 44–51.

45. Ajilore O, Vizueta N, Walshaw P, et al. Connectome signatures of neurocognitive abnormalities in euthymic bipolar I disorder. *J Psychiatr Res*. 2015; **68**: 37–44.

46. Gadelkarim JJ, Ajilore O, Schonfeld D, et al. Investigating brain community structure abnormalities in bipolar disorder using path length associated community estimation. *Hum Brain Mapp*. 2014; **35**(5): 2253–2264.

47. van den Heuvel MP, Sporns O. An anatomical substrate for integration among functional networks in human cortex. *J Neurosci*. 2013; 33(36): 14489–14500.

48. Van Erp TGM, Hibar DP, Rasmussen JM, et al. Subcortical brain volume abnormalities in 2028 individuals with schizophrenia and 2540 healthy controls via the ENIGMA consortium. *Mol Psychiatry*. 2016; **21**(4): 547–553.

49. Schmaal L, Veltman DJ, van Erp TGM, et al. Subcortical brain alterations in major depressive disorder: Findings from the ENIGMA Major Depressive Disorder working group. *Mol Psychiatry*. 2016; **21**(6): 806–812.

50. van Erp TG, Walton E, Hibar DP, et al. Cortical brain abnormalities in 4474 individuals with schizophrenia and 5098 controls via the ENIGMA consortium. *Biol Psychiatry*. 2018 November 1; **84**(9): 644–654.

51. Schmaal L, Hibar DP, Sämann PG, et al. Cortical abnormalities in adults and adolescents with major depression based on brain scans from 20 cohorts worldwide in the ENIGMA major depressive disorder working group. *Mol Psychiatry*. 2017; **22**(6): 900–909.

52. Maggioni E, Crespo-Facorro B, Nenadic I, et al. Common and distinct structural features of schizophrenia and bipolar disorder: The European network on psychosis, affective disorders and cognitive trajectory (ENPACT) study. *PLoS One*. 2017; **12**(11): 1–22.

53. Wise T, Radua J, Via E, et al. Common and distinct patterns of grey-matter volume alteration in major depression and bipolar disorder: Evidence from voxel-based meta-analysis. *Mol Psychiatry*. 2016 October; 22(10): 1455–1463.

54. Kempton M, Salvador Z, R Munafò M, et al. Structural neuroimaging studies in major depressive disorder: Meta-analysis and comparison with bipolar disorder. *Archives of General Psychiatry*. 2011; **68**: 675–690

55. Sussmann JE, Lymer GKS, McKirdy J, et al. White matter abnormalities in bipolar disorder and schizophrenia detected using diffusion tensor magnetic resonance imaging. *Bipolar Disord*. 2009 February; **11**(1): 11–18.

56. Skudlarski P, Schretlen DJ, Thaker GK, et al. Diffusion tensor imaging white matter endophenotypes in patients with schizophrenia or psychotic bipolar disorder and their relatives. *Am J Psychiatry*. 2013; **170**(8): 886–898.

57. Kumar J, Iwabuchi S, Oowise S, et al. Europe PMC Funders Group. Shared white matter dysconnectivity in schizophrenia and bipolar disorder with psychosis. *Psychoogical Medicine*. 2015; **45**(4): 759–770.

58. Squarcina L, Bellani M, Rossetti MG, et al. Similar white matter changes in schizophrenia and bipolar disorder: A tract-based spatial statistics study. *PLoS One*. 2017; **12**(6): 1–17.

59. O'Donoghue S, Holleran L, Cannon DM, et al. Anatomical dysconnectivity in bipolar disorder compared with schizophrenia: A selective review of structural network analyses using

diffusion MRI. *J Affect Disord.* 2017; **209**: 217–228.

60. Liberg B, Rahm C, Panayiotou A, et al. Brain change trajectories that differentiate the major psychoses. *Eur J Clin Invest.* 2016; **46**(7): 658–674.

61. Quiroz JA, MacHado-Vieira R, Zarate CA, et al. Novel insights into lithium's mechanism of action: Neurotrophic and neuroprotective effects. *Neuropsychobiology.* 2010; **62**(1): 50–60.

62. Sun YR, Herrmann N, Scott CJM, et al. Global grey matter volume in adult bipolar patients with and without lithium treatment: A meta-analysis. *J Affect Disord.* 2018; **225**: 599–606.

63. Abramovic L, Boks MPM, Vreeker A, et al. The association of antipsychotic medication and lithium with brain measures in patients with bipolar disorder. *Eur Neuropsychopharmacol.* 2016; **26**(11): 1741–1751.

64. Yucel K, McKinnon MC, Taylor VH, et al. Bilateral hippocampal volume increases after long-term lithium treatment in patients with bipolar disorder: A longitudinal MRI study. *Psychopharmacology.* 2007; **195**(3): 357–367.

65. Lyoo IK, Dager SR, Kim JE, et al. Lithium-induced gray matter volume increase as a neural correlate of treatment response in bipolar disorder: A longitudinal brain imaging study. *Neuropsychopharmacology.* 2010; **35**(8): 1743–1750.

66. Selek S, Nicoletti M, Zunta-Soares GB, et al. A longitudinal study of fronto-limbic brain structures in patients with bipolar I disorder during lithium treatment. *J Affect Disord.* 2013; **150**(2): 629–633.

67. Hafeman DM, Chang KD, Garrett AS, et al. Effects of medication on neuroimaging findings in bipolar disorder: An updated review. *Bipolar Disord.* 2012; **14**(4): 375–410.

68. McDonald C. Brain structural effects of psychopharmacological treatment in bipolar disorder. *Curr Neuropharmacol.* 2015; **13**(4): 445–457.

69. Vernon AC, Natesan S, Modo M, et al. Effect of chronic antipsychotic treatment on brain structure: A serial magnetic resonance imaging study with ex vivo and postmortem confirmation. *Biol Psychiatry.* 2011; **69**(10): 936–944.

70. Ho B-C, Andreasen N, Ziebel S, et al. Long-term antipsychotic treatment and brain volumes: A longitudinal study of first-episode schizophrenia. *Arch Gen Psychiatry.* 2012; **68**(2): 128–137.

71. Abramovic L, Boks MPM, Vreeker A, et al. White matter disruptions in patients with bipolar disorder. *Eur Neuropsychopharmacol.* 2018; **28**(6): 743–751.

72. Cropley VL, Klauser P, Lenroot RK, et al. Accelerated gray and white matter deterioration with age in schizophrenia. *Am J Psychiatry.* 2017; **174**(3): 286–295.

73. Nenadić I, Dietzek M, Langbein K, et al. BrainAGE score indicates accelerated brain aging in schizophrenia, but not bipolar disorder. *Psychiatry Res – Neuroimaging.* 2017; **266**: 86–89.

74. Amelia Versace, Almeida Jorge RC, Stefanie Hassel, et al. Elevated left and reduced right orbitomedial prefrontal fractional anisotropy in adults with bipolar disorder revealed by tract-based spatial statistics. *Arch Gen Psychiatry.* 2008 September; **65**(9): 1041–1052. DOI:10.1001/archpsyc.65.9.1041.

75. Schneider MR, Delbello MP, McNamara RK, et al. Neuroprogression in bipolar disorder. *Bipolar Disord.* 2012; **14**(4):356–374.

76. Lim CS, Baldessarini RJ, Vieta E, et al. Longitudinal neuroimaging and neuropsychological changes in bipolar disorder patients: Review of the evidence. *Neurosci Biobehav Rev.* 2013; **37**(3): 418–435.

77. Kozicky JM, McGirr A, Bond DJ, et al. Neuroprogression and episode recurrence in bipolar I disorder: A study of gray matter volume changes in first-episode mania and association with clinical outcome. *Bipolar Disord.* 2016; **18**(6): 511–519.

78. Abé C, Ekman CJ, Sellgren C, et al. Manic episodes are related to changes in frontal cortex: A longitudinal neuroimaging study of bipolar disorder 1. *Brain.* 2015; **138**(11): 3440–3448.

Chapter 4

Neuroimaging Biomarkers in Pediatric Mood Disorders

Mary Melissa Packer, Whitney Tang, and Manpreet K. Singh

Mood disorders, including bipolar disorder (BD) and major depressive disorder (MDD), are serious and often-recurring psychiatric conditions that commonly first manifest during childhood or adolescence (1, 2). Youth with mood disorders are four times more likely to attempt suicide (32% vs. 8% in the general population) (3), are at elevated risk for developing co-occurring psychiatric disorders (4), and frequently experience family maladjustment and exposure to significant early-life stress (5, 6). Pediatric mood disorders are also associated with academic impairment and reduced global functioning (7). Despite advances in accurately diagnosing and treating pediatric mood disorders, objective diagnostic and therapeutic biomarkers anchored in neurophysiological underpinnings of these psychiatric conditions are only beginning to emerge.

Neuroimaging studies in humans hold promise for a mechanistic understanding of aberrant structure and function in brain regions that contribute to the onset, persistence, and recurrence of mood disorders that start in childhood. For example, studies thus far have revealed altered interactions between prefrontal and subcortical brain regions that are central to mood disorders and putatively result in dysfunctional regulation of emotion and cognition over time (8) (Figure 4.1).

Brain regions and circuits that subserve core symptoms in pediatric mood disorders may function pathologically or may function to compensate prevention of pathology when compared to healthy control (HC) youth. For example, aberrant emotion salience and regulation, reward processing, and cognition in mood disorders may result from anomalous reciprocal connections between the amygdala and dorsal and ventral prefrontal areas (8, 9), which may further result in anatomical differences compared to healthy

youth, including amygdala volume reductions (10). These anomalies may further generate susceptibilities toward dysfunction in other brain regions related to emotion, including the anterior cingulate cortex (ACC), ventrolateral prefrontal cortex (VLPFC), striatum, thalamus, cerebellar vermis, and hippocampus (11). Alternatively, structural abnormalities, such as reductions in the amygdala and hippocampal volumes, may characterize mood disorders independently of functional abnormalities, including the subgenual anterior cingulate cortex (sgACC), dorsolateral prefrontal cortex (DLPFC), amygdala, and ventral striatum. Understanding variations in structure–function interactions in the brain over development may be critical to the pathophysiology of underlying mood disorders.

We subsequently review functional and structural magnetic resonance imaging (MRI) data that demonstrate aberrant responses to stress and reward and maladaptive developmental trajectories in pediatric BD and MDD. We conclude with implications of these neuroimaging markers for treatment of pediatric mood disorders.

4.1 Aberrant Responses to Stress and Reward

Acute stress causes a natural effect on attention, motivation, mood, perception, and other aspects of mental function. Although these brain responses to stress may be adaptive for most, in youth with BD and MDD, they may adversely affect the stress-response pathway and lead to maladaptive behaviors and outcomes. Similarly, mood disorders are centrally conceptualized by aberrant responses to reward- or goal-directed stimuli (9). Aberrant stress and reward responses can biologically interact, especially in the context of early exposures to trauma or adversity (6), and

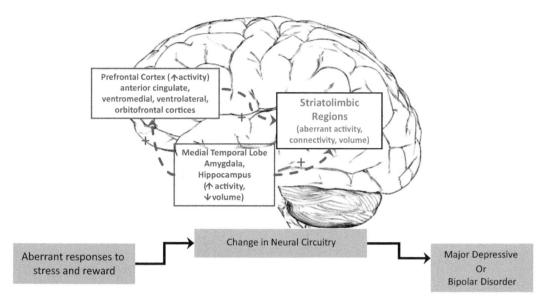

Figure 4.1 Candidate brain regions and circuits associated with aberrant responses to stress and reward in youth with or at risk for a major mood disorder. A black and white version of this figure will appear in some formats. For the colour version, refer to the plate section.

reveal themselves through key biomarkers. Selected biomarkers are outlined subsequently and summarized in Table 4.1.

In pediatric BD, the most notable brain biomarker of aberrant response to stress is reduced medial temporal lobe volumes in the amygdala and hippocampus. Reduced amygdala volume in pediatric versus adult populations with BD is consistently supported by metanalytic data (10). Indeed, amygdala and hippocampal volumes are highly sensitized to stress exposure, as evident in studies of adults with BD with and without exposures to traumatic life events, so the prevalence of these biomarkers in pediatric BD, which commonly involves onsets of mania that may be associated with or triggered by a stressful life event, follows logically (12, 13).

It is reassuring that prefrontal cortical activation has been found to be relatively intact in children, compared to adults, with BD. In the context of exposure to stress, intact prefrontal function is critical for effective emotion regulation. In some studies, euthymic children with BD have exhibited prefrontal *over*activation (e.g., in the ACC) during emotional paradigms, such as a 2-back visuospatial working memory task and an affective task involving the visualization of positively, neutrally, or negatively valenced pictures (1), suggesting that emotion dysregulation may interrupt typical cognitive function during times of stress.

Neuroimaging studies also show a statistical trend for decrease in hippocampal volume in youth with BD (14). Through inhibitory connections with other subcortical structures, the hippocampus is involved in the appraisal and regulation of stress and the generation of emotion and memory, indicating that youth with BD who have a smaller hippocampus may be more susceptible to stress. Reduced hippocampal volume is typically interpreted as resultant of enhanced cortisol release in response to hyperarousal, but might also be a preexistent risk factor (6). Of note, adversity may also contribute to reduced hippocampal volume, thus enhancing the likelihood of developing BD. In addition to volumetric comparisons, studies have also found that connectivity between the right laterobasal amygdala and right hippocampus is positively correlated with levels of anxiety (15). This further supports the role of the hippocampus in stress processing.

Reduced hippocampal volume is a recurring finding in youth with MDD. Reductions in hippocampal volume are a consequence of depressive symptoms detected as early as preschool (16). As with BD, this implicates an aberrant response to stress in adolescents with MDD and may represent a preexisting risk factor. Because of the significant role of the hippocampus in emotion regulation, the impact of decreased volume signifies a blunted

Table 4.1 Selected brain biomarkers of aberrant responses to stress and reward likely leading to mood disorders in youth

Region/network	Major depressive disorder (MDD)/ bipolar disorder (BD)	Specificity/implication for mood disorder	Reference
		Stress	
Medial temporal lobe	BD	Reductions in amygdala and hippocampal volume*	(10, 45)
		Connectivity between the right laterobasal amygdala and right hippocampus positively correlate with anxiety levels	(15)
	MDD	Reductions in gray matter	(16)
Anterior cingulate cortex (ACC), ventral medial prefrontal cortex (vmPFC), orbitofrontal cortex (OFC), amygdala	MDD	Across tasks assessing emotion processing, cognitive control, affective cognition, reward-processing, and resting state, elevated neural activity in ACC, vmPFC and OFC, and the amygdala	(26)
		Reward	
Striatum	BD	Increased putamen volume	(8)
		Increased caudate volume	(8)
		Bilateral caudate and left putamen volumes related inversely to age and pubertal status	
		Increased left nucleus accumbens (NAcc)	(48)
		Smaller NAcc	(49)
	MDD	Reductions in overall striatal volume	(22)
		Decreased striatal activity during reward feedback	(22)
		Decreased activity in right caudate (body and head) and left caudate body during reward feedback	(22)
		Decreased activity during reward anticipation bilaterally at caudate head and left putamen. Stronger blunting of activity in younger age studies	(22)
		Decreased activity in caudate, putamen, and globus pallidus	(22)
		Increased connectivity of ventral striatum predicts depression	(51)

* Some studies observed no difference in hippocampal volumes between youth with BD versus healthy subjects (8, 37).

response during emotion processing. Studies show that GM reductions in hippocampal volume are associated with an increased number of depressive episodes, greater symptom severity, and longer illness duration (17). Advancements in imaging resolution and processing have helped delineate amygdala–hippocampal boundaries, morphology, and subfields (18, 19), which provide additional granularity to explain progressive deficits in structure and function of the amygdala and hippocampus in relation to illness duration.

Similar to stress processing, reward processing activates limbic, striatal, and prefrontal systems in the brain. For healthy individuals, activity in the nucleus accumbens (NAcc) shell, ventral pallidum, parabrachial nucleus, orbitofrontal cortex (OFC), and insular cortex commonly instantiate reward-related pleasure. In youth with MDD and BD, however, a different neuroanatomical map is observed.

Reward processing in pediatric BD. BD is defined by aberrant emotion and motivation that may lead to prompt risk-taking behaviors, and may be characterized by fluctuating experiences of hyperhedonia and anhedonia (20). Studies demonstrate that youth with BD compared with HCs report increased reward reactivity, greater arousal in reward conditions, and greater satisfaction with winning (21). These reports are substantiated in the pediatric brain through increased striatal volume and striatal hyperactivity, including enlargement of the putamen, caudate, and NAcc.

Youth with BD with higher levels of manic symptoms have decreased NAcc activation during reward anticipation compared to those with fewer manic symptoms (20), perhaps indicating that errors in reward prediction signaling may come from NAcc desensitization during reward activation. Together, these patterns of activation may clinically manifest in BD as grandiosity and dysregulated goal pursuit (20). In healthy youth offspring of parents with BD, increased OFC activation and increased pregenual anterior cingulate connectivity to the VLPFC while anticipating rewards suggest pre–illness-specific prefrontal regulatory mechanisms that may be deployed to mitigate reward activation and to keep mania symptoms at bay. Notably, in high-risk but not low-risk children, novelty seeking was associated with increased striatal and amygdalar activation in the anticipation of losses, and impulsivity was associated with increased striatal and insula activation in the receipt of rewards, suggesting potential targets for preventive intervention.

Reward processing in pediatric MDD. Depression is also characterized by an inability to modulate behavior in response to intermittent rewards, possibly due to blunted phasic dopaminergic signaling critically implicated in reward learning (9). Recent findings indicate that ventral striatal (VS) blunting might constitute a risk factor for depression. Specifically, reduced reward-related VS activation predicted increased depressive symptoms over two years among adolescents (22).

Youth with MDD show decreased volumes in the striatum and decreased activation in the caudate, putamen, and globus pallidus during reward responses (22). This suggests decreased brain sensitivity to anticipating and consuming rewards, which is a defining characteristic of anhedonia and a core feature of MDD. Structural abnormalities in key prefrontal subregions, including the VLPFC, the DLPFC, the ACC and sgACC, and the OFC (23), may result in impairments in executive functions, emotion regulation, and reward processing in MDD.

In youth with MDD, abnormal limbic processing is attributed to decreased regulatory control of dorsal cortical regions (24) and altered functional activation and connectivity in extended medial prefrontal network regions, including the ACC, OFC, ventromedial PFC, and closely linked subcortical areas that include the amygdala (elevated amygdala activation) (25) and striatal regions. These prefrontal–limbic network findings have been observed in both medicated and unmedicated youth with MDD, and cover various domains of brain functioning, including tasks of cognitive control, emotional processing, affective cognition, stress, and reward-based decision-making (26). Similar to adults, depressed youth have been found to have alterations in prefrontal activation, including the medial and ventral subregions, resulting in impaired regulation of emotion during depression (26).

The neural network dysfunction observed in depression has interactive or consequent effects with multiple regulatory systems that may manifest through co-occurring conditions. For example, recent evidence suggests that a shared brain motivational network underpins the co-occurrence of depression and obesity among youth (27). Reward neural circuits (including regions such as the ACC and hippocampus) may underlie dysfunctional behavioral responses and increased sensitivity to rewarding aspects of ingesting high-calorie food that lead to disinhibitory behavior toward eating despite satiation. Youth with greater levels of insulin resistance (IR) show higher levels of anhedonia and food-seeking behaviors, reduced hippocampal and ACC volumes, and greater levels of ACC and hippocampal dysconnectivity to fronto-limbic reward networks at rest. Moreover, for youth with high levels of IR, thinner ACC and smaller hippo-campal volumes were associated with more severe depressive symptoms. The opposite was found for youth with low levels of IR. The ACC–hippocampal motivational network that underlies depression and IR separately may signify an important neural collaboration that connects these two syndromes to each other. Reward neural systems are also perturbed by early-life stress such that in youth with depression and obesity, higher levels of abuse moderate the relation between reward network connectivity in the amygdala, insula, and NAcc and IR (28).

Collectively, these neuroimaging findings support mechanistic formulations of pediatric mood disorders as having aberrant responses to stress and reward mapped along abnormal structure and function of prefrontal–limbic and prefrontal–striatal networks. Stress-related reductions in medial temporal neuroanatomy and overactivity of striatal and limbic networks during tasks of emotion and reward processing are consistent across BD and MDD youth. Whereas reduced-reward system task activation and resting-state connectivity may represent a dimensional phenotype of depression severity common to bipolar and unipolar depression, categorical differences in reward system resting-state connectivity between unipolar and bipolar depression may represent a differential risk for mania. The biomarkers that emerge from these mechanisms hold promise for the development of novel and targeted interventions matched to individual profiles of stress and reward response.

4.2 Maladaptive Developmental Trajectories

Cortical GM maturation in childhood has been marked by early neuronal development and volume increases culminating in puberty, followed by discriminatory removal and myelination, and volume loss and thinning. This inverted-U-shaped course, in addition to cortical thickness, has been mapped to the evolution of emotion and cognitive regulation of emotion (29). Because many major psychiatric illnesses are viewed as neurodevelopmental, research on how mood disorders affect developmental trajectories is critical.

Disturbances in prefrontal–subcortical circuits in pediatric BD may manifest partly from structural volumetric deviations within regions in these circuits or come from distinct networks in BD that

may result in less glial or neuronal support for specific brain structures (1). These interconnected functional and structural differences may contribute to the development or exacerbation of mood symptoms or represent markers of resilience in youth at familial risk for BD and MDD. For example, when compared with youth with a family history of BD or MDD who developed a mood disorder, those who were resilient had higher left inferior parietal lobe connectivity with visual cortical regions while processing happy faces and higher inferior frontal gyrus connectivity with frontal, temporal, and limbic regions while processing fearful faces (30). Through prospective evaluation of youth at risk for mood disorders, markers of conversion to a mood disorder versus resilience from developing a mood disorder may be delineated. Indeed, cortical GM loss that is typical during adolescence has been observed to occur at an accelerated rate in children with BD, suggesting disorder-related disruptions in typical neurodevelopment (31).

In a longitudinal study of youth with MDD, Luby and colleagues found that global reduction in GM volume, as indexed by cortical thinning, was directly associated with depression severity (29). Given that the age range covered in the study (preschool to adolescence) is characterized by a reduction in GM volume, putatively indicating synaptic pruning, this study suggests accelerated synaptic pruning in individuals who have experienced depressive symptoms (2). Moreover, their findings showing depression-related changes in volume and thickness of cortical GM present as early as middle childhood add to an expanding body of neuroimaging data in youth with MDD.

BD and MDD are often recurrent, and it is possible that an initial mood episode in youth may trigger key biological processes, in turn leading to subsequent mood episodes that may also be exacerbated by life stressors. Future investigation could use longitudinal modeling to examine precisely how the accumulation and timing of stressors along with the experience of mood symptoms influence brain development (2) or compare youth at familial risk for depression to those who have already developed depression (32). Table 4.2 summarizes studies that suggest maladaptive developmental trajectories, though additional longitudinal studies are needed to understand mood disorder onset and persistence over time, especially into adulthood.

Table 4.2 Selected brain biomarkers of maladaptive developmental trajectories likely leading to mood disorders in youth

Region/ network	Impact	Major depressive disorder (MDD)/ bipolar disorder (BD)	Specificity/implication for mood disorder	Reference
Whole brain	Drives functional deficits during critical periods of neurodevelopment	BD	Volumetric reductions in GM and white matter in the cerebrum, but not in cerebrospinal fluid	(8, 45)
			Parietal and temporal lobe volume reductions in regions pertaining to face recognition, attentional control, and memory	(45)
			Significant reductions in superior temporal gyrus in the temporal lobe	(52)
		MDD	Bilateral reductions in cortical GM thickness and in the volume of the right hemisphere, but needs further replication	(29)
			Cortical thinning in anterior, subgenual, and posterior cingulate, and medial orbitofrontal cortex of the right hemisphere	(53)
			Thinning in right pericalcarine gyrus, postcentral gyrus, superior parietal gyrus, and left supramarginal gyrus	(54)
			Larger lateral ventricular volume, but smaller frontal lobe volume	(55)
			General reductions in whole brain volumes	(56)
Prefrontal cortex (PFC)	Impairment in executive functions, processing of rewards and motivation, and regulation of emotion and attention (1)	BD	Reductions in dorsolateral prefrontal cortex (DLPFC) volumes	(48)
			Reductions in ventrolateral PFC volumes	(57)
			Reductions in ACC	(58)
			Bilateral anterior and subgenual ACC reductions most pronounced after illness onset	(59)
			Subgenual anterior cingulate cortex (sgACC) volume reductions observed in the left hemisphere**	(60)
			Amplified bilateral posterior sgACC volumes with past mood stabilizer exposure	(36)
		MDD	Aberrations in rostral ACC (rACC) volume for boys**	(61)

Table 4.2 (cont.)

Region/network	Impact	Major depressive disorder (MDD)/ bipolar disorder (BD)	Specificity/implication for mood disorder	Reference
			Decreased GM rACC volumes in patients with comorbid MDD and borderline personality disorder***	(62)
			Reductions in GM volume in bilateral DLPFC	(63)
Amygdala	Impairment to perception and emotional valence, memory, and learning	BD	Decreased amygdala volume#	(8, 45)
		MDD	Bilateral reductions of GM in the caudate nucleus	(64)
Thalamus and other regions	Impairments in learning, processing, and regulating social emotions (e.g., guilt)	MDD	Reduced GM in right superior and middle temporal gyri and in the thalamus	(64)
			Decreased left and right anterior insula volumes in school-age children previously diagnosed with preschool-onset MDD	(65)
		BD	None	(8, 45)

* Studies mixed contingent upon specific region/hemisphere examined and sex of participants.

** More significant with familial risk.

*** rACC volume correlated with BD symptom severity and suicide attempts, not with depressive symptom severity.

\# Possibly a developmental finding specific to youth with BD versus adults (10)

4.3 Implications of Neurobiological Markers for Treatment

Brain characteristics which represent behavioral and cognitive aberrations that are evident in youth with mood disorders can be utilized to clarify overlapping and distinct characteristics in MDD and BD that may shed light on etiologic underpinnings, suitable diagnostic classification structures, and the assignment of appropriate treatment. Brain-responsive biomarkers in pediatric mood disorders have been described with pharmacological and psychotherapeutic interventions (33). Reassuringly, most studies reviewed have suggested that intervention has an overall normalizing effect on brain structure and function, particularly in the prefrontal, limbic, and striatal regions and networks that are critical for emotional functioning and regulation.

4.4 Pediatric BD Treatment Implications

Medications used to treat BD symptoms may restore volumetric deficits and improve functional activity in ventrolateral and medial prefrontal regions critical for emotional functioning and regulation (33). Indeed, the neurotrophic effects of lithium on amygdala and hippocampal volumes also correlate with symptom improvement. Moreover, there appears to be normalization of structure and functional activations while performing a wide array of neurocognitive tasks after treatments with antidepressants, atypical antipsychotics, and mood stabilizers. For example, response to lithium treatment in pediatric BD is associated with normalization of white matter microstructure in regions associated with emotion processing (34), larger right hippocampal volumes (35), and greater posterior sgACC (36) and amygdala (37) volumes.

In other cases, treatment studies with neuroimaging may yield novel interpretations of early studies. For example, the neuroimaging study with the longest follow-up period for patients with pediatric BD after an intervention found that DLPFC activation normalized by sixteen weeks, but the VLPFC, ACC, amygdala, and striatum did not normalize until the three-year follow-up (38). This study suggested that medication has the earliest effect on DLPFC function than any other region tested. Additional information is needed to better understand when the benefit from interventions is optimal, and how they compare relative to one another. Longitudinal studies that track youth into adulthood may clarify long-term effects of treatment.

Nonpharmacological treatment also has normalizing effects on the developing brain in youth with or at-risk for BD. Specifically, youth with BD exhibiting depressive symptoms show increased activation in the hippocampus and thalamus (39) following psychotherapy. Family-focused therapy and mindfulness-based cognitive therapy have proven brain benefits for youth with and at-risk for BD, restoring prefrontal (DLPFC) regulatory function that corresponds to improvement in mania symptom severity (40), and increased activation of the insula and anterior cingulate (41) corresponding to improved anxiety, respectively.

4.5 Pediatric MDD Treatment Implications

In pediatric depression, emotion regulation processes are central to cognitive behavioral therapy (CBT), which is the most studied and first-line psychotherapeutic intervention for youth with MDD (26). Psychotherapy has pronounced neurobiological effects on MDD youth. Moreover, treatment effects are observed to be sustained beyond the acute phase of treatment. Depressed patients who had increased activation in the left anterior hippocampus/amygdala, sgACC, and medial prefrontal cortex (mPFC) before treatment with psychodynamic psychotherapy showed a reduction in activation in these areas and improved depression symptoms after fifteen months of treatment (42). CBT seems to have selective effects on the functioning of specific limbic and cortical regions (43). Together, these results suggest that neuroimaging can identify treatment-specific biomarkers.

In the only fMRI study to examine changes in brain activity with treatment in pediatric MDD, overactivation in prefrontal and temporal regions in depressed youth normalized after eight weeks of fluoxetine treatment (44). Subsequent region-of-interest analyses of the areas implicated in emotion processing signified that, prior to treatment, the youth exhibited significantly greater activations to fearful versus neutral facial expressions than did HC subjects in the OFC, amygdala, and subgenual ACC bilaterally. Fluoxetine treatment reduced activations in these three emotion regulatory regions.

Longitudinal controlled studies are needed to understand the relations between mood disorders and neuroimaging findings to identify neurobiomarkers. Such studies are emerging, and will aid in developing rational treatment strategies in individuals with and at-risk for developing mood disorders, to determine whether there are particular windows during development that would be optimal (or deleterious), and to elucidate the mechanisms that contribute to illness onset and progression.

4.6 Conclusion

Cumulative research suggests that there are early neural markers and events that predispose youth for the development of major mood disorders. Aberrant stress reactivity and reward processing, and maladaptive developmental trajectories predispose mood symptom development and suggest prefrontal-subcortical mechanisms that underpin the pathophysiology of pediatric mood disorders. Some extant studies, however, have been limited by confounding illness-related variables, such as co-occurring conditions, exposures to psychotropic medications, or recreational drugs, that can make it challenging to clarify the etiology of mood disorders in youth. Newly advanced MRI and computational tools will help clarify neural biomarkers while prospective cortical thickness and other advanced, multimodal brain mapping approaches will aid in deeper characterization of structural anomalies. Novel functional and resting-state connectivity studies that clarify functional relations among brain networks involved in complex and transdiagnostic symptoms are also being developed. Neuroimaging studies directly comparing high-risk youth and youth with BD or MDD over time are important to elucidate risk factors for, versus consequences of,

BD and MDD. High-risk and longitudinal neu-roimaging studies can shed light on the hetero-geneity in these processes and the etiologic pathways to disorder (32). With additional research, the multifactorial etiology of pediatric-onset mood disorders may be elucidated so that young patients diagnosed with these disorders may be more accurately diagnosed and more effectively treated at the earliest opportunity.

References

1. Strakowski SM (ed.). *The Bipolar Brain: Integrating Neuroimaging with Genetics.* New York: Oxford University Press; 2012.

2. Gotlib IH, Ordaz SJ. The importance of assessing neural trajectories in pediatric depression. *JAMA Psychiatry.* 2016; **73**(1): 9–10.

3. Centers for Disease Control and Prevention. CDC/National Center for Health Statistics [Internet]. 2017; available from: www.cdc.gov/datastatistics/index.html

4. Axelson D, Birmaher B, Strober M, et al. Phenomenology of children and adolescents with bipolar spectrum disorders. *Arch Gen Psychiatry.* 2006; **63**(10): 1139–1148.

5. Strawn JR, Adler CM, Fleck DE, et al. Post-traumatic stress symptoms and trauma exposure in youth with first episode bipolar disorder. *Early Interv Psychiatry.* 2010; **4**(2): 169–173.

6. Rao U, Chen L-A, Bidesi AS, et al. Hippocampal changes associated with early-life adversity and vulnerability to depression. *Biol Psychiatry.* 2010; **67**(4): 357–364.

7. Verboom CE, Sijtsema JJ, Verhulst FC, Penninx BWJH, Ormel J. Longitudinal associations between depressive problems, academic performance, and social functioning in adolescent boys and girls. *Dev Psychol.* 2014; **50**(1): 247–257.

8. DelBello MP, Zimmerman ME, Mills NP, Getz GE, Strakowski SM. Magnetic resonance imaging analysis of amygdala and other subcortical brain regions in adolescents with bipolar disorder. *Bipolar Disord.* 2004; **6**(1): 43–52.

9. Whitton AE, Treadway MT, Pizzagalli DA. Reward processing dysfunction in major depression, bipolar disorder and schizophrenia. *Curr Opin Psychiatry.* 2015; **28**(1): 7–12.

10. Pfeifer JC, Welge J, Strakowski SM, Adler CM, DelBello MP. Meta-analysis of amygdala volumes in children and adolescents with bipolar disorder. *J Am Acad Child Adolesc Psychiatry.* 2008; **47**(11): 1289–1298.

11. Caetano SC, Olvera RL, Glahn D, et al. Fronto-limbic brain abnormalities in juvenile onset bipolar disorder. *Biol Psychiatry.* 2005; **58**(7): 525–531.

12. Usher J, Leucht S, Falkai P, Scherk H. Correlation between amygdala volume and age in bipolar disorder – a systematic review and meta-analysis of structural MRI studies. *Psychiatry Res.* 2010; **182** (1): 1–8.

13. Janiri D, Sani G, Rossi PD, et al. Amygdala and hippocampus volumes are differently affected by childhood trauma in patients with bipolar disorders and healthy controls. *Bipolar Disord.* 2017; **19**(5): 353–362.

14. Frazier JA, Breeze JL, Makris N, et al. Cortical gray matter differences identified by structural magnetic resonance imaging in pediatric bipolar disorder. *Bipolar Disord.* 2005; **7**(6): 555–569.

15. Singh MK, Kelley RG, Chang KD, Gotlib IH. Intrinsic amygdala functional connectivity in youth with bipolar I disorder. *J Am Acad Child Adolesc Psychiatry.* 2015; **54**(9): 763–770.

16. Caetano SC, Fonseca M, Hatch JP, et al. Medial temporal lobe abnormalities in pediatric unipolar depression. *Neurosci Lett.* 2007; **427**(3): 142–147.

17. Videbech P, Ravnkilde B. Hippocampal volume and depression: a meta-analysis of MRI studies. *Am J Psychiatry.* 2004; **161**(11): 1957–1966.

18. Kelley R, Chang KD, Garrett A, et al. Deformations of amygdala morphology in familial pediatric bipolar disorder. *Bipolar Disord.* 2013; **15** (7): 795–802.

19. Tannous J, Amaral-Silva H, Cao B, et al. Hippocampal subfield volumes in children and adolescents with mood disorders. *J Psychiatr Res.* 2018; **101**: 57–62.

20. Singh MK, Chang KD, Kelley RG, et al. Reward processing in adolescents with bipolar I disorder. *J Am Acad Child Adolesc Psychiatry.* 2013; **52**(1): 68–83.

21. Rich BA, Schmajuk M, Perez-Edgar KE, et al. The impact of reward, punishment, and frustration on attention in pediatric bipolar disorder. *Biol Psychiatry.* 2005; **58**(7): 532–539.

22. Keren H, O'Callaghan G, Vidal-Ribas P, et al. Reward processing in depression: a conceptual and meta-analytic review across fMRI and EEG studies. *Am J Psychiatry.* 2014 January; **9**(1): 94–108. DOI:10.1177/1745691613513469.

23. Salvadore G, Quiroz JA, Machado-Vieira R, et al. The neurobiology of the switch process in bipolar disorder: a review. *J Clin Psychiatry.* 2010; **71**(11): 1488–1501.

24. Gotlib IH, Joormann J, Foland-Ross LC. Understanding familial risk for depression: a 25-year perspective. *Perspect Psychol Sci.* 2014; **9**(1): 94–108.

25. Pagliaccio D, Luby J, Gaffrey M, et al. Anomalous functional brain activation following negative mood induction in children with pre-school onset major depression. *Dev Cogn Neurosci.* 2012; **2**(2): 256–267.

26. Kerestes R, Davey CG, Stephanou K, Whittle S, Harrison BJ. Functional brain imaging studies of youth depression: a systematic review. *NeuroImage: Clin.* 2014; **4**: 209–231.

27. Singh MK, Leslie SM, Packer MM, et al. Brain and behavioral correlates of insulin resistance in youth with depression and obesity. *Hormones and Behavior.* [Internet] 2018 [cited 2018 September 11]; available from: https://linkinghub.elsevier.com/retrieve/pii/S0018506X17305019

28. Sun KL, Watson KT, Angal S, et al. Neural and endocrine correlates of early life abuse in youth with depression and obesity. *Front Psychiatry.* 2018; **9**: 721.

29. Luby JL, Belden AC, Jackson JJ, Lessov-Schlaggar CN, Harms MP, Tillman R, et al. Early childhood depression and alterations in the trajectory of gray matter maturation in middle childhood and early ddolescence. *JAMA Psychiatry.* 2016; **73**(1): 31.

30. Nimarko AF, Garrett AS, Carlson GA, Singh MK. Neural correlates of emotion processing predict resilience in youth at familial risk for mood disorders. *Dev Psychopathol.* 2019 August; **31**(3): 1037–1052. DOI:10.1017/S0954579419000579.

31. Gogtay N, Rapoport JL. Childhood-onset schizophrenia: Insights from neuroimaging studies. *J Am Acad Child Adolesc Psychiatry.* 2008; **47**(10): 1120–1124.

32. Singh MK, Leslie SM, Packer MM, Weisman EF, Gotlib IH. Limbic intrinsic connectivity in depressed and high-risk youth. *Journal of Am Acad Child Adolesc Psychiatry.* 2018 October; **57**(10): 775–785.e3. DOI:10.1016/j.jaac.2018.06.017.

33. Singh MK, Garrett AS, Chang KD. Using neuroimaging to evaluate and guide pharmacological and psychotherapeutic treatments for mood disorders in children. *CNS Spectr.* 2015; **20**(4): 359–368.

34. Kafantaris V, Spritzer L, Doshi V, Saito E, Szeszko PR. Changes in white matter microstructure predict lithium response in adolescents with bipolar disorder. *Bipolar Disord.* 2017; **19**(7): 587–594.

35. Baykara B, Inal-Emiroglu N, Karabay N, et al. Increased hippocampal volumes in lithium treated adolescents with bipolar disorders: A structural MRI study. *J Affect Disord.* 2012; **138**(3): 433–439.

36. Mitsunaga MM, Garrett A, Howe M, et al. Increased subgenual cingulate cortex volume in pediatric bipolar disorder associated with mood stabilizer exposure. *J Child Adolesc Psychopharmacol.* 2011; **21**(2): 149–155.

37. Chang K, Barnea-Goraly N, Karchemskiy A, et al. Cortical magnetic resonance imaging findings in familial pediatric bipolar disorder. *Biological Psychiatry.* 2005; **58**(3): 197–203.

38. Yang H, Lu LH, Wu M, et al. Time course of recovery showing initial prefrontal cortex changes at 16 weeks, extending to subcortical changes by 3 years in pediatric bipolar disorder. *J Affect Disord* 2013; **150**(2): 571–577.

39. Diler RS, Segreti AM, Ladouceur CD, et al. Neural correlates of treatment in adolescents with bipolar depression during response inhibition. *J Child Adolesc Psychopharmacol.* 2013; **23**(3): 214–221.

40. Garrett AS, Miklowitz DJ, Howe ME, et al. Changes in brain activation following psychotherapy for youth with mood dysregulation at familial risk for bipolar disorder. *Prog Neuropsychopharmacol Biol Psychiatry.* 2015; **56**: 215–220.

41. Strawn JR, Cotton S, Luberto CM, et al. Neural function before and after mindfulness-based cognitive therapy in anxious adolescents at risk for developing bipolar disorder. *J Child Adolesc Psychopharmacol.* 2016; **26**(4): 372–379.

42. Buchheim A, Viviani R, Kessler H, et al. Changes in prefrontal-limbic function in major depression after 15 months of long-term psychotherapy. *PLoS ONE.* 2012; **7**(3): e33745.

43. Goldapple K, Segal Z, Garson C, et al. Modulation of cortical-limbic pathways in major depression: treatment-specific effects of cognitive behavior therapy. *Arch Gen Psychiatry.* 2004; **61**(1): 34–41.

44. Tao R, Calley CS, Hart J, et al. Brain activity in adolescent major depressive disorder before and after fluoxetine treatment. *Am J Psychiatry.* 2012; **169**(4): 381–388.

45. Frazier JA, Breeze JL, Makris N, et al. Cortical gray matter differences identified by structural magnetic resonance imaging in pediatric bipolar disorder. *Bipolar Disord.* 2005; **7**(6): 555–569.

46. Bearden CE, Thompson PM, Dutton RA, et al. Three-dimensional mapping of hippocampal anatomy in unmedicated and lithium-treated patients with bipolar disorder. *Neuropsychopharmacology.* 2008; **33**(6): 1229–1238.

47. Ahn W-Y, Rass O, Fridberg DJ, et al. Temporal discounting of rewards in patients with bipolar disorder and schizophrenia. *J Abnorm Psychol*. 2011; **120**(4): 911–921.

48. Dickstein DP, Leibenluft E. Emotion regulation in children and adolescents: Boundaries between normalcy and bipolar disorder. *Development and Psychopathology*. 2006; **18**(4): 1105–1131.

49. Geller B, Tillman R, Bolhofner K, Zimerman B. Child bipolar I disorder: Prospective continuity with adult bipolar I disorder; characteristics of second and third episodes; predictors of 8-year outcome. *Arch Gen Psychiatry*. 2008; **65**(10): 1125–1133.

50. Matsuo K, R Rosenberg D, C Easter P, et al. Striatal volume abnormalities in treatment-naïve patients diagnosed with pediatric major depressive disorder. *Journal of Child and Adolescent Psychopharmacology*. 2008; **18**: 121–131.

51. Pan PM, Sato JR, Salum GA, et al. Ventral striatum functional connectivity as a predictor of adolescent depressive disorder in a longitudinal community-based sample. *AJP*. 2017; **174**(11): 1112–1119.

52. Chen HH, Nicoletti MA, Hatch JP, et al. Abnormal left superior temporal gyrus volumes in children and adolescents with bipolar disorder: A magnetic resonance imaging study. *Neurosci Lett*. 2004; **363**(1): 65–68.

53. Peterson BS, Warner V, Bansal R, et al. Cortical thinning in persons at increased familial risk for major depression. *PNAS*. 2009; **106**(15): 6273–6278.

54. Fallucca E, MacMaster FP, Haddad J, et al. Distinguishing between major depressive disorder and obsessive-compulsive disorder in children by measuring regional cortical thickness. *Arch Gen Psychiatry*. 2011; **68**(5): 527–533.

55. Steingard RJ, Renshaw PF, Yurgelun-Todd D, et al. Structural abnormalities in brain magnetic resonance images of depressed children. *J Am Acad Child Adolesc Psychiatry*. 1996; **35**(3): 307–311.

56. Steingard RJ, Renshaw PF, Hennen J, et al. Smaller frontal lobe white matter volumes in depressed adolescents. *Biological Psychiatry*. 2002; **52**(5): 413–417.

57. Blumberg HP, Krystal JH, Bansal R, et al. Age, rapid-cycling, and pharmacotherapy effects on ventral prefrontal cortex in bipolar disorder: A cross-sectional study. *Biol Psychiatry*. 2006; **59**(7): 611–618.

58. Chiu S, Widjaja F, Bates M, et al. Anterior cingulate volume in pediatric bipolar disorder and autism. *Journal of Affective Disorders*. 2008; **105**: 93–99.

59. Gogtay N, Ordonez A, Herman DH, et al. Dynamic mapping of cortical development before and after the onset of pediatric bipolar illness. *J Child Psychol Psychiatry*. 2007; **48**(9): 852–862.

60. Baloch HA, Hatch JP, Olvera RL, et al. Morphology of the subgenual prefrontal cortex in pediatric bipolar disorder. *J Psychiatr Res*. 2010; **44**(15): 1106–1110.

61. Boes AD, McCormick LM, Coryell WH, Nopoulos P. Rostral anterior cingulate cortex volume correlates with depressed mood in normal healthy children. *Biol Psychiatry*. 2008; **63**(4): 391–397.

62. Goodman M, Hazlett EA, Avedon JB, et al. Anterior cingulate volume reduction in adolescents with borderline personality disorder and co-morbid major depression. *Journal of Psychiatric Research*. 2011; **45**(6): 803–807.

63. Nolan CL, Moore GJ, Madden R, et al. Prefrontal cortical volume in childhood-onset major depression: Preliminary findings. *Arch Gen Psychiatry*. 2002; **59**(2): 173–179.

64. Shad MU, Muddasani S, Rao U. Gray matter differences between healthy and depressed adolescents: A voxel-based morphometry study. *J Child Adolesc Psychopharmacol*. 2012; **22**(3): 190–197.

65. Belden AC, Irvin K, Hajcak G, et al. Neural correlates of reward processing in depressed and healthy preschool-age children. *Journal of the American Academy of Child & Adolescent Psychiatry*. 2016; **55**(12): 1081–1089.

Chapter

5

Brain Imaging of Reward Dysfunction in Unipolar and Bipolar Disorders

Poornima Kumar, Yueyi Jiang, and Alexis E. Whitton

5.1 Introduction

In recent years, there has been tremendous support for working toward the RDoC goals of identifying the neurobiological mechanisms that cut across or are common to multiple psychiatric disorders. Identifying the pathophysiological mechanisms underlying transdiagnostic symptoms will improve the validity of disease classifications by grouping individuals based on multiple dimensions of behavior and biology. This could potentially account for heterogeneity and comorbidity observed among DSM diagnostic categories. One of the constructs that provides an excellent opportunity for transdiagnostic research is reward processing, as reward-related dysfunction is reported across several psychiatric disorders including schizophrenia and addiction, but especially mood disorders. Current research suggests that abnormal reward sensitivity is involved across the entire mood disorder spectrum, with blunted reward-related functioning observed as a risk for major depression, whereas abnormally elevated reward-related functioning reported as a risk for bipolar disorders (BDs). However, the results are mixed and there is considerable debate regarding the degree to which shared or distinct profiles of reward system dysfunction contribute to the motivational deficits observed across unipolar and bipolar mood disorders. This is due to the fact that reward processing is not a unitary construct, but multifaceted, and comprises subcomponents with distinct and overlapping neurobiological underpinnings. For example, different components of reward processing are suggested to include reward anticipation, reward consumption, and reward learning. In addition, both unipolar depression and BDs are highly heterogeneous. Consequently, considerable research has focused on understanding if these discrete components of reward processing could explain the heterogeneity observed across mood disorders and lead to finer parcellation of symptom clusters.

This will further lead to identification of homogeneous subgroups based on symptomatology, a prerequisite process to the development of targeted prevention and treatment strategies.

The primary focus of this chapter is to review the neural mechanisms underlying different reward processing components, including reward anticipation, reward consumption, and reward learning, in major depressive disorder (MDD) and BD. The chapter will also review evidence for these neural mechanisms acting as state-like versus trait-like markers of mood pathology. In addition, we will comment on future analytical approaches that are needed to understand the complex reward-related disruptions observed across mood disorders.

5.2 Neurobiology of Reward Processing and Its Components

The components of reward processing mentioned here – reward anticipation, reward consumption, and learning map onto the core reward components (reward responsiveness, reward valuation, and reward learning) of reward processing outlined in the Positive Valence Systems Matrix of the National Institute of Mental Health's (NIMH's) Research Domain Criteria (1–3). Reward responsiveness (or anticipation) is associated with the ability to anticipate or represent future incentives. In contrast, reward valuation refers to the processes by which the value of a reinforcer is computed as a function of its magnitude, predictability, time to expected delivery, and the effort required to obtain it. Finally, reward learning incorporates the process by which an organism acquires information about reward-predictive cues and by which novel reward outcomes subsequently shape behavior.

Evidence suggests that these processes map onto partially distinct neural circuitry (for a review, see 4). Briefly, the reward system has been linked to the frontal–striatal circuit that responds to stimuli involving the anticipation and receipt of rewards (e.g., 5). The ventral striatum is thought to play a central role in reward anticipation and is involved in processing both primary (e.g., food) and secondary (e.g., monetary) rewards. In contrast, studies examining reward consumption implicate "hedonic hotspots" in the ventral pallidum and nucleus accumbens that are the site of endogenous opioid receptors (6), as well as the encoding of reward value in the orbitofrontal cortex (OFC; 7). In the past decade there has been a burgeoning interest in applying computational algorithms to dissect reward learning in healthy and psychiatric populations. Using these models, individual differences can be estimated by measuring trial-by-trial variability in learning. Learning occurs when there is a deviation between the expected and actual outcome, quantified as a prediction error which is then used to update value estimates that support better prediction of future rewards. Nonhuman primate findings have shown that phasic firing of dopamine (DA) neurons in the ventral tegmental area (VTA) encodes reward prediction error (RPE). These midbrain DA RPE signals are then transmitted to the striatum and cortex and used to update stimulus-action values and guide goal-directed behavior (8, 9). Consistent with this, human fMRI studies have described RPE signals in cortico-striatal circuits including the striatum, midbrain, and prefrontal cortex (10, 11), and these signals have been found to be disrupted under conditions that affect phasic DA signaling (e.g., DA antagonists) (12–14).

5.3 Major Depressive Disorder

5.3.1 Neural Correlates of Reward Anticipation

Several fMRI studies have found that compared to psychiatrically healthy individuals, individuals with MDD show evidence of blunted striatal activation during anticipation of monetary rewards. For example, a recent meta-analysis of thirty-eight fMRI studies found that when both whole-brain effects as well as effects in targeted regions of interest were examined, individuals with MDD exhibited reduced activation in the ventral striatum during anticipation of reward (15). Furthermore, evidence suggests that this neural abnormality may

be a trait-like marker of MDD that precedes depression onset. For example, reduced striatal activation during reward anticipation has been observed in adolescents who are at increased familial risk for MDD relative to their low-risk peers (16–18). Reduced anticipation-related ventral striatum activation also appeared to predict clinical course, with one study showing that blunted anticipation-related activation in this region predicted transition to subthreshold or clinical depression in healthy adolescents, and also predicted concurrent anhedonia in adolescents with depression at a two-year follow-up (19). In the context of treatment, changes in reward anticipation-related ventral striatum activation observed following treatment with a selective serotonin reuptake inhibitor (SSRI) were found to track changes in depressive symptom severity (20). Taken together, these findings indicate that disturbances in anticipation-related striatal function may underlie to the pathogenesis of MDD and may have important implications for the development of new interventions for the disorder.

In addition to disturbances in striatal function, several studies have found evidence for abnormal activation in cortical regions during reward anticipation in individuals with MDD, particularly in parts of the anterior cingulate cortex (ACC) and insula. For example, one study found evidence of increased activation in the ACC during anticipation of gains, along with reduced discrimination of gain versus non-gain outcomes, in unmedicated individuals with MDD (21). Additionally, relative to healthy controls, adolescents at increased familial risk for MDD exhibited both reduced and increased reward anticipation-related activation in the left and right insula, respectively (22). Furthermore, when comparing adolescents at increased familial risk for MDD who did and did not experience a depressive episode, Fischer and colleagues (16) found that although both groups showed evidence of blunted striatal activation during reward anticipation relative to adolescents who were not at familial risk for MDD, those who did not experience depression (i.e., those who appeared to be resilient despite having increased familial risk) showed greater activation in the middle frontal gyrus during reward anticipation relative to those who did go on to develop depression. These findings are again consistent with the hypothesis that attenuation of reward anticipation-related neural responses may be a trait-like marker of risk for depression. However, they also suggest that resilient individuals show changes in neural activation in cortical regions that may compensate for these deficits and thereby confer protective effects on mood and motivation.

5.3.2 Neural Correlates of Reward Consumption

In addition to disturbances in anticipation-related neural activation, MDD has been associated with abnormal patterns of neural activation during the receipt or "consumption" of rewards. For example, in the context of fMRI studies, the same meta-analysis that showed significantly reduced anticipation-related activation in the ventral striatum in MDD also found evidence for consistent reductions in striatal activation during reward feedback (15). Specifically, studies examining patterns of whole-brain activation during reward consumption found decreased activation in the left and right caudate in individuals with MDD relative to controls, whereas studies employing a region-of-interest approach found significantly reduced consumption-related activation in the caudate as well as the putamen and globus pallidus (15).

Evidence for disrupted consumption-related neural activation in MDD is not solely restricted to fMRI studies. For example, several event-related potential (ERP) studies have shown that individuals with MDD show a more blunted reward positivity (RewP) amplitude in response to reward feedback relative to healthy controls (for a review, see 23). The RewP is a fronto-central positive-going deflection in the scalp-recorded ERP that occurs approximately 250–350 ms following receipt of reward feedback (note that this component is often referred to as the feedback-related negativity [FRN] in cases where neural responses to reward and loss feedback are directly contrasted; 24). Although the precise origin of the RewP signal remains a topic of debate, it is thought to reflect the indirect effect of reward-related striatal activation on other regions, particularly the ACC (25). A meta-analysis of twelve ERP studies found that individuals with MDD had significantly more blunted RewP amplitudes in response to reward feedback relative to healthy controls, with the magnitude of this effect being largest for studies using adolescent MDD samples (15). Several studies have also highlighted links between blunted RewP amplitudes and increased risk for MDD. For example, a blunted RewP/FRN amplitude has been found to predict the onset of a first depressive episode longitudinally (26), and has been found to moderate the association between maternal depression and future depressive symptoms in offspring (27). Blunted RewP amplitudes have also been observed in individuals who are in remission from a depressive episode (28, 29). Taken together, findings from the fMRI and ERP literature suggest that disruption in reward consumption-related neural activation may also be a trait-like risk marker for MDD.

5.3.3 Neural Correlates of Reward Learning

In addition to anticipation and consumption, another domain of reward processing that is reported to be impaired in MDD is reward learning. Prior fMRI studies have highlighted blunted RPE signals in the striatum (30–33) but intact RPE signal in the VTA (which are the hypothesized source of striatal RPE signals) during learning in individuals with MDD. This suggests that, in MDD, RPE signals might be accurately encoded in the VTA but are not appropriately transmitted to the striatum potentially due to abnormal connectivity between these two regions, thereby causing reduced downstream RPE signaling and impaired reward learning. Supporting this interpretation, a recent study observed intact VTA RPE signals but reduced functional connectivity between the VTA and striatum during reward feedback in individuals with MDD. (33) This weakened VTA–striatal connectivity in the MDD group points to a downstream DA signaling deficit (as observed by reduced RPE signals in the striatum), which then leads to impaired reward learning (34).

Another study reported that the striatal RPE signals correlated with self-reported depression severity suggesting that higher depression severity scores exhibit lower reward learning. Further, supporting the importance of these learning signals in a healthy sample, individuals with a higher genetic risk exhibited higher stress-induced reduction in RPE in the striatum. These studies together suggest these RPE signals may be a trait-marker of MDD, but future studies investigating learning in at-risk individuals are warranted.

5.4 Is Reward Dysfunction a Potential Endophenotype of MDD?

According to Gottesman and Gould (35), endophenotypes (or intermediate phenotypes) are measurable components (e.g., neurophysiological, biochemical, neuroanatomical, cognitive, or neuropsychological) that exist between the behavioral symptoms of a disease and genes. To be considered an endophenotype, a reward dysfunction should meet the following criteria (35): (a) specificity (i.e., reward dysfunction is strongly associated to a given condition); (b) heritability; (c) state independent (i.e., reward dysfunction is stable over time and independent from clinical state and treatment); (d) cosegregation (i.e., reward dysfunction occurs more frequently in affected compared to non-affected relatives of an ill individual); (e) familial association (i.e., reward dysfunction is more frequent in relatives of ill individuals than the general population); and (f) biological and clinical plausibility (36). Because endophenotypes are presumed to be more proximal to genes than clinical diagnoses, they may help us identify genetic variants and associated genes with small samples. Identification of genetic variants and associated genes using small samples. Endophenotypes are thought to be to be disorder-specific. Blunted striatal response to both anticipation and consumption has been suggested as an endophenotype of MDD, as blunted striatal response to rewards has been reported in individuals with current depression, remitted MDD, and non-affected family members of individuals with MDD. Next, endophenotypes must be heritable and although no studies have investigated the heritability of striatal reward responses, behavioral response to rewards and reward-related ERPs is reported to be heritable. In addition, blunted striatal response to reward response has been observed within never-depressed offspring of depressed versus healthy parents (37, 38). This blunted striatal response to both anticipation (39) and consumption (40, 41) prospectively predicted worsening of depressive symptoms over two years among adolescents, even after controlling for baseline symptoms. Furthermore, reduced FRN amplitude – a deflection in the ERP thought to

originate from RPE activity in the dorsal ACC and striatum, predicted first onset of MDD in a two-year follow-up among never-depressed adolescent girls (26). Finally, the reliability of striatal response to rewards has been poor to moderate (17). Nevertheless, taken together, these studies suggest that neural markers of altered reward processing are a promising endophenotype for MDD risk. However, future studies will need to replicate these findings over a broad developmental range and to investigate the specificity and reliability of such findings.

5.5 Bipolar Disorder

5.5.1 Neural Correlates of Reward Anticipation

One prominent theory of BD proposes that the hyper-hedonic symptoms observed in (hypo)mania (e.g., sensation-seeking, spending sprees, hypersexuality) may arise due to hypersensitivity in the fronto-striatal circuits that support reward processing (e.g., see 42). A number of studies have yielded findings consistent with this theory. For example, Nusslock and colleagues (43) used a card-guessing paradigm to examine reward-related neural activation in euthymic BD versus healthy control participants. They found that relative to controls, the BD group displayed greater ventral striatal, medial OFC, and left lateral OFC activation during anticipation, but not during receipt, of monetary reward. This finding appeared to be specific to reward, as no group differences in neural activation were observed in response to anticipation or receipt of monetary loss. Increased left lateral OFC (particularly left ventrolateral prefrontal cortex; vlPFC) activation during reward anticipation appears to be one of the most consistent findings in fMRI studies of BD. Increased anticipation-related left lateral OFC/vlPFC activation has been observed across all mood states, including mania (44), depression (45), and euthymia (43), and has been observed in samples with BD type I (43–45) and BD type II (46). Similar findings have also been observed in unaffected first-degree relatives of individuals with BD (47). These findings suggest that abnormal left lateral OFC activation during reward anticipation may be a risk marker for BD.

However, not all studies have yielded findings consistent with the reward hypersensitivity theory of BD (hypo)mania. For example, using the monetary incentive delay task, Schreiter and colleagues (48) found that euthymic individuals with BD had decreased, rather than increased, activation in the bilateral ventral striatum during reward anticipation relative to controls. Other studies have found evidence for decreased striatal activation during reward anticipation in samples that include individuals with BD not otherwise specified (49). Furthermore, although Caseras and colleagues (46) found greater anticipation-related activation in the ventral striatum in individuals with BD type II relative to controls, no abnormalities in anticipation-related striatal activation were observed for individuals with BD type I, who are at risk for more severe (hypo)manic symptoms than are individuals with BD type II. These findings have raised the question of whether BD can be characterized by increased or decreased activity in reward-related regions. In an attempt to reconcile these conflicting findings, Mason and colleagues (50) proposed a model wherein mood strongly biases reward perception in individuals with BD, such that patients might exhibit hypersensitivity to rewards when mood is high and hyposensitivity to rewards when mood is low. Future studies examining the association between changes in mood state and changes in neural responses to reward in individuals with BD are needed to fully test this hypothesis.

5.5.2 Neural Correlates of Reward Consumption

Consistent with the reward sensitivity hypothesis of BD, several studies have reported increased activation in the ventral striatum and medial OFC in response to reward outcome in individuals with subthreshold hypomania or euthymic BD (51, 52). These abnormal patterns of neural activation have been observed in response to a range of reward types. For example, using monetary and social incentive delay tasks, euthymic individuals with BD type I have been found to show increased striatal activation during receipt of both monetary and social rewards, suggesting that hypersensitivity to reward consumption may be evident across a variety of contexts in individuals with BD (53). Several ERP studies examining RewP/FRN amplitudes in response to reward

feedback have also found abnormalities in reward consumption-related neural activation in individuals at risk for BD. For example, individuals with elevated scores on the hypomanic personality scale were found to show elevated FRN amplitudes in response to reward feedback relative to individuals with moderate or low scores on this measure (54). Similar findings have also been observed in individuals meeting full criteria for BD (55).

Although many of these findings appear to align with the reward hypersensitivity model of BD, not all studies have yielded consistent findings. For example, one study found that individuals with BD mania had reduced, rather than increased, striatal activation during receipt of monetary rewards relative to controls (56). Furthermore, another study found that reduced ventral striatal activation during receipt of social rewards correlated with the severity of depressive symptoms in depressed individuals with BD, despite there being no differences in overall neural activation between the BD group and controls (57). Compared to the growing literature on the neural correlates of reward processing in MDD, the relative paucity of studies in BD samples makes it difficult to determine the precise role that abnormal reward circuit activation plays in BD. Future studies are needed to determine the direction and extent of reward processing abnormalities that are evident across different BD subtypes and across different BD mood states.

5.6 Heritability of Reward Dysfunction in BD

BD is a highly heritable disorder, with an estimated heritability of 60–80% (47). The offspring of patients are reported to have a tenfold risk of developing BD relative to the general population. Therefore, identifying endophenotypes (or intermediate phenotypes) based on biological constructs that are associated with BD and reported in individuals at risk of BD could elucidate the pathophysiology of BD. Consistent with this, abnormalities in reward-related neural responses have been reported in healthy offspring of parents with BD. For example, similar to BD patients, healthy offspring of parents with BD also had elevated vlPFC activation during reward consumption (47, 58). Similarly, they also show elevated vlPFC–striatal functional connectivity during reward processing that was specific to offspring of parents with BD and not observed in healthy controls or offspring of parents with non-BD psychopathology (59), underscoring the specificity of these findings to BD and a potential "intermediate phenotype" for risk of BD.

5.7 Studies Comparing MDD to BD

Given the significant clinical utility of biomarkers that are able to distinguish MDD from BD, a handful of studies have directly compared the neural correlates of reward processing in both samples. These studies have mostly focused on comparing MDD samples to BD samples in the depressive phase of illness, since the overlap in symptom profiles makes it especially difficult to distinguish the two conditions. One study examining differences in reward anticipation-related neural activation in individuals with MDD and individuals with BD depression with comparable degrees of illness severity found evidence of significantly increased anticipation-related activation in the left vlPFC in the BD group relative to the MDD group (45). This finding is consistent with the findings of several other studies in BD (43, 44, 46), which have suggested that heightened anticipation-related activation in the left vlPFC/ left lateral OFC may be a unique marker of BD. Studies comparing reward consumption-related neural activation in MDD and BD have yielded mixed findings. For example, Redlich and colleagues (60) found that compared to individuals with MDD, individuals with BD depression showed significantly reduced activation in the striatum, thalamus, insula, and prefrontal cortex during reward consumption. This contrasts with other studies that have found no differences between MDD and depressed BD samples in terms of consumption-related neural activation (61).

In light of the significant symptomatic overlap between MDD and BD, and the growing recognition that subsyndromal hypomanic states are present in up to 40% of individuals with recurrent MDD, a growing literature has come to conceptualize these two conditions as occurring along a spectrum, rather than having clear-cut diagnostic boundaries. Accordingly, some studies have focused on examining dimensional associations between hypomanic traits and aspects of reward processing, rather than directly comparing

categorically defined diagnostic groups. For example, a recent ERP study examined dimensional associations between RewP amplitude in response to reward feedback, and hypomanic and unipolar depressive traits, in an undergraduate sample (62). This study used a task in which the RewP was examined in response to rewards that were delivered immediately or after a delay. The results showed that proneness to hypomania was associated with an increased RewP amplitude in response to immediate rewards as well as an increased P3 amplitude (a later component reflecting motivational salience) in response to delayed rewards. The reverse pattern of findings was observed for proneness to depression, where increasing depressive tendencies were associated with more blunted RewP and P3 amplitudes in response to immediate and delayed rewards, respectively. These findings suggest that reward consumption-related neural activation, as measured using scalp-recorded ERPs, may represent biomarkers that can separate risk for bipolar spectrum from unipolar depressive disorders. Future studies in clinical samples are needed in order to more fully evaluate this hypothesis.

5.8 Future Directions: Transdiagnostic Mechanisms and Multimodal Imaging

As reviewed in this chapter, abnormal reward processing appears to be centrally involved in both MDD and BD, supporting a transdiagnostic approach. Transdiagnostic studies can therefore provide us with the opportunity to uncover endophenotypes or intermediate phenotypes that may be more reliable indicators of illness trajectory. Although the number of studies relevant to testing vulnerability or illness prediction based on abnormal reward functioning are sparse, the current literature suggests that blunted striatal reward response and elevated vlPFC activation to rewards may indicate vulnerability to onset and worsening of unipolar depression and BD, respectively.

Aberrant reward functioning in both MDD and BD has been characterized by both abnormal fMRI and ERP signals during reward processing. For example, both blunted striatal fMRI response and reduced RewP ERP amplitude to rewards have both been reported, although results originating from separate studies. It would be more informative to integrate critical information about the shared contribution of these multimodal deficits to the illness by adopting a multimodal data fusion analytical approach that combines information from both modalities. We can then map these integrated patterns onto discrete dimensions of mood-related pathology (e.g., depression, impulsivity) that cut across diagnostic categories (63, 64). This promises to reveal important links about the heterogeneity of MDD and BD that cannot be detected by single modalities. In addition, adding structural information about the brain regions involved during abnormal reward processing in MDD and BD will provide us with more information. This is critical, as the genetic and environmental interactions modulate brain structure and function in an intrinsically multimodal manner, affecting gray and white matter, and chemistry simultaneously.

Further, to be able to identify vulnerability markers of MDD and BD, we need to conduct "true" longitudinal studies, whereby we measure these reward dysfunctions in patients over time and understand how these interact with mood and symptom change. Linking real-life behavior (measured by ecological momentary assessment) to neuroimaging can elucidate critical information about how the neural abnormalities might be manifested in real-world behaviors. One study showed that duration of the ventral striatal activation to winning money in an fMRI scanner was associated with positive affect increase to winning money in a task performed outside the lab (65). Another study showed that in healthy controls RL-induced striatal DA release was associated with daily-life reward-oriented behavior (66). Recently, it was shown that a lower striatal RPE signal during a laboratory-based RL task was associated with increased decoupling between real-life enjoyment of activities and previous anticipation of pleasure (possibly akin to real-life prediction error) in individuals with subclinical depression (67). Taken together, these studies suggest that gaining more insight into how neuroimaging links with real-life dynamics could help to improve treatment interventions aimed at normalizing these reward-related dysfunctions across mood disorders.

5.9 Conclusions

Reward-related dysfunction is central to mood disorders. As outlined in this chapter, the impairments in reward anticipation, consumption, and learning cut across diagnostic categories and pose as potential endophenotypes of mood disorders. Studying mood disorders in a transdiagnostic fashion will elucidate the underlying shared and overlapping neurobiological mechanisms that will pave the way for improved treatment and prevention strategies.

References

1. Insel T, Cuthbert B, Garvey M, et al. Research domain criteria (RDoC): Toward a new classification framework for research on mental disorders. *The American Journal of Psychiatry*. 2010; **167**(7): 748751. https://doi.org/10.1176/appi.ajp.2010.09091379

2. Positive Valence systems workshop proceedings - National Institute of Mental Health. (2011b). Positive valence systems: Workshop proceedings. Retrieved from www.nimh.nih.gov/research/research-funded-by-nimh/rdoc/positive-valence-systems-workshop-proceedings.shtml

3. Sanislow CA, Pine DS, Quinn KJ, et al. Developing constructs for psychopathology research: Research domain criteria. *Journal of Abnormal Psychology*. 2010; **119**(4): 631–639. https://doi.org/10.1037/a0020909

4. Der-Avakian A, Markou A, The neurobiology of Anhedonia and other reward-related deficits. *Trends Neurosci*. 2012 January; **35**(1): 68–77. DOI:10.1016/j.tins.2011.11.005. Epub 2011 December 15.

5. Haber Suzanne N, Knutson Brian, The reward circuit: Linking primate anatomy and human imaging. *Neuropsychopharmacology*. 2010 January; **35**(1): 4–26. DOI:10.1038/npp.2009.129.

6. Peciña Susana, Berridge Kent C., Hedonic hot spot in nucleus accumbens shell: Where do μ-Opioids cause increased hedonic impact of sweetness? *Journal of Neuroscience*. 2005 December 14; **25**(50): 11777–11786.

7. O'Doherty John P, Deichmann Ralf, Critchley Hugo D, Dolan Raymond J, Neural responses during anticipation of a primary taste reward. *Neuron*. 2002 February 28; **33**(5): 815–826. DOI:10.1016/s0896-6273(02)00603-7.

8. Schultz. Neural substrate of prediction and reward. *Science*. 1997 March 14; **275**(5306): 1593–1599.

9. Stauffer William R., Yang Aimei, Borel Melodie, et al. Dopamine neuron-specific optogenetic stimulation in rhesus macaques. *Cell*. 2016 September 8; **166**(6): 1564–1571.e6.

10. Chase Henry W, Kumar Poornima, Eickhoff Simon B, Dombrovski Alexandre Y, Reinforcement learning models and their neural correlates: An activation likelihood estimation meta-analysis. *Cogn Affect Behav Neurosci.* 2015 June; 15(2): 435–459.

11. Garrison Kathleen A, Santoyo Juan F, Davis Jake H, et al. Effortless awareness: using real time neurofeedback to investigate correlates of posterior cingulate cortex activity in meditators' self-report. *Front Hum Neurosci.* 2013; 7: 440. Published online 2013 August 6.

12. Diederen Kelly M.J., Ziauddeen Hisham, Vestergaard Martin D., et al. Dopamine modulates adaptive prediction error coding in the human midbrain and striatum. *Journal of Neuroscience.* 2017 February 15; 37(7): 1708–1720;

13. Jocham Gerhard, Klein Tilmann A, Ullsperger Markus, Dopamine-mediated reinforcement learning signals in the striatum and ventromedial prefrontal cortex underlie value-based choices. *J Neurosci.* 2011 February 2; 31(5): 1606–1613. DOI:10.1523/JNEUROSCI.3904-10.

14. Pessiglione Mathias, Seymour Ben, Flandin Guillaume, Dolan Raymond J, Frith Chris D, Dopamine-dependent prediction errors underpin reward-seeking behaviour in humans. *Nature.* 2006 August 31; 442(7106): 1042–1045. DOI:10.1038/nature05051. Epub 2006 August 23.

15. Keren H, O'Callaghan G, Vidal-Ribas P, et al. Reward processing in depression: A conceptual and meta-analytic review across fMRI and EEG studies. *American Journal of Psychiatry.* 2018; 175(11): 1111–1120.

16. Fischer AS, Ellwood-Lowe ME, Colich NL, et al. Reward-circuit biomarkers of risk and resilience in adolescent depression. *Journal of Affective Disorders.* 2019; 246: 902–909.

17. Luking KR, Pagliaccio D, Luby JL, Barch DM. Depression risk predicts blunted neural responses to gains and enhanced responses to losses in healthy children. *Journal of the American Academy of Child & Adolescent Psychiatry.* 2016; 55(4): 328–337.

18. Olino TM, McMakin DL, Morgan JK, et al. Reduced reward anticipation in youth at high-risk for unipolar depression: A preliminary study. *Developmental Cognitive Neuroscience.* 2014; 8: 55–64.

19. Stringaris A, Vidal-Ribas Belil P, Artiges E, et al. The brain's response to reward anticipation and depression in adolescence: Dimensionality, specificity, and longitudinal predictions in a community-based sample. *American Journal of Psychiatry.* 2015; 172(12): 1215–1223.

20. Takamura M, Okamoto Y, Okada G, et al. Patients with major depressive disorder exhibit reduced reward size coding in the striatum. *Progress in Neuro-Psychopharmacology and Biological Psychiatry.* 2017; 79: 317–323.

21. Knutson B, Bhanji JP, Cooney RE, Atlas LY, Gotlib IH. Neural responses to monetary incentives in major depression. *Biological Psychiatry.* 2008; 63(7): 686–692.

22. Gotlib IH, Hamilton JP, Cooney RE, et al. Neural processing of reward and loss in girls at risk for major depression. *Archives of General Psychiatry.* 2010; 67(4): 380–387.

23. Proudfit GH. The reward positivity: From basic research on reward to a biomarker for depression. *Psychophysiology.* 2015; 52(4): 449–459.

24. Foti D, Hajcak G. Depression and reduced sensitivity to non-rewards versus rewards: Evidence from event-related potentials. *Biological Psychology.* 2009; 81(1): 1–8.

25. Foti D, Weinberg A, Bernat EM, Proudfit GH. Anterior cingulate activity to monetary loss and basal ganglia activity to monetary gain uniquely contribute to the feedback negativity. *Clinical Neurophysiology.* 2015; 126(7): 1338–1347.

26. Bress JN, Foti D, Kotov R, Klein DN, Hajcak G. Blunted neural response to rewards prospectively predicts depression in adolescent girls. *Psychophysiology.* 2013; 50(1): 74–81.

27. Kujawa A, Hajcak G, Klein DN. Reduced reward responsiveness moderates the effect of maternal depression on depressive symptoms in offspring: Evidence across levels of analysis. *Journal of Child Psychology and Psychiatry.* 2019; 60(1): 82–90.

28. Whitton AE, Kakani P, Foti D, et al. Blunted neural responses to reward in remitted major depression: A high-density event-related potential study. *Biol Psychiatry Cogn Neurosci Neuroimaging.* 2016; 1(1): 87–95.

29. Weinberg A, Shankman SA. Blunted reward processing in remitted melancholic depression. *Clinical Psychological Science.* 2017; 5(1): 14–25.

30. Dombrovski AY, Szanto K, Clark L, Reynolds CF, Siegle GJ. Reward signals, attempted suicide, and impulsivity in late-life depression. *JAMA Psychiatry Chic Ill.* 2013; 70(10). DOI:10.1001/jamapsychiatry.2013.75.

31. Gradin VB, Kumar P, Waiter G, et al. Expected value and prediction error abnormalities in depression and schizophrenia. *Brain.* 2011; 134 (Pt 6): 1751–1764. DOI:10.1093/brain/awr059.

32. Kumar P, Waiter G, Ahearn T, et al. Abnormal temporal difference reward-learning signals in major depression. *Brain*. 2008; **131** (Pt 8): 2084–2093. DOI:10.1093/brain/awn136.

33. Kumar P, Goer F, Murray L, et al. Impaired reward prediction error encoding and striatal-midbrain connectivity in depression. *Neuropsychopharmacology*. 2018; **43**(7): 1581–1588. DOI:10.1038/s41386-018-0032-x.

34. Rutledge RB, Moutoussis M, Smittenaar P, et al. Association of neural and emotional impacts of reward prediction errors with major depression. *JAMA Psychiatry*. 2017; **74**(8): 790–797.

35. Gottesman II, Gould TD. The endophenotype concept in psychiatry: Etymology and strategic intentions. *Am J Psychiatry*. 2003; **160**(4): 636–645. DOI:10.1176/appi.ajp.160.4.636.

36. Pizzagalli DA. Depression, stress, and anhedonia: Toward a synthesis and integrated model. *Annu Rev Clin Psychol*. 2014; **10**(1): 393–423. DOI:10.1146/annurev-clinpsy-050212-185606.

37. Olino TM, Silk JS, Osterritter C, Forbes EE. Social reward in youth at risk for depression: A preliminary investigation of subjective and neural differences. *J Child Adolesc Psychopharmacol*. 2015; **25**(9): 711–721. DOI:10.1089/cap.2014.0165.

38. Luking KR, Pagliaccio D, Luby JL, Barch DM. Reward processing and risk for depression across development. *Trends Cogn Sci*. 2016; **20** (6): 456–468. DOI:10.1016/j.tics.2016.04.002.

39. Stringaris A, Vidal-Ribas Belil P, Artiges E, et al. The brain's response to reward anticipation and depression in adolescence: Dimensionality, specificity, and longitudinal predictions in a community-based sample. *Am J Psychiatry*. 2015; **172**(12): 1215–1223. DOI:10.1176/appi.ajp.2015.14101298.

40. Morgan JK, Olino TM, McMakin DL, Ryan ND, Forbes EE. Neural response to reward as a predictor of increases in depressive symptoms in adolescence. *Neurobiol Dis*. 2013; **52**: 66–74. DOI:10.1016/j.nbd.2012.03.039.

41. Telzer EH, Fuligni AJ, Lieberman MD, Galván A. Neural sensitivity to eudaimonic and hedonic rewards differentially predict adolescent depressive symptoms over time. *Proc Natl Acad Sci*. 2014; **111**(18): 6600–6605. DOI:10.1073/pnas.1323014111.

42. Alloy LB, Nusslock R. Future directions for understanding adolescent bipolar spectrum disorders: A reward hypersensitivity perspective. *Journal of Clinical Child & Adolescent Psychology*. 2019; **48**(4): 669–683.

43. Nusslock R, Almeida JR, Forbes EE, et al. Waiting to win: Elevated striatal and orbitofrontal cortical activity during reward anticipation in euthymic bipolar disorder adults. *Bipolar Disorders*. 2012; **14**(3): 249–260.

44. Bermpohl F, Kahnt T, Dalanay U, et al. Altered representation of expected value in the orbitofrontal cortex in mania. *Human Brain Mapping*. 2010; **31**(7): 958–969.

45. Chase HW, Nusslock R, Almeida JR, et al. Dissociable patterns of abnormal frontal cortical activation during anticipation of an uncertain reward or loss in bipolar versus major depression. *Bipolar Disorders*. 2013; **15**(8): 839–854.

46. Caseras X, Lawrence NS, Murphy K, Wise RG, Phillips ML. Ventral striatum activity in response to reward: Differences between bipolar I and II disorders. *American Journal of Psychiatry*. 2013; **170**(5): 533–541.

47. Cattarinussi G, Di Giorgio A, Wolf RC, Balestrieri M, Sambataro F. Neural signatures of the risk for bipolar disorder: A meta-analysis of structural and functional neuroimaging studies. *Bipolar Disorders*. 2019; **21**(3): 215–227.

48. Schreiter S, Spengler S, Willert A, et al. Neural alterations of fronto-striatal circuitry during reward anticipation in euthymic bipolar disorder. *Psychological Medicine*. 2016; **46**(15): 3187–3198.

49. Yip SW, Worhunsky PD, Rogers RD, Goodwin GM. Hypoactivation of the ventral and dorsal striatum during reward and loss anticipation in antipsychotic and mood stabilizer-naive bipolar disorder. *Neuropsychopharmacology*. 2015; **40**(3): 658.

50. Mason L, Eldar E, Rutledge RB. Mood instability and reward dysregulation—a neurocomputational model of bipolar disorder. *JAMA Psychiatry*. 2017; **74**(12): 1275–1276.

51. Linke J, King AV, Rietschel M, et al. Increased medial orbitofrontal and amygdala activation: Evidence for a systems-level endophenotype of bipolar I disorder. *American Journal of Psychiatry*. 2012; **169**(3): 316–325.

52. O'Sullivan N, Szczepanowski R, El-Deredy W, Mason L, Bentall RP. fMRI evidence of a relationship between hypomania and both increased goal-sensitivity and positive outcome-expectancy bias. *Neuropsychologia*. 2011; **49**(10): 2825–2835.

53. Dutra SJ, Cunningham WA, Kober H, Gruber J. Elevated striatal reactivity across monetary and social rewards in bipolar I disorder. *Journal of Abnormal Psychology*. 2015; **124**(4): 890.

54. Mason L, O'Sullivan N, Blackburn M, Bentall R, El-Deredy W. I want it now! Neural correlates of

hypersensitivity to immediate reward in hypomania. *Biological Psychiatry.* 2012; **71**(6): 530–537.

55. Mason L, Trujillo-Barreto NJ, Bentall RP, El-Deredy W. Attentional bias predicts increased reward salience and risk taking in bipolar disorder. *Biological Psychiatry.* 2016; **79**(4): 311–319.

56. Abler B, Greenhouse I, Ongur D, Walter H, Heckers S. Abnormal reward system activation in mania. *Neuropsychopharmacology.* 2008; **33**(9): 2217.

57. Sharma A, Satterthwaite TD, Vandekar L, et al. Divergent relationship of depression severity to social reward responses among patients with bipolar versus unipolar depression. *Psychiatry Research: Neuroimaging.* 2016; **254**: 18–25.

58. Singh MK, Kelley RG, Howe ME, et al. Reward processing in healthy offspring of parents with bipolar disorder. *JAMA Psychiatry.* 2014; **71**(10): 1148–1156. DOI:10.1001/jamapsychiatry.2014.1031.

59. Manelis A, Almeida JRC, Stiffler R, et al. Anticipation-related brain connectivity in bipolar and unipolar depression: A graph theory approach. *Brain J Neurol.* 2016; **139**(Pt 9): 2554–2566. DOI:10.1093/brain/aww157.

60. Redlich R, Dohm K, Grotegerd D, et al. Reward processing in unipolar and bipolar depression: A functional MRI study. *Neuropsychopharmacology.* 2015; **40**(11): 2623.

61. Satterthwaite TD, Kable JW, Vandekar L, et al. Common and dissociable dysfunction of the reward system in bipolar and unipolar depression. *Neuropsychopharmacology.* 2015; **40**(9): 2258.

62. Glazer JE, Kelley NJ, Pornpattananangkul N, Nusslock R. Hypomania and depression associated with distinct neural activity for immediate and future rewards. *Psychophysiology.* 2019; **56**(3): e13301.

63. Groves AR, Beckmann CF, Smith SM, Woolrich MW. Linked independent component analysis for multimodal data fusion. *Neuroimage.* 2011; **54**: 2198–2217.

64. Calhoun VD, Sui J. Multimodal fusion of brain imaging data: a key to finding the missing link(s) in complex mental illness. *Biol. Psychiatry Cogn. Neurosci. Neuroimaging 1,* 2016; 230–244. DOI:10.1016/j.bpsc.2015.12.005.

65. Heller AS, Fox AS, Wing EK, et al. The Neurodynamics of affect in the laboratory predicts persistence of real-world emotional responses. *J Neurosci.* 2015; **35**(29): 10503–10509. DOI:10.1523/JNEUROSCI.0569-15.

66. Kasanova Z, Ceccarini J, Frank MJ, Amelsvoort TA van, Myin-Germeys I. Striatal dopaminergic modulation of reinforcement learning predicts reward—oriented behavior in daily life. *Biol Psychol.* Published online 2017. DOI:10.1016/j.biopsycho.2017.04.014.

67. Bakker JM, Goossens L, Kumar P, et al. From laboratory to life: Associating brain reward processing with real-life motivated behaviour and symptoms of depression in non-help-seeking young adults. *Psychol Med.* 2019; **49**(14): 2441–2451. DOI:10.1017/S0033291718003446.

Chapter

6

Resting-State Functional Connectivity in Unipolar Depression

Ziqi Chen and Qiyong Gong*

6.1 Background

Unipolar depression, also known as unipolar or major depressive disorder (MDD), is a globally prevalent psychiatric disorder characterized by persistent sadness and a loss of interest in normally enjoyable activities, accompanied by an inability to carry out daily activities, for at least two weeks. Furthermore, patients with unipolar depression usually exhibit some of the following symptoms: loss of energy, sleeping more or less, anxiety, change in appetite, reduced concentration, indecisiveness, feeling of worthlessness, guilt, hopelessness, and thoughts or acts of self-harm or suicide. The lifetime risk of depression is approximately 10–20%, with rates being almost doubled in women. There have been 76.4 million years lost to disability due to depression worldwide, which is 10.3% of the total burden of diseases (1). Unipolar depression causes significant individual suffering and impairs social functioning, resulting in major public health and economic burden. Therefore, studying the pathogeny and neuromechanism of depression is important for early detection, treatment, and prognosis of this disease. Except for neurochemical, genetic, and molecular theories, brain circuit models in unipolar depression have also been research hotspots with the development of functional neuroimaging, which provides a versatile platform to discover brain circuit dysfunction underlying specific syndromes and changes associated with antidepressant treatment.

Multimodal MR techniques, including structural, functional, and molecular imaging, may provide "radiological signs" for the discovery of circuitry in depressed patients and other psychiatric disorders. As a result, a new field of radiology, termed psychoradiology (http://radiopeadia.org/articles/psychoradiology)(2)), seems to play a major clinical role in guiding diagnostic and treatment planning decisions in patients with psychiatric disorders. In functional neuroimaging, resting-state functional MRI (R-fMRI) is one of the most commonly used functional imaging techniques to map intrinsic functional brain connectivity without the constraints of task-dependent paradigms. Functional connectivity (FC) is suggested to describe temporal correlations between spatially remote brain regions, reflecting the level of functional communication between regions. Among the huge number of techniques for analyzing resting-state brain function, seed-based analysis (3), independent component analysis (ICA)(4), and graph theory analysis (5) are most commonly used.

In this chapter, we will mainly discuss the resting-state MRI findings of functional connectivity abnormalities in brain circuits and networks related to symptomatology and antidepressant treatment in unipolar depression.

6.2 MRI Neurocircuitry Findings

6.2.1 Limbic-Cortical-Striatal-Pallidal-Thalamic Circuit

Evidence from neuroimaging, neuropathology, and lesion analysis studies demonstrated that the limbic–cortical–striatal–pallidal–thalamic (LCSPT) circuit is involved in the pathophysiology of unipolar depression. The LCSPT circuit is related to emotional behavior based on its anatomical connectivity with visceral control structures that mediate emotional expression and regulation, such as the hypothalamus and periaqueductal gray. This circuit has two branches: one is the limbic–thalamic–cortical branch composed of the hippocampus, amygdala, mediodorsal nucleus of thalamus, and medial and ventrolateral prefrontal cortex, and another is the limbic–striatal–pallidal–thalamic branch(6). The caudate and putamen (striatum) and globus pallidus (pallidum) are organized in parallel to connect with limbic and cortical regions. The importance of LCSPT circuit alterations in the pathophysiology of MDD has recently been confirmed in a catecholamine depletion study(7). In a randomized, double-blind and placebo-controlled catecholamine depletion study, fifteen unmedicated MDD patients in full remission and thirteen healthy controls were included. The remitted MDD subjects showed increased metabolism of the LCSPT circuit in response to catecholamine depletion. But the healthy subjects showed decreased metabolism of this circuit or remained unchanged. This study demonstrated catecholaminergic dysfunction as a trait abnormality in MDD and the depressive and anhedonic symptoms resulting from decreased catecholaminergic neurotransmission may be related to increased activity within the LCSPT circuitry. Volumetric alterations have also been reported in this circuitry. A voxel-based morphometry study revealed significantly increased gray matter volume in the left paracentral lobule, left superior frontal gyrus, bilateral cuneus, and thalamus, which form LCSPT circuitry in first-episode, drug-naive MDD patients(8). These findings were out of confounding effects of the course of illness and treatment effects that may impact anatomic measurements and provided important insight into the early neurobiology of MDD. Lui and colleagues used resting-state seed-based functional connectivity MRI to evaluate functional connectivity alterations in patients with refractory and non-refractory MDD(9). These researchers found that refractory depression is associated with altered functional connectivity mainly in thalamo–cortical circuits, while non-refractory depression is associated with more distributed decreased connectivity in the limbic–striatal–pallidal–thalamic circuit. These results suggested that refractory and non-refractory depression were characterized by distinct functional alterations in distributed brain circuits. Though there is some imaging evidence suggesting the important role of the LCSPT circuit in the pathology of MDD, functional communications within this brain circuit and its regulatory effects on other regions of the brain are too complex and more work is required. Nevertheless, based on the currently available evidence, it has been hypothesized that the balance among the brain regions within the LCSPT circuit is disrupted in depression. This may be caused by decreased activity in the prefrontal cortex that impairs its regulatory

(inhibitory) action on the limbic structures which, in turn, are overactive. This dysregulation may be responsible for clinical depressive symptoms, autonomic and neuroendocrine alterations, and other visceral functions. However, this hypothesis could explain some symptoms in MDD, but could not explain other cognitive functions, such as decreased attention and impairment in executive control(10). Thus, impairments within the LCSPT structures or in the interconnections among them could result in dysfunctions predisposing a man to depression, but it is difficult to explain all of the manifestations of depression.

6.2.2 Functional Connectivity Findings Related to Suicide in Depression

Suicide is a major global public health and social problem. MDD patients have a 2–12% risk of committing suicide in the lifetime(11). Suicide attempts, typically defined as self-destructive acts with some intent to end life, are strongly correlated with depression, and a history of attempts is one of the strongest predictors of completed suicide. Thus, studying the neurobiology of depressed patients with a history of suicide attempts or suicidal ideation (SI) is a promising strategy for learning about neurobiological factors that may confer risk for suicidal behavior and potentially for identifying an objective neurobiological marker of risk. Using the fractional amplitude of low-frequency fluctuation (fALFF) approach, Cao and colleagues (12) reported that MDD patients with a history of suicide attempt (SA) showed increased fALFF in the right superior temporal gyrus, left middle temporal gyrus, and left middle occipital gyrus compared with MDD patients without such history (nSA) and healthy controls (HC). Additionally, the SA group showed decreased fALFF in the left superior frontal gyrus and the left middle frontal gyrus compared with the nSA group. By conducting ROC (receiver operating characteristic) analysis, the authors claimed that fALFF in these two regions could serve as a potential predisposition to suicidal behavior in depression. In an ICA study, Zhang and colleagues explored resting-state functional connectivity changes in the default mode network (DMN) comparing thirty-five suicidal, eighteen non-suicidal depressed adolescents, and twenty-seven healthy controls(13).

Compared with the healthy controls, all the depressed patients showed increased functional connectivity in DMN regions. Compared to the non-suicidal patients, the suicidal patients showed increased connectivity in the left cerebellum, left lingual gyrus and decreased connectivity in the right precuneus. These results highlighted the important role of the DMN in the pathophysiology of depression and suggested that abnormal functional connectivity in the DMN may be related to suicidal behavior in depressed adolescents. Since the amygdala is the key brain region involved in emotional and cognitive processing, Wei and colleagues compared whole-brain amygdala resting-state functional connectivity among first-episode MDD patients with SI, first-episode MDD patients without SI, and healthy controls (14). Compared with the non-SI and HC groups, the SI group showed altered resting-state FC between the amygdala and precuneus/cuneus. They suggested that the abnormal functional connectivity between amygdala and precuneus/cuneus might present a trait feature for suicide in first-episode MDD. Similarly, a resting-state FC analysis of the rostral anterior cingulate cortex (rACC) reported decreased FC between the rACC, the orbitomedial prefrontal cortex, and the right middle temporal pole (TP) in MDD patients with SI (15). Using network-based statistics (NBS) and graph-theoretical methods, Kim and colleagues (16) found decreased functional connectivity in a characterized subnetwork in MDD patients with SI. The subnetwork included the brain regions in the fronto-thalamic circuit, suggesting dysfunctions of decision-making and information integration in MDD patients with SI.

6.3 Core Brain Networks in Depression

6.3.1 Default Mode Network

Within the last decade, many imaging studies on MDD-related alterations in brain network function have used different methodologies to clarify the dysfunction of these networks themselves and their interactions with other brain regions (17). One of the core networks involved in MDD is the DMN. The DMN (also known as the "task-negative network") was initially identified as brain regions that showed consistently synchronized deactivation during tasks and prominent activation during rest(18). As research continues, researchers divided the DMN into an anterior subnetwork that centers on the medial prefrontal cortex (mPFC) and a posterior subnetwork that centers on the precuneus cortex (PCu) and posterior cingulate cortex (PCC)(19, 20). Both the anterior and posterior parts of DMN are implicated in spontaneous or self-generated cognition. However, the anterior DMN is correlated with self-referential processing and emotional regulation, partly through its connections with limbic areas, such as the amygdala. The posterior DMN is more related to consciousness and memory processing through the connections to the hippocampal formation(21–23). Except for the core regions, the DMN also includes the inferior parietal lobule (IPL), lateral temporal cortex (LTC), subgenual anterior cingulate cortex (sgACC), and the hippocampal formation (hippocampus and parahippocampal gyrus)(20, 24).

One of the most commonly used seed regions in seed-based analyses investigating the DMN is the mPFC in anterior DMN. One study found decreased functional connectivity of the dmPFC with the posterior subnetwork of DMN in MDD patients, which was consistent with the hypothesis of a dissociation between the anterior and posterior DMN in depression(25). Sheline and colleagues found that each of three networks (the central executive network, the DMN, and the affective network) showed increased connectivity to the bilateral dorsal medial prefrontal cortex in depressed patients (26). They suggested that this region, which they termed the "dorsal nexus," is a functional hub with increased functional connectivity. These findings provided a potential mechanism to explain how symptoms of major depression arise concurrently from distinct networks, such as poor performance on cognitive tasks; rumination; excessive self-focus; increased vigilance; and emotional, autonomic, and visceral dysfunction.

Some brain regions such as the PCC or PCu in the posterior DMN were also commonly used as seed regions. Zhou and colleagues (27) reported increased connectivity of the PCC with other posterior DMN regions and the mPFC and OFC. Similarly, Alexopoulos and colleagues (28) found increased connectivity of the PCC with both anterior (sgACC, vmPFC) and posterior (PCu) regions of the DMN in medicated patients with late-onset depression. Further evidence was reported by another study in a larger group of unmedicated elderly MDD patients (29). The patients showed increased connectivity of the PCC with other nodes in the posterior DMN but decreased connectivity with the medial frontal gyrus before treatment. The functional connectivity with both the bilateral medial frontal gyrus and the dorsal ACC was increased after twelve weeks of antidepressant treatment, suggesting that antidepressant treatment could modulate the functional connectivity between anterior and posterior DMN regions.

Except for seed-based analysis, some studies used ICA analysis, which does not require a selection of regions of interest, to study brain functional connectivity in MDD. Many ICA studies focusing on the DMN have reported increased connectivity within several regions of the anterior DMN in MDD compared to healthy controls. One ICA study investigating the role of the DMN reported increased network functional connectivity in the subgenual cingulate, thalamus, orbitofrontal cortex, and precuneus in medicated depressed subjects(30). They also found that the subgenual cingulate was a prominent region in the network of depressed patients but not in the control group, suggesting that the presence of the subgenual cingulate in the DMN may be a finding unique to depression. Another ICA study included thirty-five first-episode, treatment-naive young adults with MDD and thirty-five matched healthy controls(31). They identified increased functional connectivity in the anterior DMN (dmPFC, vmPFC, pregenual ACC, and medial OFC) in MDD patients without the influence of disease course or medication. The results of the functional connectivity changes within posterior part of DMN in depression may be inconsistent. Two studies reported increased connectivity of the PCC/PCu in the posterior DMN in MDD (32, 33). However, Zhu et al. (31) found decreased functional connectivity in the PCC, PCu, and angular gyrus in depression. The inconsistent findings may be related to the sample size, characteristics of patients, such as age and symptom severity. The connections between anterior and posterior DMN have also been investigated using ICA. The researchers identified anterior and posterior subnetworks that were spatially independent and showed asynchronous activity patterns in depression. Furthermore, the

antidepressant treatment normalized the increased connectivity in the posterior DMN but not in the anterior DMN(32).

6.3.2 Central Executive Network

The central executive network (CEN, also known as the "cognitive control network" or "cognitive executive network") includes the dorsolateral prefrontal cortex (dlPFC), dorsal ACC, posterior parietal cortex, inferior temporal gyrus, and precentral gyrus(34, 35). The CEN is involved in attention-demanding cognitive tasks and shows increased activity in frontal and parietal regions associated with top-down modulation of attention and working memory tasks. The DMN and the CEN are often seen as opposite networks as the CEN is most active during cognitive tasks.

In the CEN, the dlPFC is important in the top-down regulation of emotional processing. Many studies used the dlPFC as a seed region to investigate functional connectivity changes in MDD. Ye and colleagues (36) reported increased functional connectivity with the right dlPFC in the left ACC, left parahippocampal gyrus, thalamus, and precentral gyrus in first-episode MDD patients. However, another study found decreased FC between right dlPFC and left cuneus, left lingual gyrus, and right ACC within the CEN in MDD patients, and the altered FC between dlPFC and right ACC was positively correlated with the executive function in MDD (37). Similarly, Alexopoulos and colleagues reported decreased connectivity of the dlPFC in the CEN in unmedicated late-life depression, and the resting functional connectivity in the CEN predicted poor remission rate after antidepressant treatment and persistence of depression, apathy, and dysexecutive behavior at the end of the treatment (28). Liston and colleagues (38) used resting-state fMRI to measure functional connectivity within and between the DMN and CEN in depressed patients before and after a five-week course of repetitive transcranial magnetic stimulation (TMS). Before treatment, depressed patients showed increased FC in the DMN and decreased FC in the CEN, and altered connectivity between these two networks. After treatment, TMS normalized depression-related subgenual cingulate hyperconnectivity in the DMN but did not modify connectivity in the CEN. TMS also induced anticorrelated connectivity between the dlPFC and medial prefrontal DMN nodes. They suggested that TMS selectively modulated functional connectivity both within and between the CEN and DMN, highlighting the potential role of the subgenual cingulate as a psychoradiological biomarker for predicting treatment response. Stange and colleagues (39) studied the functional connectivity changes within the CEN in remitted MDD using the dlPFC, inferior parietal lobule, and dorsal ACC as seeds. They reported that decreased connectivity in the entire CEN in remitted MDD patients was stable and reliable over time and was most pronounced from the right dlPFC and right inferior parietal lobule to the three bilateral CEN seeds. This study demonstrated that reduced connectivity within the CEN in MDD was stable over a short period of time, was present even in the remitted state. The use of a remitted MDD sample in this study allowed for increased confidence that CEN connectivity may act as a relatively trait-like factor that is not attributable to state-dependent depressed mood.

6.3.3 Salience Network

The salience network (SN) typically consists of the fronto-insular cortex, the dorsal ACC, the amygdala, and the temporal pole, and is involved in interceptive awareness, task-set maintenance, and detection of salient stimuli from the environment(40).

Neuroimaging, more specifically, the psychoradiological studies have reported abnormal functional connectivity in the SN in MDD patients. Manoliu and colleagues (33) performed ICA analysis of resting-state fMRI data to identify DMN, SN, and CEN in MDD patients. The MDD patients showed decreased connectivity of the right anterior insula in the SN. Moreover, decreased connectivity of the right anterior insula in the SN was associated with severity of symptoms and aberrant DMN–CEN interactions. These results suggested a link between altered salience mapping and abnormal coordination of DMN–CEN-based cognitive processes, which was in line with the insula's involvement in switching between the DMN and the CEN reported by other studies(41, 42). The insular cortex and amygdala were the commonly used seed regions in the SN. Seed-based analyses investigating the insula reported that its connectivity was increased with the pregenual ACC(43) and the medial OFC(44). This increased connectivity to brain nodes of the anterior DMN is consistent with hyperconnectivity of the anterior DMN and supported the

insula's role in coordinating interactions between networks(41, 42, 45). One study also reported increased resting-state FC of the right anterior insula to right dlPFC and right PCC in depressed elderly patients with high apathy compared to non-apathetic depressed elderly, suggesting a biological signature of the apathy in late-life depression(46). The amygdala is another important node in the SN and is highly related to MDD. Many studies have reported decreased connectivity of the amygdala with various brain regions, including the hippocampus, parahippocampus, and precuneus in adolescent depression(47) and frontal areas, postcentral gyrus, and middle occipital gyrus in late-onset depression(48). Two studies also reported decreased resting-state FC between the amygdala and insula(49, 50), which was consistent with the uncoupling of the amygdala and insula from the SN as reported by ICA studies(33, 51).

6.3.4 Between-Network Connectivity

In addition to functional connectivity changes within brain networks, researchers have also investigated the functional interaction between brain networks in depression. Jiang and colleagues (52) evaluated the functional connectivity and Granger causal connectivity across the DMN, SN, and CEN in depressed patients. They found that MDD patients showed abnormal causal connectivity between key regions of the DMN and SN, and opposing altered FC of the DMN–CEN and SN–CEN. Compared to HC, the FC of DMN–CEN was decreased and the FC of SN–CEN was increased in MDD patients. Similarly, Manoliu and colleagues (33) investigated between-network connectivity of three DMN subnetworks (anterior, inferior–posterior, and superior–posterior), three CEN subnetworks (left ventral, right ventral, and dorsal), and the SN. They found that MDD patients exhibited decreased inter-FC between inferior–posterior DMN and dorsal CEN, and between superior–posterior DMN and dorsal CEN, supporting a decreased functional connectivity between the DMN and CEN. Furthermore, MDD patients showed increased inter-FC between SN and inferior–posterior DMN, suggesting increased functional connectivity between the SN and DMN. Decreased connectivity between posterior DMN and the CEN (dlPFC) has also been reported in

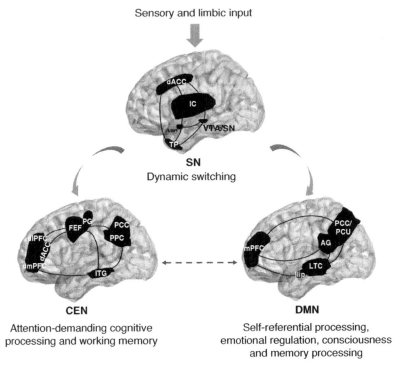

Sensory and limbic input

SN
Dynamic switching

CEN
Attention-demanding cognitive
processing and working memory

DMN
Self-referential processing,
emotional regulation, consciousness
and memory processing

Figure 6.1 The salience network (SN) plays a central role in switching between the default mode network (DMN) and central executive network (CEN), and abnormalities of the SN could lead to weak salience mapping and give rise to dysfunctions of the CEN and DMN

treatment-resistant depressed patients. This between-network connectivity changed from negative to positive following electroconvulsive therapy, providing a potential biomarker of recovery from a depressive episode(53). Mulders and colleagues reviewed the functional connectivity studies in MDD and proposed a model that incorporates changes in functional connectivity with current hypotheses of network dysfunction in MDD. These researchers summarized the findings as (1) increased connectivity within the anterior DMN, (2) increased connectivity between the SN and anterior DMN, (3) changed connectivity between the anterior and posterior DMN, and (4) decreased connectivity between the posterior DMN and CEN(54). In this context, dysfunction in one network may affect the other networks. The SN, DMN, and CEN carry out distinct functions, and their interactions subserve high-level cognitive operations, especially cognitive control. The SN has been involved in switching between the DMN and CEN(41, 42). The SN plays an important role in modulating network interactions, and alterations of the SN could lead to weak salience

mapping and further give rise to dysfunctions of the DMN and CEN(35, 55) (Figure 6.1). In addition, the abnormal coordination of information within and across these networks is important in linking the concomitant impaired cognitive function and emotional dysregulation in depression. Therefore, further investigations of the disruptions within and across core networks are necessary to advance the understanding of brain mechanisms that underlie depression.

6.4 Functional Connectomics in Depression

Graph theory provides a powerful mathematical framework to quantify the topological organization of the brain networks or connectomes(56). Several resting-state fMRI studies have reported aberrant topological organization, including global, modular, and nodal properties of functional networks in depressed patients. Zhang and colleagues (57) measured partial correlation coefficients of the R-fMRI signals between ninety cortical and subcortical regions in first-episode, drug-naive depressive patients. The depressed patients showed altered global properties including smaller path lengths and higher global efficiency, suggesting a shift toward randomization in their brain networks. However, the recurrent depressed patients showed the opposite pattern (increased path lengths and decreased global efficiency), where wavelet correlations were computed between 112 regions (58). Meanwhile, two additional R-fMRI studies by Lord et al. (59) and Bohr et al. (60) employed Pearson's correlations as a connectivity metric and reported no significant differences in these global measures between MDD patients and healthy controls. Notably, there were differences in the age, medication, and depressive episode in the patient samples that may contribute to these inconsistent results. For example, in the study by Meng et al. (58), the patient samples were highly heterogeneous in depressive episode number and medication type (antidepressant monotherapy, dual therapy, or triple therapy). Other potential factors contributing to inconsistency include the use of different network node and edge definitions or changes in arousal, cardiorespiratory, and motion artifacts, all of which are correlated with the global properties of brain networks(61, 62).

Tao and colleagues specifically studied the modular structure of 90-node brain networks in two depressed groups (fifteen first-episode, drug-naive and twenty-four long-term, drug-resistant) (63). Both depressed groups exhibited the uncoupling of the hate circuitry, including the superior frontal gyrus, insula, and putamen. Other changes were located in circuitry related to emotion, risk-taking, and processing reward. These findings may be correlated with the dysfunctional cognitive control over negative feelings in depression. Another study reported increased nodal centralities, mainly in the caudate nucleus and default-mode regions, and decreased nodal centralities in the occipital, frontal (orbital part), and temporal regions in drug-naive, first-episode adult MDD patients (57). Similarly, Jin and colleagues (64) found higher nodal degree in the DMN, dlPFC, insula, and amygdala in first-episode, drug-naive adolescent MDD patients and a positive correlation between the degree of connectivity of the amygdala and illness duration. These findings supported the notion that symptoms of depression

in adolescents may be an early sign of adult depressive disorders(65). Overall, these above-mentioned R-fMRI studies suggested abnormal topological organization of brain functional networks in depression.

6.5 Conclusions

The human brain is composed of complex networks of functionally linked brain regions. These spatially distributed but functionally correlated brain regions continuously share information with each other, together forming interconnected resting-state networks(66). With the development of R-fMRI, we have identified altered functional connections of the brain networks in depression using seed-based, ICA-based methods and connectome-based approaches. These findings of altered resting-state FC are related to the neuropathology of depression and relatively heterogeneous in many brain regions, such as frontal, parietal, temporal, basal ganglia, limbic system, and cerebellum, and important functional networks, including the DMN, CEN, and SN. The heterogeneity may be related to the complex functional interactions of brain regions and the inconsistent characteristics of depressed samples, such as MDD phenotypes and symptomatology. Other sources of the inconsistence include the various methods, data acquisition, boundary determination, and statistical models.

In summary, there is considerable evidence that functional connectivity between multiple brain regions within and between brain networks is altered in MDD. Some of these alterations could be modulated or normalized by antidepressant treatment. To identify reliable and robust functional connectivity changes in MDD and develop personalized treatments, future studies should find a common strategy for similar data acquisition and data analysis that would lead to better comparability and interpretation of the results. The large data sets with comparable methods could provide reliable and specific imaging markers related to depression symptomatology, treatment response, and personal risk for developing depression. Multimodal imaging studies should be conducted to clarify the associations between structural and functional connectivity abnormalities in depression, which could better illustrate the neuropathophysiology of abnormal connectivity in depression.

*Corresponding author

Dr Qiyong Gong, Huaxi MR Research Center (HMRRC), Department of Radiology, West China Hospital of Sichuan University, Chengdu, Sichuan Province, China. Tel/Fax: ++86(0)28 8542 3503; Email: qiyonggong@hmrrc.org.cn

Acknowledgment

The cited work from HMRRC was supported by the National Natural Science Foundation (Grant Nos. 81621003, 81820108018) and Program for Changjiang Scholars and Innovative Research Team in University (PCSIRT, Grant No. IRT16R52) of China, and the Functional and Molecular Imaging Key Laboratory of Sichuan Province (FMIKLSP, Grant No. 019JDS0044) and Psychoradiology Research Unit of Chinese Academy of Medical Sciences (Grant No. 2018RU011)

References

1. Smith K. Mental health: A world of depression. *Nature.* 2014; **515**: 181.

2. Lui S, Zhou XJ, Sweeney JA, et al. Psychoradiology: The frontier of neuroimaging in psychiatry. *Radiology.* 2016; **281**: 357–372.

3. Cordes D, Haughton VM, Arfanakis K, et al. Mapping functionally related regions of brain with functional connectivity MR imaging. *AJNR Am J Neuroradiol.* 2000; **21**: 1636–1644.

4. Beckmann CF, DeLuca M, Devlin JT, et al. Investigations into resting-state connectivity using independent component analysis. *Philos Trans R Soc Lond B Biol Sci.* 2005; **360**: 1001–1013.

5. Bullmore E, Sporns O. Complex brain networks: Graph theoretical analysis of structural and functional systems. *Nat Rev Neurosci* 2009; **10**: 186–198.

6. Sheline YI. Neuroimaging studies of mood disorder effects on the brain. *Biol Psychiatry.* 2003; **54**: 338–352.

7. Hasler G, Fromm S, Carlson PJ, et al. Neural response to catecholamine depletion in unmedicated subjects with major depressive disorder in remission and healthy subjects. *Arch Gen Psychiatry.* 2008; **65**: 521–531.

8. Qiu L, Lui S, Kuang W, et al. Regional increases of cortical thickness in untreated, first-episode major depressive disorder. *Transl Psychiatry.* 2014; **4**: e378.

9. Lui S, Wu Q, Qiu L, et al. Resting-state functional connectivity in treatment-resistant depression. *Am J Psychiatry.* 2011; **168**: 642–648.

10. Degl'Innocenti A, Agren H and Backman L. Executive deficits in major depression. *Acta Psychiatr Scand.* 1998; **97**: 182–188.

11. Nock MK, Borges G, Bromet EJ, et al. Cross-national prevalence and risk factors for suicidal ideation, plans and attempts. *Br J Psychiatry.* 2008; **192**: 98–105.

12. Cao J, Chen X, Chen J, et al. Resting-state functional MRI of abnormal baseline brain activity in young depressed patients with and without suicidal behavior. *J Affect Disord* 2016; **205**: 252–263.

13. Zhang S, Chen JM, Kuang L, et al. Association between abnormal default mode network activity and suicidality in depressed adolescents. *BMC Psychiatry.* 2016; **16**: 337.

14. Wei S, Chang M, Zhang R, et al. Amygdala functional connectivity in female patients with major depressive disorder with and without suicidal ideation. *Ann Gen Psychiatry.* 2018; **17**: 37.

15. Du L, Zeng J, Liu H, et al. Fronto-limbic disconnection in depressed patients with suicidal ideation: A resting-state functional connectivity study. *J Affect Disord.* 2017; **215**: 213–217.

16. Kim K, Kim SW, Myung W, et al. Reduced orbitofrontal-thalamic functional connectivity related to suicidal ideation in patients with major depressive disorder. *Scientific Reports.* 2017; **7**: 15772.

17. Iwabuchi SJ, Krishnadas R, Li C, et al. Localized connectivity in depression: a meta-analysis of resting state functional imaging studies. *Neurosci Biobehav Rev.* 2015; **51**: 77–86.

18. Raichle ME, MacLeod AM, Snyder AZ, et al. A default mode of brain function. *Proc Natl Acad Sci U S A.* 2001; **98**: 676–682.

19. Andrews-Hanna JR, Reidler JS, Sepulcre J, et al. Functional-anatomic fractionation of the brain's default network. *Neuron.* 2010; **65**: 550–562.

20. Buckner RL, Andrews-Hanna JR, Schacter DL. The brain's default network: anatomy, function, and relevance to disease. *Ann N Y Acad Sci.* 2008; **1124**: 1–38.

21. Cavanna AE, Trimble MR. The precuneus: A review of its functional anatomy and behavioural correlates. *Brain.* 2006; **129**: 564–583.

22. Andrews-Hanna JR, Smallwood J, Spreng RN. The default network and self-generated thought: Component processes, dynamic control, and clinical relevance. *Ann N Y Acad Sci.* 2014; **1316**: 29–52.

23. Leech R, Sharp DJ. The role of the posterior cingulate cortex in cognition and disease. *Brain*. 2014; **137**: 12–32.

24. Greicius MD, Krasnow B, Reiss AL, et al. Functional connectivity in the resting brain: a network analysis of the default mode hypothesis. *Proc Natl Acad Sci U S A*. 2003; **100**: 253–258.

25. van Tol MJ, Li M, Metzger CD, et al. Local cortical thinning links to resting-state disconnectivity in major depressive disorder. *Psychol Med*. 2014; **44**: 2053–2065.

26. Sheline YI, Price JL, Yan Z, et al. Resting-state functional MRI in depression unmasks increased connectivity between networks via the dorsal nexus. *Proc Natl Acad Sci U S A*. 2010; **107**: 11020–11025.

27. Zhou Y, Yu C, Zheng H, et al. Increased neural resources recruitment in the intrinsic organization in major depression. *J Affect Disord*. 2010; **121**: 220–230.

28. Alexopoulos GS, Hoptman MJ, Kanellopoulos D, et al. Functional connectivity in the cognitive control network and the default mode network in late-life depression. *J Affect Disord*. 2012; **139**: 56–65.

29. Andreescu C, Tudorascu DL, Butters MA, et al. Resting state functional connectivity and treatment response in late-life depression. *Psychiatry Res* 2013; **214**: 313–321.

30. Greicius MD, Flores BH, Menon V, et al. Resting-state functional connectivity in major depression: Abnormally increased contributions from subgenual cingulate cortex and thalamus. *Biol Psychiatry*. 2007; **62**: 429–437.

31. Zhu, X Wang X, Xiao J, et al. Evidence of a dissociation pattern in resting-state default mode network connectivity in first-episode, treatment-naive major depression patients. *Biol Psychiatry*. 2012; **71**: 611–617.

32. Li B, Liu L, Friston KJ, et al. A treatment-resistant default mode subnetwork in major depression. *Biol Psychiatry*. 2013; **74**: 48–54.

33. Manoliu A, Meng C, Brandl F, et al. Insular dysfunction within the salience network is associated with severity of symptoms and aberrant inter-network connectivity in major depressive disorder. *Front Hum Neurosci*. 2013; **7**: 930.

34. Smith SM, Fox PT, Miller KL, et al. Correspondence of the brain's functional architecture during activation and rest. *Proc Natl Acad Sci U S A*. 2009; **106**: 13040–13045.

35. Menon V. Large-scale brain networks and psychopathology: A unifying triple network model. *Trends Cogn Sci*. 2011; **15**: 483–506.

36. Ye T, Peng J, Nie B, et al. Altered functional connectivity of the dorsolateral prefrontal cortex in first-episode patients with major depressive disorder. *Eur J Radiol*. 2012; **81**: 4035–4040.

37. Wang YL, Yang SZ, Sun WL, et al. Altered functional interaction hub between affective network and cognitive control network in patients with major depressive disorder. *Behav Brain Res*. 2016; **298**: 301–309.

38. Liston C, Chen AC, Zebley BD, et al. Default mode network mechanisms of transcranial magnetic stimulation in depression. *Biol Psychiatry*. 2014; **76**: 517–526.

39. Stange JP, Bessette KL, Jenkins LM, et al. Attenuated intrinsic connectivity within cognitive control network among individuals with remitted depression: Temporal stability and association with negative cognitive styles. *Hum Brain Mapp*. 2017; **38**: 2939–2954.

40. Seeley WW, Menon V, Schatzberg AF, et al. Dissociable intrinsic connectivity networks for salience processing and executive control. *J Neurosci*. 2007; **27**: 2349–2356.

41. Sridharan D, Levitin DJ, Menon V. A critical role for the right fronto-insular cortex in switching between central-executive and default-mode networks. *Proc Natl Acad Sci U S A*. 2008; **105**: 12569–12574.

42. Goulden N, Khusnulina A, Davis NJ, et al. The salience network is responsible for switching between the default mode network and the central executive network: replication from DCM. *Neuroimage*. 2014; **99**: 180–190.

43. Horn DI, Yu C, Steiner J, et al. Glutamatergic and resting-state functional connectivity correlates of severity in major depression – the role of pregenual anterior cingulate cortex and anterior insula. *Front Syst Neurosci*. 2010 July 15; **4**: 33.

44. Avery JA, Drevets WC, Moseman SE, et al. Major depressive disorder is associated with abnormal interoceptive activity and functional connectivity in the insula. *Biol Psychiatry*. 2014; **76**: 258–266.

45. Hamilton JP, Chen MC, Gotlib IH. Neural systems approaches to understanding major depressive disorder: an intrinsic functional organization perspective. *Neurobiol Dis*. 2013; **52**: 4–11.

46. Yuen GS, Gunning-Dixon FM, Hoptman MJ, et al. The salience network in the apathy of late-life depression. *Int J Geriatr Psychiatry*. 2014; **29**: 1116–1124.

47. Cullen KR, Westlund MK, Klimes-Dougan B, et al. Abnormal amygdala resting-state functional connectivity in adolescent depression. *JAMA Psychiatry*. 2014; **71**: 1138–1147.

48. Yue Y, Yuan Y, Hou Z, et al. Abnormal functional connectivity of amygdala in late-onset depression was associated with cognitive deficits. *PLoS One.* 2013; **8**: e75058.

49. Ramasubbu R, Konduru N, Cortese F, et al. Reduced intrinsic connectivity of amygdala in adults with major depressive disorder. *Front Psychiatry.* 2014; **5**: 17.

50. Tahmasian M, Knight DC, Manoliu A, et al. Aberrant intrinsic connectivity of hippocampus and amygdala overlap in the fronto-insular and dorsomedial-prefrontal cortex in major depressive disorder. *Front Hum Neurosci.* 2013; 7: 639.

51. Veer IM, Beckmann CF, van Tol MJ, et al. Whole brain resting-state analysis reveals decreased functional connectivity in major depression. *Front Syst Neurosci.* 2010 September 20; **4**: 41.

52. Jiang Y, Duan M, Chen X, et al. Common and distinct dysfunctional patterns contribute to triple network model in schizophrenia and depression: A preliminary study. *Prog Neuropsychopharmacol Biol Psychiatry.* 2017; **79**: 302–310.

53. Abbott CC, Lemke NT, Gopal S, et al. Electroconvulsive therapy response in major depressive disorder: A pilot functional network connectivity resting state fMRI investigation. *Front Psychiatry.* 2013; **4**: 10.

54. Mulders PC, van Eijndhoven PF, Schene AH, et al. Resting-state functional connectivity in major depressive disorder: A review. *Neurosci Biobehav Rev.* 2015; **56**: 330–344.

55. Palaniyappan L, Liddle PF. Does the salience network play a cardinal role in psychosis? An emerging hypothesis of insular dysfunction. *J Psychiatry Neurosci.* 2012; **37**: 17–27.

56. Gong Q, He Y. Depression, neuroimaging and connectomics: A selective overview. *Biol Psychiatry.* 2015; **77**: 223–235.

57. Zhang J, Wang J, Wu Q, et al. Disrupted brain connectivity networks in drug-naive, first-episode major depressive disorder. *Biol Psychiatry.* 2011; **70**: 334–342.

58. Meng C, Brandl F, Tahmasian M, et al. Aberrant topology of striatum's connectivity is associated with the number of episodes in depression. *Brain.* 2014; **137**: 598–609.

59. Lord A, Horn D, Breakspear M, et al. Changes in community structure of resting state functional connectivity in unipolar depression. *PLoS One.* 2012; **7**: e41282.

60. Bohr IJ, Kenny E, Blamire A, et al. Resting-state functional connectivity in late-life depression: Higher global connectivity and more long distance connections. *Front Psychiatry.* 2012; **3**: 116.

61. Wang J, Wang L, Zang Y, et al. Parcellation-dependent small-world brain functional networks: a resting-state fMRI study. *Hum Brain Mapp.* 2009; **30**: 1511–1523.

62. Zalesky A, Fornito A, Harding IH, et al. Whole-brain anatomical networks: does the choice of nodes matter? *Neuroimage.* 2010; **50**: 970–983.

63. Tao H, Guo S, Ge T, et al. Depression uncouples brain hate circuit. *Mol Psychiatry.* 2013; **18**: 101–111.

64. Jin C, Gao C, Chen C, et al. A preliminary study of the dysregulation of the resting networks in first-episode medication-naive adolescent depression. *Neurosci Lett.* 2011; **503**: 105–109.

65. Pine DS, Cohen E, Cohen P, et al. Adolescent depressive symptoms as predictors of adult depression: Moodiness or mood disorder? *Am J Psychiatry.* 1999; **156**: 133–135.

66. van den Heuvel MP, Hulshoff Pol HE. Exploring the brain network: A review on resting-state fMRI functional connectivity. *Eur Neuropsychopharmacol.* 2010; **20**: 519–534.

Functional Connectome in Bipolar Disorder

Jungwon Cha and Amit Anand

7.1 Introduction

Bipolar disorder (BD) is a major psychiatric illness which is thought to have strong biological underpinnings. A biological basis for BD is exemplified by a strong heritability of the disorder (1), occurrence of mood periods of mania (BPM), and depression (BPD), which may or may not be precipitated by environmental factors and dramatic improvement with specific medication treatment such as lithium(2). Therefore, with the augment of brain imaging techniques to study brain metabolism and task-induced activation there is an expectation that a brain state or trait abnormalities specific to BD will be identified. Indeed, regional brain abnormalities in the orbitofrontal cortex, anterior cingulate cortex, striatum, thalamus, and amygdala have been identified in BD; however, no particular abnormality has been consistently reported. In light of this state of affairs, it has been proposed that the abnormality in BD may lie in the functional connectivity (FC) between brain regions rather than in a particular region (3).

7.2 The Functional Connectome

The concept of functional connectome has been developed recently to denote the functional connectivity between brain regions. Functional connectivity is a correlation of neuronal activity between brain regions during task-induced activation or at rest. The former is, however, more accurately labeled as task-related co-activation or coupling of activation as only that activity which changes in response to an active task versus a control task is measured. Functional connectivity is a correlation between two brain regions and as such does not provide any direct knowledge of the effect of one region or the other. Functional connectivity between two regions can occur because of one region influencing the activity of the other or vice versa or both or even by another

factor or region simultaneously affecting both the regions in question (4). Effective connectivity, on the other hand, implies the effect of the activity of one region over that of another region (4). Techniques such as dynamic causal modeling (5) have been developed to measure effective connectivity; however, they are more cumbersome to measure and have not been as much investigated as functional connectivity. The most commonly used methods to study the functional connectome are described later.

7.2.1 Methods to Study the Functional Connectome in Brain Imaging Studies

Task-Based Functional Connectivity: A number of studies have investigated the coupling of activation while subjects perform an activation task. As noted earlier, this is not strictly a measure of functional connectivity as activation depends on the baseline level of activity of a region that can influence whether a higher or lower BOLD change is observed. Therefore, mere correlation of time series during an activation task should not be done. A more accurate measure of co-activation is pathophysiological interaction (PPI) in which activation in two regions is correlated in the context of a task (6). Several studies have used PPI to investigate functional connectivity in BD.

Brain task-related functional connectome findings in bipolar disorders are depicted in Table 7.1.

Resting-State Low-Frequency BOLD Fluctuations Correlation (Connectivity): As discussed earlier, computing functional connectivity from task-induced co-activation has some limitations. Resting-state low-frequency BOLD fluctuations (LFBF) correlation has provided a much more powerful and relatively easy to measure method to deduce functional connectivity between brain regions. Resting-state functional connectivity (RSFC) has been empirically shown to correlate

Table 7.1 Brain task-related functional connectome findings in bipolar disorders

Task	Study	Subjects	Medication	Area	BPE/BP vs. HC	BPM vs. BPD vs. BPE vs. HC	BPD vs. MDD
Emotional regulation task Emotional Stroop task	Caseras (7) Favre (8)	16 BPE I, 19 BPE II, and 20 HC 14 BPE and 13 HC	Combinations Combinations	dlPFC-amygdala	↑ BPE compared with HC	↑ BP II compared with BPE I and HC	
Facial emotion identification/ matching tasks Emotional regulation task	Tseng (9) Townsend (10)	14 BP and 14 HC30 BPE I and 26 HC	Combinations Combinations	vPFC-amygdala	↓ BP compared with HC (+)		
Facial emotion identification/ matching tasks	Wang (81)	33 BP and 31 HC	Combinations	pACC-amygdala	↓ BP compared with HC		
CPT-END task	Cerullo (11)	15 BP I and 15 HC	Combinations	IFC-amygdala		↑BPM	
CPT-END task	Cerullo (11)	15 BP I and 15 HC	Combinations	insula-right amygdala		↑ Transition from BPM to BPD	
During sad experiment, facial emotion identification/ matching tasks	Versace (12)	31 BP and 24 HC	Combinations	OFC-amygdala	↑ BP compared with HC		
During happy experiment, facial emotion identification/ matching tasks	Versace (12)	31 BP and 24 HC	Combinations	OFC-amygdala	↓ BP compared with HC		
Verbal working memory task	Stegmayer (13)	18 BPE and 18 HC	Combinations	right hemispheric-amygdala	↓ BPE compared with HC		
2-Back working memory task	Goikolea (14)	31 FEM and 31 HC	Combinations	vmPFC-SFG		↑ BPM compared with HC	
Motor activation paradigm	Marchand (15)	19 BPE II and 18 HC	Combinations	within SFG	↑ BPE compared with HC		

During reward receipt reward processing task	Dutra (16)	24 BP I and 25 HC	Combinations	OFC-VS	↑ BP compared with HC
During reward omission reward processing task	Dutra (16)	24 BP I and 25 HC	Combinations	PFC-VS	↓ BP compared with HC (+)
Reward anticipation task	Schreiter (17)	20 BPE and 20 HC	Combinations		
Card-guessing paradigm	Redlich (18)	33 BP, 33 MDD, and 34 HC	Combinations	VTA-VS	↑ MDD compared with HC (Classification between MDD and BP: 66.6% accuracy)
Distraction and reappraisal emotion regulation task	Lois (19)	21 BP, 21 MDD, and 23 HC	Combinations	within DMN, between DMN and CCN	↑ Both BPD and MDD

Symbols: +, more than one report from different investigators; negative or contrary finding reported; ↑, increased functional connectivity; ↓, decreased functional connectivity

Disorders: BP, bipolar; BPE, euthymic bipolar; BPM, manic bipolar; BPD, depressive bipolar; MDD, major depressive disorder; HC, healthy control; BP I, bipolar type I; BP II, bipolar type II; BPE I, euthymic bipolar type I; BPE II, euthymic bipolar type II; FEM, first episode mania

Brain regions: PFC, prefrontal cortex; dlPFC, dorsolateral PFC; vPFC, ventral PFC; vlPFC, ventrolateral PFC; vmPFC, ventromedial PFC; aPFC, anterior PFC; mPFC, medial PFC; IFC, inferior frontal cortex; OFC, orbitofrontal cortex; mOFC, medial OFC; ACC, anterior cingulate cortex; pACC, perigenual ACC; sgACC, subgenual ACC; PCC, posterior cingulate cortex; IFG, inferior prefrontal gyrus; ITG, inferior temporal gyrus; SFG, superior frontal gyrus; VTA, ventral tegmental area; SMA, supplementary motor area; VS, ventral striatum

Brain networks: DMN, default mode network; CCN, cognitive control network; SMN, sensorimotor network; CEN, central executive network; SN, salience network

Analysis: ICA, independent component analysis

Task: CPT-END, continuous performance task with emotional and neutral distractors

Table 7.2 Brain resting-state functional connectome findings in bipolar disorders

Study	Subjects	Medication	Area	BPE/BP vs. HC	BPM vs. BPD vs. BPE vs. HC	BPD vs. MDD
Anand (3)	6 BDM, 5 BDD, 15 MDD and 15 HC	Unmedicated	ACC-amygdala	↑ BPE compared with HC	↓ BPM compared with BPE	
Rey (23)	15 BPE, 12 Non-Euthymic BP, and 27 HC	Combinations			↓ Both BPD and BPM compared with HC	
Brady (24)	26 BPM, 21 BPE, and 10 across Both mood states	Combinations				
Brady (24)	26 BPM, 21 BPE, and 10 across Both mood states	Combinations	dlPFC-amygdala	↓ BP compared with HC	↑ BPM compared with BPE	
Anticevic (25)	68 BP I and 51 HC	Combinations				
Anticevic (25)	68 BP I and 51 HC	Combinations	(v or m)PFC-amygdala	↑ BP compared with HC (+)	↓ Both BPM and BPD	
Favre (26)	20 BPE and 20 HC	Combinations				
Wei (27)	16 BDD, 16 BPD, 13 BPM and 30 HC1	Combinations		↑ BPE compared with HC (+)		
Chepenik (28)	15 BP and 10 HC	Combinations				
Torrisi (30)	20 BPE and 20 HC	Combinations				
Li (30)	18 BPM, 10 BPD and 28 HC	Combinations	OFC-amygdala		↓ Both BPM and BPD compared with HC	
Brady (24)	26 BPM, 21 BPE, and 10 across Both mood states	Combinations			↓ BPM compared with BPD	
Singh (31)	20 BP I, 23 HC	Combinations	preceuneus-amygdala	↓ BP I compared to HC		
Li (32)	21 BPE and 28 HC	Lamotrigine for BPE	SMA-amygdala	↓ BPE compared with HC		
Chen (33)	43 BP II, 36 MDD and 47 HC	Unmedicated	ACC-OFC			↓ Both MDD and 3PD compared with HC
Magioncalda (34) Gong (35)	40 BP and 40 HC; 96 BP II and 100 HC	Combinations; Unmedicated	pACC-ITG	↓ BP compared with HC (+)		
Martino (36)	21 BPM, 20 BPE, and 42 HC	Combinations	ACC-PCC	↓ BP compared with HC	↓ BPM compared with Both BPD and HC	
Magioncalda (34)	40 BP and 40 HC	Combinations				

Study	Sample	Medication	Connectivity/Region	Finding		
He (38)	32 BP, 33 MDD, and 43 HC	Combinations	dlPFC-cerebellar			↓ BPD compared with Both MDD and HC (Classification between BPD and MDD : 69% accuracy)
Favre (26)	20 BPE and 20 HC	Combinations	mPFC-dlPFC	↑ BP compared with HC		
Gong (35)	96 BP II and 100 HC	Unmedicated	mPFC-PCC	↓ BP compared with HC		
Minuzzi (39)	32 right-handed BPE women and 36 HC	Combinations	OFC-IFG	↑ BPE compared with HC		
Wang (40)	36 BP II, 32 MDD, and 40 HC	Combinations	inter-hemispheric	↓ BP II compared with HC		
Yasuno (41)	16 BP and 22 MDD	Combinations	inter-hemispheric			↓ BPD compared with HC
Reinke (42)	21 BPE and 20 HC	Combinations	IFG-Insula	↑ BP compared with HC		
Li (32)	18 BPD, 10 BPD and 28 HC, 26 BPM, 21 BPE	Combinations	IFG-lingual gyrus		↓ Both BPM and BPD	
Pang (43)	30 BP, 30 MDD, and 30 HC	Combinations	insula-inferior parietal lobe			↑ BPD compared with MDD (–)
Ellard (44)	35 MDD, 24 BP, and 39 HC	Combinations				
Minuzzi (39)	32 right-handed BPE women and 36 HC	Combinations	insular-somatosensory cortex	↑ BPE compared with HC		
Marchand (45)	14 BPD and 26 MDD	Combinations	PCC-inferior parietal lobule, precentral gyrus and insula			↑ BPD compared with MDD
Yin (46)	21 BP, 40 MDD and 70 HC	Combinations	SFG-insula			↓ BPD compared with HC
Pang (43)	30 BP, 30 MDD, and 30 HC	Combinations	dlPFC-insula			↑ BPD compared with MDD

Table 7.2 (cont.)

Study	Subjects	Medication	Area	BPE/BP vs. HC	BPM vs. BPD vs. BPE vs. HC	BPD vs. MDD
Liu (47)	17 BP and 17 MDD	Combinations	IFG-hippocampal			↑ BPD compared with MDD, ↑ Both BPD and MDD compared with HC
Fateh (48)	30 BPD, 29 MDD, 30 HC	Combinations	lingual gyrus-hippocampal			↑ BPD compared with MDD
Chen (33)	43 BP II, 36 MDD and 47 HC	Unmedicated	SFG-hippocampal			↓ MDD compared with HC
Oertel-Knochel (49)	21 BP and 21 HC	Combinations	IFG-hippocampal	↑BP compared with HC		
Dandash (50)	61 FEM and 30 HC	Combinations	in the dorsal and caudal cortico-striatal systems		↓ BPM compared with HC	
Anand (3)	6 BDM, 5 BDD, 15 MDD and 15 HC	Unmedicated	pACC-striatum		↓ Both BPM and BPD	
Anand (3)	6 BDM, 5 BDD, 15 MDD and 15 HC	Unmedicated	pACC-thalamus		↓ Both BPM and BPD	
He (51)	25 BPD, 25 MDD, and 34 HC	Combinations	dlPFC-striatum			↑ BPD compared with MDD
Altinay (52)	30 BDD, 30 BDM, and 30 HC	Unmedicated	left dorsal caudate and midbrain regions		↑ BPM	
Altinay (52)	30 BDD, 30 BDM, and 30 HC	Unmedicated	caudate-midbrain region		↑ BPM	
Ambrosi (53) Singh (31)	36 BD, 40 MDD and 40 HC 20 BP I, 23 HC	Combinations Combinations	hippocampus-amygdala	↑ BP I compared with HC		↓ MDD compared with Both BPD and HC
Teng (54)	15 BP I, 16 HC	Combinations	thalamic-hippocampus	↑ BP I		
Dandash (50)	61 FEM and 30 HC	Combinations	VS-thalamus		↑ BPM	
Lv (55) Reinke (42)	42 BP and 28 HC 21 BPE and 20 HC	Combinations Combinations	language areas	↑ BP compared with HC	↓ BPD compared to BPE	
Luo (56)		Unmedicated				

Reference	Sample	Medication	Brain region	Findings
Chen (57)	94 BP II depression and 100 HC	Unmedicated	the cerebellar crus and lobules with areas of the frontal cortex	↓ BP II compared with HC (++)
Wang (58)	90 BP II and 100 HC, 25 remitted BP II and 25 HC	Combinations		
Shi (60)	66 BPD and 40 HC	Combinations	VTA-VS	↓ BPD compared with MDD (Classification between BPD and MDD: 70% accuracy)
Han (61)	40 BPD, 54 MDD and 44 HC	Combinations	raphe nucleus with subcortical regions	↓ BPD

Symbols: +, more than one report from different investigators; −, negative or contrary finding reported; ↑, increased functional connectivity; ↓, decreased functional connectivity

Disorders: BP, bipolar; BPE, euthymic bipolar; BPM, manic bipolar; BPD, depressive bipolar; MDD, major depressive disorder; HC, healthy control; BP I, bipolar type I; BP II, bipolar type II; BPE I, euthymic bipolar type I; BPE II, euthymic bipolar type II; FEM, first-episode mania

Brain regions: PFC, prefrontal cortex; dlPFC, dorsolateral PFC; vPFC, ventral PFC; vlPFC, ventrolateral PFC; vmPFC, ventromedial PFC; aPFC, anterior PFC; mPFC, medial PFC; IFC, inferior frontal cortex; OFC, orbitofrontal cortex; mOFC, medial OFC; ACC, anterior cingulate cortex; pACC, perigenual ACC; sgACC, subgenual ACC; PCC, posterior cingulate cortex; IFG, inferior prefrontal gyrus; ITG, inferior temporal gyrus; SFG, superior frontal gyrus; VTA, ventral tegmental area; SMA, supplementary motor area; VS, ventral striatum

Brain networks: DMN, default mode network; CCN, cognitive control network; SMN, sensorimotor network; CEN, central executive network; SN, salience network

Analysis: ICA, independent component analysis

Task: CPT-END, continuous performance task with emotional and neutral distractors

Table 7.3 Brain functional connectome findings in bipolar disorders analyzed by independent component analysis

Study	Subjects	Medication	Area	BPE/ BP vs. HC	BPM vs. BPD vs. BPE vs. HC	BPD vs. MDD
Ishida (66)	22 BP and 24 HC	Combinations	In two clusters in the SMN (right and left primary somatosensory areas)	↓ BP compared with HC		
Syan (67)	32 BPE women and 36 HC	Combinations	PCC-angular gyrus	↑ BPE		
Lois (68)	30 BDEI and 35 HC	Combinations	Between the meso/paralimbic and the right frontoparietal network	↑ BPE compared with HC		
Lois (68)	30 BDEI and 35 HC	Combinations	Across the bilateral insula and putamen and across a temporo-insular network	↑ BP II		
Martino (37)	20 BPD, 20 BPM, 20 BPE, and 40 HC	Combinations	Within the DMN and SMN		↑ BPD compared with BPM	
Ford (69)	15 BPD and 15 MDD	Combinations	In ICA components			↓ Both BPD and MDD
Wang (59)	38 BPD, 35 MDD, and 47 HC	Unmedicated	Intra-network FC within the DMN			↓ Both the BPD and MDD
Wang (59)	38 BPD, 35 MDD, and 47 HC	Unmedicated	Inter-network FC between the CEN and SN			↑ BPD compared with either the MDD or HC
He (70)	13 BP, 40 MDD, and 33 HC	Unmedicated	Within sensory, motor and cognitive networks			↓ BP compared with MDD (Classification between BP and MDD : 99% accuracy)

| Goya-Maldonado (71) | 20 BPD, 20 MDD, and 20 HC | Combinations | In the frontoparietal network | ↑ BPD |
| Goya-Maldonado (71) | 20 BPD, 20 MDD, and 20 HC | Combinations | in the DMN | ↑ MDD |

Symbols: +, more than one report from different investigators; −, negative or contrary finding reported; ↑, increased functional connectivity; ↓ decreased functional connectivity

Disorders: BP, bipolar; BPE, euthymic bipolar; BPM, manic bipolar; BPD, depressive bipolar; MDD, major depressive disorder; HC, healthy control; BP I, bipolar type I; BP II, bipolar type II; BPE I, euthymic bipolar type I; BPE II, euthymic bipolar type II; FEM, first-episode mania

Brain regions: PFC, prefrontal cortex; dlPFC, dorsolateral PFC; vPFC, ventral PFC; vlPFC, ventrolateral PFC; vmPFC, ventromedial PFC; aPFC, anterior PFC; mPFC, medial PFC; IFC, inferior frontal cortex; OFC, orbitofrontal cortex; mOFC, medial OFC; ACC, anterior cingulate cortex; pACC, perigenual ACC; sgACC, subgenual ACC; PCC, posterior cingulate cortex; IFG, inferior prefrontal gyrus; ITG, inferior temporal gyrus; SFG, superior frontal gyrus; VTA, ventral tegmental area; SMA, supplementary motor area; VS, ventral striatum

Brain networks: DMN, default mode network; CCN, cognitive control network; SMN. sensorimotor network; CEN, central executive network; SN, salience network

Analysis: ICA, independent component analysis

Task: CPT-END, continuous performance task with emotional and neutral distractors

Table 7.4 Brain functional connectome findings in bipolar disorders analyzed by graph-theory method

Study	Subjects	Medication	Area	BPE/ BP vs. HC	BPM vs. BPD vs. BPE vs. HC	BPD vs. MDD
Doucet (73)	78 BP, 64 unaffected siblings, and 41 HC	78 BP, 64 unaffected siblings, and 41 HC	Global cohesiveness and their unaffected siblings	↓ BP and their unaffected siblings compared with HC		
Wang (74)	37 BP II and 37 HC	Unmedicated	DMN	↓ BP compared with HC		
Wang (74)	37 BP II and 37 HC	Unmedicated	Limbic regions	↑ BP II compared with HC		
Spielberg (75)	30 BPM, 30 BPD and 30 HC	Unmedicated	Amygdala centrality		↑BPM	
Spielberg (75)	30 BPM, 30 BPD and 30 HC	Unmedicated	OFC centrality		↓BPD	
He (76)	13 BP, 40 MDD and 33 HC	Unmedicated	ICA components			↑ BPD compared with MDD
Wang (77)	31 BP II depressed, 32 MDD, and 43 HC	Unmedicated	In the bilateral precuneus			↓ Both BPD and MDD short range FCS
Wang (77)	31 BP II depressed, 32 MDD, and 43 HC	Unmedicated	In the bilateral cerebellum			↑ BPD compared with MDD long-range FCS and short range FCS
Wang (77)	31 BP II depressed, 32 MDD, and 43 HC	Unmedicated	In the DMN, limbic network and cerebellum			↓ Both the MDD and BP II nodal characteristics (nodal strength and nodal efficiency)

Symbols: +, more than one report from different investigators; negative or contrary finding reported; ↑, increased functional connectivity; ↓ decreased functional connectivity

Disorders: BP, bipolar; BPE, euthymic bipolar; BPM, manic bipolar; BPD, depressive bipolar; MDD, major depressive disorder; HC, healthy control; BP I, bipolar type I; BP II, bipolar type II; BPE I, euthymic bipolar type I; BPE II, euthymic bipolar type II; FEM, first-episode mania

Brain regions: PFC, prefrontal cortex; dlPFC, dorsolateral PFC; vPFC, ventral PFC; vlPFC, ventrolateral PFC; vmPFC, ventromedial PFC; aPFC, anterior PFC; mPFC, medial PFC; IFC, inferior frontal cortex; OFC, orbitofrontal cortex; mOFC, medial OFC; ACC, anterior cingulate cortex; pACC, perigenual ACC; sgACC, subgenual ACC; PCC, posterior cingulate cortex; IFG, inferior prefrontal gyrus; ITG, inferior temporal gyrus; SFG, superior frontal gyrus; VTA, ventral tegmental area; SMA, supplementary motor area; VS, ventral striatum

Brain networks: DMN, default mode network; CCN, cognitive control network; SMN, sensorimotor network; CEN, central executive network; SN, salience network

Analysis: ICA, independent component analysis

Task: CPT-END, continuous performance task with emotional and neutral distractors

between brain regions known to have functional or anatomical connections (20–22). Three commonly used methods to quantify results from the resting-state LFBF correlation analysis are to study the functional connectome in health and disease – seed-based analysis, independent component analysis, and graph-theory analysis.

Brain resting-state functional connectome findings in bipolar disorders are depicted in Table 7.2.

Seed-Based Functional Connectivity Analysis: For this method, a reference area of interest is first identified and then the mean resting-state BOLD fluctuations of this region are correlated with the mean of BOLD fluctuations in one or more target regions of interest (ROIs) or all of the voxels of the whole brain. A majority of studies that have hypothesized an a priori reference ROI have been conducted using the ROI approach.

Independent Component Analysis (ICA): Independent component analysis of the resting-state BOLD signal has revealed several components comprising correlated brain regions which have been named according to their purported neuropsychiatric function – default mode, salience, executive function, and others (62, 63). The ACC and PCC connectivity is part of a default mode network (DMN) that shows high connectivity during rest, and these areas get deactivated when any task is conducted (64). The default mode circuit has been related to consciousness and vigilance to external and internal milieus while no task is being conducted (65). The salience network (SN) comprising the insula and other cortical areas is thought to be involved in the assessment of the internal mental and emotional state, while executive motor network (EMN) comprises correlated motor areas.

Brain functional connectome findings in bipolar disorders analyzed by independent component analysis are depicted in Table 7.3.

Graph-Theory Analysis: Graph-theory metrics provide measures of network-wide properties to provide insights into network function rather than the strength of connectivity between seed regions (72). Nodes and edges (connections) between nodes are measured in terms of network organization patterns related to network *Resilience* (e.g., assortativity), *Segregation* (e.g., clustering coefficient, transitivity), *Integration* (e.g., diffusion

efficiency), and Centrality (e.g., pageRank centrality, subgraph Centrality).

Brain functional connectome findings in bipolar disorders analyzed by graph-theory method are depicted in Table 7.4.

7.2.2 The Functional Connectome in Bipolar Disorder

7.2.2.1 Study Designs for Investigationof Functional Connectome in Bipolar Disorder

Since we published the first report of abnormalities of resting-state functional connectivity in major depression (MDD) and BD (3, 22), the number of reports of FC abnormalities in BD has exponentially increased. Various studies have used several different experimental strategies to investigate the functional connectome pathophysiology in BD. Comparison with healthy controls (HCs) and BD subjects is one straightforward strategy. Studies of euthymic subjects versus HCs provide evidence for trait-related abnormalities in BD. However, it is challenging to study truly euthymic bipolar subjects particularly in the absence of confounds such as medication load effects. Another strategy to study trait-related abnormalities is to study affected and unaffected relatives of BD subjects.

Studies investigating mania or depression provide information regarding state-related connectome abnormalities, though technically BPM and BPD have a combination of state- and trait-related abnormalities. Abnormalities common to both BPD and BPM could be thought of as trait-related abnormalities, or they could be common state-related abnormalities that can give rise to both mania and depression, for example, a general emotional dysregulation. A powerful strategy is to compare the different states rather than comparison with healthy subjects as other confounds related to bipolar illness can be controlled. An even more attractive approach is to study the various states within the same subject, though in this design, it is difficult to control for changes in confounding factors such as environmental, biological, and therapeutic factors as a subject transitions from one state to the other. The comparison with unipolar major depression (MDD) is not only a powerful strategy to isolate abnormalities related to bipolarity but also a highly clinical relevant distinction for which a biomarker is critically needed.

69

For the purpose of this review, we examined all reports in which trait and state-related abnormalities of the FC have been investigated. Pediatric BD and comparison with schizophrenia and other non-mood disorders studies are not included as that is beyond the scope of this review. Several findings related to different brain regions have been reported; therefore we have organized them into the major categories of hypothesized FC abnormalities in BD – cortico-limbic, cortico-cortical, and subcortical for reference ROI methodology, ICA component abnormalities, and graph-theory property abnormalities. We discuss each of these abnormalities reported in the context of the comparison group experimental paradigm used.

7.2.2.2 ROI Based Analysis

7.2.2.2a Cortico-Limbic Connectivity

The study of cortico-limbic connectivity implies that investigators studied the relationship between cortical mood-regulating areas, for example, anterior cingulate cortex (ACC), orbitofrontal cortex (OFC), and subcortical or limbic mood-generating areas such as the amygdala (AMYG) and ventral striatum (VS). This hypothesis is derived from the Jacksonian view of neural architecture, which models the brain in terms of hierarchical structures with the higher structures influencing the activity of the lower structures (79). The influence of mood-regulating regions on the mood-generating regions also harkens back to the Freudian model of the psyche in which the superego and ego control the expression of the instinctual drives of the id. It should be noted though that despite being a neurologist, Freud did not propose a neuroanatomical model for his model of the organization of the psyche (80). As BD involves impairments in inhibition of emotional responses and impulsive behavior, it is thought that cortico-limbic emotion regulatory mechanisms have become impaired in some way leading to unregulated mood symptomatology. As noted earlier, functional connectivity does not give any information regarding the effect of one region over the other but coherence of activity between brain regions has been thought to provide some information regarding whether two brain areas are working simultaneously or not. The findings of altered cortico-limbic functional connectivity in BD are summarized later.

Task-Related Cortico-Limbic Psychophysiological Interaction (PPI) Studies: Using facial emotion identification/matching tasks, several studies have reported decreased connectivity between amygdala and areas of the frontal cortex such as the ventromedial prefrontal cortex (vmPFC) (9) and posterior anterior cingulate cortex (pACC) (81). On a verbal working memory task, euthymic BD subjects (BPE) exhibited decreased PPI right-sided cortico-amygdalar connectivity compared to HC (13). Other studies have reported increased cortico-limbic connectivity: increased PPI dlPFC-amygdalar connectivity in BPE versus HC using an emotional Stroop task (8) and during an emotion regulation task, PPI cortico-limbic connectivity has been reported to be less decreased in BPE I subjects compared to HC (7, 10). Still, other studies have reported both an increase and a decrease depending on the emotional task used: using a face processing task, increased pACC-amygdala connectivity during processing of sad faces versus decreased OFC-amygdala connectivity during processing of happy faces was reported in remitted/depressed BD subjects compared to HCs (12). During a reward-processing task, increased FC between VS and mPFC during reward receipt and decreased FC during reward omission in BD I subjects compared to controls(16), while in a reward anticipation task decreased FC between VS and anterior prefrontal cortex (aPFC) was seen (17).

In a study that investigated state-related differences, subjects who transitioned from BPM to BPD after treatment, BPM at baseline had increased frontal gyri (IFC)-amygdala correlation of activations during continuous performance task (CPT-END) while when they transition to a BPD state, this connectivity was decreased but right amygdala-insula connectivity increased(11). In another study in which BPE I and BPE II were directly compared in terms of PPI FC during an emotion regulation task, BPE I subjects exhibited a decreased inverse correlation between cortico-amygdalar connectivity while BP-II subjects exhibited increased inverse correlation suggesting a difference between the two subtypes (7).

In studies that investigated differences between BPD and MDD, the following cortico-limbic FC abnormalities have been reported: Redlich and colleagues using PPI during a card-guessing reward-processing task reported increased FC between the VS and ventral tegmental area (VTA) in the MDD group compared to HC, but no differences with BPD group were found compared to HC (18). In a study that investigated effective connectivity differences in amygdala-OFC connectivity in BD and MDD subjects, Almeida and colleagues reported top-down left-sided amygdala-OMPFC abnormality in MDD and right-sided bottom-up abnormality in BD (82).

Resting-State Reference ROI-Based Cortico-Limbic Connectivity Studies: Anand and colleagues first reported decreased resting-state LFBFs correlation with perigenual ACC-limbic connectivity in medication-free subjects compared to HCs in both BPD and BPM groups compared to HCs (3). Since the first report, several studies have studied cortico-limbic, particularly cortico-amygdalar connectivity in BD and in general have reported decreased amygdala connectivity with dorsal PFC areas but increased amygdala and other limbic areas with the ventral PFC in BD. Chepenik and colleagues reported increased vPFC correlations with amygdala (28). Increased amygdala-mPFC but decreased amygdala-dlPFC connectivity was also reported in remitted BD patients with and without psychosis (25). Increased frontal-hippocampal and vlPFC-VS FC has also been reported in BD subjects compared to HCs (49). Studies that have specifically looked at differences between BPE and HC to identify trait-related abnormalities have reported hyperconnectivity between right amygdala and right vlPFC (29), decreased amygdala connectivity with supplementary more area (32), greater connectivity between mPFC and right amygdala compared to HS, which was also correlated with the duration of the disease (26), and increased amygdala connectivity to the subgenual ACC (23).

A number of cortico-limbic RSFC studies have looked at state-related differences between bipolar mood states. In general, both BPD and BPM have been found to share cortico-limbic connectivity abnormalities, but some differences were also found. Decreased pregenual ACC connectivity with the striatum and thalamus (3), decreased amygdala connectivity with inferior frontal orbital gyrus and lingual gyrus (30), decreased FC between the amygdala and left middle frontal cortex (27), and widespread common cortico-striatal connectivity abnormalities (52) have been reported in both states. Decreased FC between right OFC and amygdala in BPM compared to BPD and in a study comparing BPM with BPE subjects, decreased connectivity between amygdala and ACC in BPM has been reported (24). Conversely, increased

connectivity between the amygdala and dorsal frontal cortical structures involved in emotion regulation has also been observed (24). Cortico-striatal connectivity has been reported to be different in BPM and BPD subjects. In a relatively large study comparing medication-free subjects, BPD showed increased connectivity of the dorsal caudal putamen with somatosensory areas such as the insula and temporal gyrus while BPM showed unique increased connectivity between left dorsal caudate and midbrain regions as well as increased connectivity between VS and thalamus (52). Another study reported similar findings in first episode manic patients regarding reduced connectivity in the dorsal and caudal cortico-striatal systems and increased connectivity in a circuit linking the VS with the medial orbitofrontal cortex, cerebellum, and thalamus when compared to HCs (50).

Studies with an aim to distinguish between BPD and MDD have reported significant differences in hippocampal and striatal FC. In an FDG PET study, Benson and colleagues (83) reported an increased correlation between hippocampus and prefrontal areas in MDD versus BPD. In resting-state LFBF studies also, hippocampal connectivity abnormalities have been found in both BPD and MDD with some differences. In BPD patients, increased FC of the bilateral anterior/posterior hippocampus with lingual gyrus and inferior frontal gyrus (IFG) relative to MDD patients was observed while in comparison to HCs, both groups had an increased FC between the right anterior hippocampus and lingual gyrus and a decreased FC between the right posterior hippocampus and right IFG (47). Increased FC between IFG and lingual gyrus with the hippocampus in BPD compared to MDD (48) was also observed. Increased FC of the striatum in BPD versus MDD has also been reported in a few studies. Increased positive metabolic correlations between prefrontal and ventral striatal areas(83), increased FC between VS and ACC (84), and increased dlPFC connectivity with the striatum in BPD compared to MDD in a PET cerebral blood flow study (51) have been reported.

7.2.2.2b Cortico-Cortical Connectivity

Connection between cortical regions is involved in emotion perception, evaluation, and expression. In that regard, the OFC is thought to be the main area where emotional stimuli are evaluated and processed. Connection of the OFC to the subgenual ACC is thought to be important in emotional expression. The dlPFC through its connection with the ACC and OFC is further involved in regulating their function. The insular cortex is involved in processing the emotional salience of both external and internal stimuli and has extensive connections with both other cortical regions involved in emotion as well as subcortical regions. Several studies have investigated cortico-cortical connections in BD.

Task-Related Cortico-Cortical Psychophysiological Interaction (PPI) Studies: Using a cognitive interference task in the context of emotional images, Ellard and colleagues reported abnormalities in insula connectivity with areas of the default mode and frontoparietal networks in BD subjects (44). Using a Stroop Color Word Task (SCWT), Pompei and colleagues also reported in fronto-insular connectivity abnormalities in BPE subjects compared to their unaffected relatives and HCs (85). Using a motor activation paradigm, Marchand and colleagues reported that in BPE subjects compared to HCs increased FC was found in central midline structures such as the left and right superior frontal gyri (15).

In state-related findings, first-episode BPM subjects exhibited increased PPI connectivity between vmPFC and superior frontal gyrus while performing a 2-back working memory task (14).

In regard to the comparison between BPD and MDD groups, during a distraction and reappraisal emotion regulation task, remitted BD subjects were similar to remitted MDD subjects in that both groups exhibited increased FC between regions of the default mode and between default mode and cognitive control networks during distraction compared to reappraisal task (19).

Resting-State Reference ROI-Based Cortico-Cortical Functional Connectivity Studies: Differences between BD and HCs have been reported in regard to ACC, PCC, parietal cortex, mPFC, cerebellum, and temporal lobes. Decreased connectivity has been reported between perigenual ACC and PCC as well as the inferior temporal gyrus (34). Another study also reported decreased connectivity of the left PCC to the bilateral medial prefrontal cortex (mPFC) and bilateral precuneus/PCC, and the left sgACC to the right inferior temporal gyrus (ITG) (35). A third study reported less variable (i.e., more rigid) over time dynamic connectivity between the mPFC and PCC in BPE, which was associated with slower processing speed and reduced cognitive set-shifting (86). Another finding reported in terms of FC of the mPFC is decreased connectivity with the dlPFC (26). In BPE subjects, increased RSFC between the somatosensory cortex and insular cortex and between inferior prefrontal gyrus and frontal-orbital cortex was observed (39). Another study also reported increased RSFC between right inferior frontal/precentral gyrus and insula in BD subjects compared to HCs (42). For language area connectivity, in BD compared to HC, decreased RSFC between Heschl's gyrus and planum temporale, the left superior and the middle temporal gyri was reported to be associated with verbal memory deficits (42); though in another study comparing BPD and BPE subjects, the decrease in connectivity in language areas appeared to be state-dependent and was not present during euthymia (55). In BP II subjects compared to HCs, three studies reported decreased connectivity of the cerebellar crus and lobules with areas of the frontal cortex (56–58). Unmedicated BPD II subjects compared to HCs have been reported to exhibit decreased interhemispheric connectivity (40).

Studies that have compared different states of BD including BPM have reported: decreased FC between ACC and PCC in BPM, which was correlated with clinical severity scores (37) and an unbiased whole-brain analysis study reported an altered connectivity between nodes found in the dorsal attention network (DAN) and DMN in BPM compared to BPE and HCs (87).

A number of studies have compared cortico-cortical RSFC in MDD and BPD subjects to elucidate the signature of bipolarity while controlling for the depressed state. Insula RSFC differences have been reported in several studies. In addition, decreased FC between right anterior insula and inferior parietal lobe (88) has been reported. In medication-naive BPD, decreased FC from ventral anterior insula to the left superior/middle frontal gyrus in BPD compared to HC and decreased v-AIN to lOFC and Lstg (46) connectivity has been observed. Furthermore, decreased FC in BPD between the left insula and left dlPFC and bilateral insula and right frontal pole (53) has been reported. On the other hand, Pang and colleagues reported increased dynamic FC (dFC) between right anterior insula and left inferior parietal lobe in BPD while MDD exhibited decreased dFC of right anterior insula and right precuneus, temporal lobe, and left dlPFC (43). In other findings, in one study both unmedicated MDD and BPD groups were observed to have decreased RSFC between the left ACC and the left OFC, but only the MDD group exhibited decreased RSFC between the left SFG and the left hippocampus compared with the HCs (33), while in another study increased connectivity of the right PCC (45) in BPD was observed. One study reported decreased inter-hemispheric FC in BPD subjects compared to HCs (41) while another study reported no differences in inter-hemispheric connectivity between BPD II subjects and HCs (40). Decreased dlPFC-cerebellar connectivity in unmedicated BPD subjects has been reported to differentiate them from both unmedicated MDD and HC subject groups (38).

7.2.2.2c Intrinsic Subcortical Connectivity

The circuit comprising the connections between the amygdala, hippocampus, globus pallidus, VS, and thalamus and back to the amygdala has been postulated as the putative mood-generating circuit. Moreover, as depression and mania are associated with decreased motor activity and hyperactivity, respectively, the motor part of the connections between striatum, thalamus, and cortical regions has also been of interest in the investigation of BD connectome pathophysiology.

Resting-State Reference ROI-Based Subcortical Functional Connectivity Studies: Intrinsic functional connectivity within the thalamic–striatal circuit and between the striatal regions and middle and posterior cingulate cortex has been reported to be decreased and thalamic–hippocampus RSFC increased in BP I subjects (54). In youth with BP I, laterobasal amygdala–hippocampus RSFC was observed to be increased while laterobasal–amygdala–precuneus connectivity was decreased (31).

Comparison of mood states has been reported to show that unique increased connectivity between left dorsal caudate and midbrain regions, as well as increased connectivity between VS inferior and thalamus, was present in BPM. Both BPD and BPM groups, however, showed widespread connectivity changes between striatal subregions and limbic regions and midbrain

structures (52). In a study of first-episode BPM, increased connectivity of the VS with the thalamus (50) was reported.

In studies differentiating between BPD and MDD – decreased FC of raphe nucleus with subcortical regions(61) in BPD and decreased FC within the reward circuit between the VTA and VS in BPD subjects compared to MDD (60) was observed but a lower RSFC between the right amygdala and the left anterior hippocampus was seen in MDD compared to BPD and HC (53).

7.2.2.3 Independent Component Analysis Studies

The DMN, ICA component of resting-state LFBFs, has been extensively studied in BD. Other components that have been commonly studied are the salience network (SN), central executive network (CEN) and the somatosensory network (SMN). Difference between groups on the strength of these networks has been studied as is the intrinsic connectivity of subregions within these circuits. In recent times, the correlation between the different ICA components has been an area of interest.

A decreased within-connectivity in two clusters of the SMN (right and left primary somatosensory areas) compared with HC (66) has been reported. In another study, no difference was seen in whole-brain ICA components in remitted women with BPE, but an increased connectivity of PCC seed region with angular gyrus was observed (67). Between-network connectivity findings include increased functional connectivity between the meso/paralimbic and the right frontoparietal network in BPE compared to HCs, possibly reflecting abnormal integration of affective and cognitive information in ventral-emotional and dorsal-cognitive networks in euthymic bipolar patients (68). Another study reported increased coherence across several brain regions in BP II subjects, including the bilateral insula and putamen and across a temporo-insular network but no between-group differences in engagement of the DMN (89) in BD subjects compared to HCs.

In a study looking at state-related findings in BD, altered topographical imbalance and variability of BOLD fluctuations within the DMN and SMN, specifically in the lowest frequency band, as calculated by the Slow5 fSD DMN/SMN ratio, was observed (increased in depression, decreased in mania; in depression increased variability in DMN but decreased in SMN and opposite in mania) (37)

Several studies using ICA have been done to look at differences between BPD and MDD. Findings include decreased variability in dynamic functional connectivity in ICA components in both unmedicated BPD and MDD, abnormalities in DMN network related to bipolarity index in a group of BPD and MDD subjects (69), and in both the BPD and MDD patients weaker intra-network FC within the DMN (58). Findings of differences between BPD and MDD include stronger inter-network FC between the CEN and SN in BPD compared with either the MDD or the control group (58), coaltered reduced gray matter density and decreased connectivity within sensory, motor, and cognitive networks in a fusion analyses differentiating BPD and MDD groups (70), and increased functional connectivity in the frontoparietal network in BPD and increased functional connectivity in the DMN but reduced connectivity of the cingulo-opercular network to default mode regions in MDD (71).

7.2.2.4   Graph-Theory Network Properties Studies

As an intermediate step before graph-theory properties of a network can be calculated, correlations between all ROIs across the whole brain need to be calculated, which itself can be investigated for network-based statistics. The graph-theory properties in terms of edges and nodes can then be calculated. The centrality of nodes, efficiency of the network, and resilience are the most frequently studied abnormalities.

In comparison between BD and HC subjects, decreased global cohesiveness in BD and their unaffected siblings compared to HC (73) and decreased functional connectivity strength (FCS) in DMN regions have been observed (74). Conversely an increased FCS in limbic regions (74) in BP II subjects versus HC was reported. Spielberg and colleagues (75) investigated graph properties of whole-brain functional network in thirty unmedicated BPM, thirty unmedicated BPD, and thirty matched HCs. BD group exhibited hyperconnectivity in a network involving the right amygdala and (hypo)manic symptoms correlated with this network as well as with disruptions in the brain's "small-world" organization. Depressive symptoms on the other hand predicted hyperconnectivity in a network involving the OFC and were associated with a less-resilient global network organization (75).

Comparison between BPD and MDD has shown that compared to unmedicated MDD, the functional network connectivity (FNC) of ICA components in BPD is more closely connected and more efficient in topological structures as assessed by graph theory (76). In both BPD and MDD patients, a decreased short-range FCS in the bilateral precuneus has been reported. In addition, the BPD patients showed increased and the MDD patients showed decreased long-range FCS and short-range FCS in the bilateral cerebellum (77). A direct comparison between BPD II and MDD subjects revealed common characteristics in both BPD II and MDD groups (78). Both the MDD and BP II patients showed increased characteristic path length, decreased global efficiency, and disrupted intramodular connectivity within the DMN and limbic system networks compared with the controls. Furthermore, decreased nodal characteristics (nodal strength and nodal efficiency) were found predominantly in brain regions in the DMN, limbic network, and cerebellum of both the MDD and BP II patients, whereas differences between the MDD and BP II patients in the nodal characteristics were observed in the precuneus and temporal pole (78).

7.2.2.5   Functional Connectome in Subjects At-Risk for Bipolar Disorder

The study of at-risk individuals, such as offspring of BD parents (OBP) who have not yet developed BD has the potential to uncover trait-related abnormalities in BD. Moreover, identification of these subjects using an imaging biomarker would have immense significance in early diagnosis and treatment of these individuals. These at-risk subjects have been compared with affected offspring. A review of FC abnormalities in pediatric BD is beyond the scope of this chapter. However, here we discuss findings in at-risk as a study design to identify trait-related abnormalities in BD.

Task-Related Psychophysiological Interaction (PPI) High-Risk Studies: The vlPFC has been studied in various studies and abnormalities reported in unaffected OBPs. Reduced vlPFC modulation of the amygdala to both the positive and negative emotional distracters (90) has been reported. OBP versus offspring of subjects with non-BD psychopathology (OCP) have also been studied and have revealed differences in right posterior insula activity (OCP>OBP) and VS-left posterior insula connectivity (OBP>OCP) on a number-guessing reward task (91). In another study, OBP had greater amygdala to left ACC functional connectivity when regulating attention to fearful faces versus OCP with increases in this measure positively correlating with increases in affective lability over follow-up (92). In a more recent study, OBP had significantly lower right VS-left caudal anterior cingulate FC to loss and greater right pars orbitalis-left and -right orbitofrontal cortex FC to reward versus OCP and OHP, respectively (93) . In another study, OBP observed to have increased negative right amygdala-anterior cingulate cortex functional connectivity to emotional faces versus shapes, and positive right amygdala-left ventrolateral prefrontal cortex functional connectivity to happy faces than OCP and HCs (94). In a study of twins at high and low risk for BD, no group differences in ventrolateral prefrontal cortex seed-based functional connectivity during reappraisal or neural response during mental imagery or emotional reactivity was found (95).

Resting-State Functional Connectivity High-Risk Studies: No group differences were seen in RSFC between IFG and target regions but within OBP, risk score negatively correlated with IFG-lingula cortex RSFC (96). Using ICA analysis as well as reference ROI-based analysis, Singh and colleagues reported increased connectivity in the vlPFC subregion of the left executive control network (ECN). ROI-based analyses revealed that high-risk versus low-risk youth had decreased connectivities between the left vlPFC and left caudate. Other findings were decreased connectivities between the left amygdala and pregenual cingulate, and between the subgenual cingulate and supplementary motor cortex (97). In another study, RSFC between the posterior cingulate (PCC) and clusters in the subcallosal cortex, amygdala, and hippocampus significantly differed among HC, BD-risk, and MDD-risk groups (98). In another study, offspring of patients with SZ (schizophrenia) showed reduced connectivity within the left basal ganglia network compared to control offspring but OBP did not show any differences with HCs (99). In studies of siblings, increased functional connectivity was seen between the NAcc and the ventromedial prefrontal cortex – comprising mainly the subgenual anterior cingulate – in patients

compared with HC subjects. Resilient-non-affected siblings showed FC values midway between the former two groups (100), and in a PET FDG study, FC in the dlPFC (right)–amygdala circuit was statistically abnormal in patients with BD and BD siblings (101). In a study of first-degree relatives of BD subjects, a small network incorporating neighboring insular regions and the anterior cingulate cortex showed weaker functional connectivity in at-risk than HC participants (102).

Graph-Theory Analysis High-Risk Studies: In comparison with offspring of SZ subjects, SZ offspring were found to show connectivity deficits of the brain's central rich club (RC) system relative to both control subjects and BD offspring (103).

7.2.2.6 Treatment Effect on the Functional Connectome in BD

Until recently, there has been a lack of studies of treatment effects and response predictors in relation to the functional connectome in BD. Recent studies have started to shed some light on the effects of treatment. Lithium monotherapy has been shown to increase amygdala-vlPFC connectivity (104), decrease amygdala centrality (105), and more rapidly be able to, compared to quetiapine, normalize abnormally increased VS functional connectivity (50). In one study, bilateral transcranial magnetic stimulation led to significantly decreased DMN strength and significant decrease in SMN connectivity in responders (106).

7.2.2.7 Psychotic Bipolar Disorder

In psychotic BD versus HC, reduced cerebero-cerebellar connectivity(107), no difference in hippocampal connectivity compared with other psychotic disorders (108), and BD with psychosis history exhibiting reduced vACC connectivity while BD without psychosis showing increased vACC connectivity compared to HC(109) has been reported. Though a number of abnormalities have been reported in BD, the diagnostic specificity in being able to differentiate between BD and other similar major psychiatric illnesses such as schizophrenia is not clear. A number of studies have been conducted for comparison with schizophrenia and schizoaffective disorder using the same functional connectome measures as described earlier. A review of the functional connectome in schizophrenia is beyond the scope of this chapter, but it is sufficient to say that many studies have reported many commonalities between schizophrenia and BD, particularly psychotic BD, while some differences have also been seen. In the future, more studies will need to be conducted using another psychiatric disorder as a control group to identify the unique functional connectome abnormality, if any, that may be present in BD.

7.3 Discussion

BD is a major psychiatric illness, and its manifestations of manic and depressive states are quite apparent and sometimes dramatic in their presentation. However, the neurobiological basis of these behavioral changes still needs to be elucidated. As is evident from the review, several investigators have studied trait- and state-related abnormalities of the functional connectome in BD. Some findings have been replicated while others have only been observed in single reports. Cortico-amygdalar and cortico-striatal connectivity findings have been most reported. In terms of amygdala connectivity, several studies indicate decreased connectivity with the dorsal frontal areas but increased connectivity with the ventral limbic areas of the prefrontal cortex. Frontostriatal abnormalities also seem to be present with abnormalities of the motor striatum possibly involved in abnormalities in motor function and ventral striatal connectivity abnormalities in the altered reward function in mania and depression, respectively. Insula connectivity also seems to be altered, and there are several studies that indicate that unipolar and bipolar depression have differences in insula FC. Finally, findings from at-risk individuals also suggest that at-risk individuals have similar changes in FC as those seen in BD subjects but possibly in a milder form.

Despite the progress made in identifying these functional connectome findings in BD, they have yet to reach a level of reliability and validity that they can be used in clinical practice as biomarkers for diagnosis and treatment. There are several reasons for this. First, the findings reported to date have been identified at the group level and not at an individual level. Though some studies have conducted classification analysis using statistical techniques or machine-learning techniques, only moderate levels of classification accuracy has been achieved. Furthermore, very few studies have conducted classification separately on training, and test data sets making their results less robust.

Even for between-group difference studies, the findings are not very strong and have been difficult to replicate. There are several reasons for this including problems with data acquisition from fMRI – the predominant method used for studying the functional connectome. Task-related data, though more constrained by the experimental conditions, suffer from the limitation of not being able to account for baseline state of activity, which determines the level of BOLD change that can be measured with fMRI. Resting-state LFBF data are inherently noisy and are affected by many confounds related to the scan as well as physiological state and motion. As a result between-subject variance is high, which decreases power to identify significant effects. This problem is compounded by the small sample size of ten to twenty subjects in each group usually included in most studies, which makes the results reported highly susceptible to outlier effects. The clinical population of patients is also susceptible to many confounds such as medication, substance abuse, and age and gender effects. These need to be controlled if the imaging findings are attributed to trait- and state-related pathophysiology in BD. Finally, the recommended thresholds for correction of multiple comparisons across all voxels in imaging software using the general linear model (GLM) have low yield for true positive findings. Voxel-wise analysis has not produced replicated corrected results for most studies. The use of machine-learning algorithms has been used to offset this limitation, but it is itself subject to false-positive findings due to overfitting of the data.

As noted earlier, some common findings have been reported across studies, but it is not clear whether that is because these studies have used the same a priori ROI for their hypothesis. For example, amygdala connectivity findings are more frequently reported, but that is an area for which there is an a priori hypothesis leading to restriction of analysis to amygdala connectivity. However, these findings are self-perpetuated because future investigations are also conducted with amygdala as an a priori ROI, further reinforcing the frequency of amygdala connectivity-related findings in the literature. However, an a priori reference or target ROI study design remains popular as it is more likely to yield multiple-comparisons corrected results. Ideally, whole-brain connectivity analysis should be conducted without an a priori ROI in mind. Very few studies have conducted whole-brain studies until present, though ICA and graph-theory techniques have made some progress in this direction.

Last, keeping in mind that the brain works as a connected network, it is more intuitive that connectivity abnormalities are more likely to be present in illnesses such as BD that are associated with abnormalities of higher-level mental function. However, connectivity analysis yields a large amount of quantitative data that is being analyzed with more and more complex mathematical analysis. For example, ICA analysis of resting-state functional data initially started with finding differences between groups on ICA components, but then led to ROI to ROI analysis of different regions of the components and furthermore to correlations of the components themselves. The more complex analysis does not necessarily make it easier to correlate FC findings to behavior and is more likely to yield nonspecific findings. Instead, more straightforward approaches, which involve data dimension reduction, may be more effective.

In conclusion, much more work needs to be done in future studies with larger sample sizes, better study design in terms of populations studied, more accurate data acquisition methods, whole-brain connectivity analysis, and better statistical techniques and machine-learning methods, to elucidate the pathophysiology of BD in terms of functional connectome abnormalities.

References

1. Nurnberger JI. Genetics of bipolar disorder: Where we are and where we are going. *Depression and Anxiety*. 2012; 29(12): 991–993.

2. Lenox RH, Watson DG, Lithium and the brain: a psychopharmacological strategy to a molecular basis for manic depressive illness. [Review] [61 refs]. *Clinical Chemistry*. 1994; 40 (2): 309–314.

3. Anand A, Li Y, Wang Y, Lowe MJ, Dzemidzic M, Resting state corticolimbic connectivity abnormalities in unmedicated bipolar disorder and unipolar depression. *Psychiatry Res*. 2009; 171(3): 189–198.

4. Horwitz, B. The elusive concept of brain connectivity. *Neuroimage*. 2003; 19(2 Pt 1): 466–470.

5. Friston KJ, Harrison L, Penny W, Dynamic causal modelling. *Neuroimage*. 2003; 19(4): 1273–1302.

6. O'Reilly JX, Woolrich MW, Behrens TEJ, Smith SM, Johansen-Berg H, Tools of the trade: Psychophysiological interactions and functional connectivity. *Social Cognitive and Affective Neuroscience*. 2012; 7(5): 604–609.

7. Caseras X, Murphy K, Lawrence NS, et al. Emotion regulation deficits in euthymic bipolar I versus bipolar II disorder: A functional and diffusion-tensor imaging study. *Bipolar Disord*. 2015; 17(5): 461–470.

8. Favre P, Polosan M, Pichat C, Bougerol T, Baciu M, Cerebral correlates of abnormal emotion conflict processing in euthymic bipolar patients: A functional MRI study. *PLoS One*. 2015; 10(8): e0134961.

9. Tseng WL, Thomas LA, Harkins E, et al. Functional connectivity during masked and unmasked face emotion processing in bipolar disorder. *Psychiatry Res Neuroimaging*. 2016; 258: 1–9.

10. Townsend JD, Torrisi SJ, Lieberman MD, et al. Frontal-amygdala connectivity alterations during emotion downregulation in bipolar I disorder. *Biol Psychiatry*. 2013; 73(2): 127–135.

11. Cerullo MA, Fleck DE, Eliassen JC, et al. A longitudinal functional connectivity analysis of the amygdala in bipolar I disorder across mood states. *Bipolar Disord*. 2012; 14(2): 175–184.

12. Versace A, Thompson WK, Zhou D, et al. Abnormal left and right amygdala-orbitofrontal cortical functional connectivity to emotional faces: state versus trait vulnerability markers of depression in bipolar disorder. *Biol Psychiatry*. 2010; 67(5): 422–431.

13. Stegmayer K, Usher J, Trost S, et al. Disturbed cortico-amygdalar functional connectivity as pathophysiological correlate of working memory deficits in bipolar affective disorder. *Eur Arch Psychiatry Clin Neurosci*. 2015; 265 (4): 303–311.

14. Goikolea JMD, Dima D, Landin-Romero R, et al. Multimodal brain changes in first-episode mania: A voxel-based morphometry, functional magnetic resonance imaging, and connectivity study. *Schizophr Bull*. 2019; 45(2): 464–473.

15. Marchand WR, Lee JN, Johnson S, Gale P, J. Thatcher J, Abnormal functional connectivity of the medial cortex in euthymic bipolar II disorder. *Prog Neuropsychopharmacol Biol Psychiatry*. 2014; 51: 28–33.

16. Dutra SJ, Man V, Kober H, Cunningham WA Gruber J Disrupted cortico-limbic connectivity during reward processing in remitted bipolar I disorder. *Bipolar Disord*. 2017; 19(8): 661–675.

17. Schreiter S, Spengler S, Willert A, et al. Neural alterations of fronto-striatal circuitry during reward anticipation in euthymic bipolar disorder. *Psychol Med.* 2016; 46(15): 3187–3198.

18. Redlich R, Dohm K, Grotegerd D, et al. Reward processing in unipolar and bipolar depression: A functional MRI study. *Neuropsychopharmacology.* 2015; 40(11): 2623–2631.

19. Lois G, Gerchen MF, Kirsch P, et al. Large-scale network functional interactions during distraction and reappraisal in remitted bipolar and unipolar patients. *Bipolar Disord.* 2017; 19(6): 487–495.

20. Biswal B, Yetkin FZ, Haughton VM, Hyde JS, Functional connectivity in the motor cortex of resting human brain. *Magnetic Resonance in Medicine.* 1995; 34(4): 537–541.

21. Lowe MJ, Dzemidzic M, Lurito JT, Mathews VP, Phillips MD, Correlations in low-frequency BOLD fluctuations reflect cortico-cortical connections. *Neuroimage.* 2000; 12(5): 582–587.

22. Anand A, Li Y, Wang Y, et al. Activity and connectivity of mood regulating circuit in depression: A functional magnetic resonance study. *Biological Psychiatry.* 2005; 15(10): 1079–1088.

23. Rey G, Piguet C, Benders A, et al. Resting-state functional connectivity of emotion regulation networks in euthymic and non-euthymic bipolar disorder patients. *Eur Psychiatry.* 2016; 34: 56–63.

24. Brady RO Jr, Masters GA, Mathew IT, et al. State dependent cortico-amygdala circuit dysfunction in bipolar disorder. *J Affect Disord.* 2016; 201: 79–87.

25. Anticevic A, Brumbaugh MS, Winkler AM, et al. Global prefrontal and fronto-amygdala dysconnectivity in bipolar I disorder with psychosis history. *Biol Psychiatry.* 2013; 73(6): 565–573.

26. Favre P, Baciu M, Pichat C, Bougerol T, Polosan M, fMRI evidence for abnormal resting-state functional connectivity in euthymic bipolar patients. *J Affect Disord.* 2014; 165: 182–189.

27. Wei S, Geng H, Jiang X, et al. Amygdala-prefrontal cortex resting-state functional connectivity varies with first depressive or manic episode in bipolar disorder. *Neurosci Lett.* 2017; 641: 51–55.

28. Chepenik LG, Raffo M, Hampson M, et al. Functional connectivity between ventral prefrontal cortex and amygdala at low frequency in the resting state in bipolar disorder. *Psychiatry Res.* 2010; 182(3): 207–210.

29. Torrisi S, Moody TD, Vizueta N, et al. Differences in resting corticolimbic functional connectivity in bipolar I euthymia. *Bipolar Disord.* 2013; 15(2): 156–166.

30. Li M, Huang C, Deng W, et al. Contrasting and convergent patterns of amygdala connectivity in mania and depression: A resting-state study. *J Affect Disord.* 2015; 173: 53–58.

31. Singh MK, Kelley RG, Chang KD, Gotlib IH, Intrinsic amygdala functional connectivity in youth with bipolar I disorder. *J Am Acad Child Adolesc Psychiatry.* 2015; 54(9): 763–770.

32. Li G, Liu P, Andari E, Zhang A, Zhang K, The role of amygdala in patients with euthymic bipolar disorder during resting state. *Front Psychiatry.* 2018; 9: 445.

33. Chen L, Wang Y, Niu C, et al. Common and distinct abnormal frontal-limbic system structural and functional patterns in patients with major depression and bipolar disorder. *Neuroimage Clin.* 2018; 20: 42–50.

34. Magioncalda P, Martino M, Conio B, et al. Functional connectivity and neuronal variability of resting state activity in bipolar disorder–reduction and decoupling in anterior cortical midline structures. *Hum Brain Mapp.* 2015; 36(2): 666–682.

35. Gong J, G. Chen G, Y. Jia Y, et al. Disrupted functional connectivity within the default mode network and salience network in unmedicated bipolar II disorder. *Prog Neuropsychopharmacol Biol Psychiatry.* 2019; 88: 11–18.

36. Martino M, Magioncalda P, Huang Z, et al. Contrasting variability patterns in the default mode and sensorimotor networks balance in bipolar depression and mania. *Proc Natl Acad Sci U S A.* 2016; 113(17): 4824–4829.

37. Martino M, Magioncalda P, Saiote C, et al. Abnormal functional-structural cingulum connectivity in mania: Combined functional magnetic resonance imaging-diffusion tensor imaging investigation in different phases of bipolar disorder. *Acta Psychiatr Scand.* 2016; 134 (4): 339–349.

38. He Y, Wang Y, Chang TT, et al. Abnormal intrinsic cerebro-cerebellar functional connectivity in un-medicated patients with bipolar disorder and major depressive disorder. *Psychopharmacology (Berl).* 2018; 235(11): 3187–3200.

39. Minuzzi L, Syan SK, Smith M, et al. Structural and functional changes in the somatosensory cortex in

euthymic females with bipolar disorder. *Aust N Z J Psychiatry.* 2018; 52(11): 1075–1083.

40. Wang Y, Zhong S, Jia Y, et al. Interhemispheric resting state functional connectivity abnormalities in unipolar depression and bipolar depression. *Bipolar Disord.* 2015; 17(5): 486–495.

41. Yasuno F, Kudo T, Matsuoka K, et al. Interhemispheric functional disconnection because of abnormal corpus callosum integrity in bipolar disorder type II. *BJPsych Open.* 2016; 2(6): 335–340.

42. Reinke B, Ven V, Matura S, Linden DE, Oertel-Knochel V, Altered intrinsic functional connectivity in language-related brain regions in association with verbal memory performance in euthymic bipolar patients. *Brain Sci.* 2013; 3(3): 1357–1373.

43. Pang Y, Chen H, Wang Y, et al. Transdiagnostic and diagnosis-specific dynamic functional connectivity anchored in the right anterior insula in major depressive disorder and bipolar depression. *Prog Neuropsychopharmacol Biol Psychiatry.* 2018; 85: 7–15.

44. Ellard KK, Gosai AK, Felicione JM, et al.Deficits in frontoparietal activation and anterior insula functional connectivity during regulation of cognitive-affective interference in bipolar disorder. *Bipolar Disord.* 2019; May; **21**(3): 244–258.

45. Marchand WR, Lee JN, Johnson S, Gale P, Thatcher J, Differences in functional connectivity in major depression versus bipolar II depression. *J Affect Disord.* 2013; 150(2): 527–532.

46. Yin Z, Chang M, Wei S, et al. Decreased functional connectivity in insular subregions in depressive episodes of bipolar disorder and major depressive disorder. *Front Neurosci.* 2018; 12: 842.

47. Liu Y, Wu X, Zhang J, et al. Altered effective connectivity model in the default mode network between bipolar and unipolar depression based on resting-state fMRI. *J Affect Disord.* 2015; 182: 8–17.

48. Fateh AA, Long Z, Duan X, et al. Hippocampal functional connectivity-based discrimination between bipolar and major depressive disorders. *Psychiatry Res Neuroimaging.* 2019; 284: 53–60.

49. Oertel-Knochel V, Reinke B, Matura S, Prvulovic D, Linden DE, van de Ven V, Functional connectivity pattern during rest within the episodic memory network in association with episodic memory performance in bipolar disorder. *Psychiatry Res.* 2015; 231(2): 141–150.

50. Dandash O, Yucel M, Daglas R, et al. Differential effect of quetiapine and lithium on functional connectivity of the striatum in first episode mania. *Transl Psychiatry.* 2018; 8(1): 59.

51. He Z, Sheng W, Lu F, et al. Altered resting-state cerebral blood flow and functional connectivity of striatum in bipolar disorder and major depressive disorder. *Prog Neuropsychopharmacol Biol Psychiatry.* 2019; 90: 177–185.

52. Altinay MI, Hulvershorn LA, Karne H, Beall EB, Anand A, Differential Resting-State Functional Connectivity of Striatal Subregions in Bipolar Depression and Hypomania. *Brain Connect.* 2016; 6(3): 255–265.

53. Ambrosi E, Arciniegas DB, Madan A, et al. Insula and amygdala resting-state functional connectivity differentiate bipolar from unipolar depression. *Acta Psychiatr Scand.* 2017; 136(1): 129–139.

54. Teng S, Lu CF, Wang PS, et al. Altered resting-state functional connectivity of striatal-thalamic circuit in bipolar disorder. *PLoS One.* 2014; 9(5): e96422.

55. Lv D, W. Lin W, Z. Xue Z, et al. Decreased functional connectivity in the language regions in bipolar patients during depressive episodes but not remission. *J Affect Disord.* 2016; 197: 116–124.

56. Luo X, Chen G, Jia Y, et al. Disrupted cerebellar connectivity with the central executive network and the default-mode network in unmedicated bipolar II disorder. *Front Psychiatry.* 2018; 9: 705.

57. Chen G, Zhao L, Jia Y, et al. Abnormal cerebellum-DMN regions connectivity in unmedicated bipolar II disorder. *J Affect Disord.* 2019; 243: 441–447.

58. Wang J, Y. Wang Y, X. Wu X, et al. Shared and specific functional connectivity alterations in unmedicated bipolar and major depressive disorders based on the triple-network model. *Brain Imaging Behav.* 2020; February; **14** (1):186–199.

59. Wang Y, Zhong S, Chen G, et al. Altered cerebellar functional connectivity in remitted bipolar disorder: A resting-state functional magnetic resonance imaging study. *Aust N Z J Psychiatry.* 2018; 52(10): 962–971.

60. Shi J, Geng J, Yan R, et al. Differentiation of transformed bipolar disorder from unipolar depression by resting-state functional connectivity within reward circuit. *Front Psychol.* 2018; 9: 2586.

61. Han S, He Z, Duan X, et al. Dysfunctional connectivity between raphe nucleus and subcortical regions presented opposite differences in bipolar disorder and major depressive disorder. *Prog Neuropsychopharmacol Biol Psychiatry.* 2018; 92: 76–82.

62. Calhoun VD, Adali T, Pearlson GD, Pekar JJ, Spatial and temporal independent component

analysis of functional MRI data containing a pair of task-related waveforms. *Hum Brain Mapp.* 2001; 13(1): 43–53.

63. Beckmann CF, DeLuca M, Devlin JT, Smith SM, Investigations into resting-state connectivity using independent component analysis. *Philos Trans R Soc Lond B Biol Sci.* 2005; 360(1457): 1001–1013.

64. Raichle ME. Modern phrenology: Maps of human cortical function. *Annals of the New York Academy of Sciences.* 1999; 882: 107–118; discussion 128–134.

65. Raichle ME, MacLeod AM, Snyder AZ, et al. A default mode of brain function. *Proc Natl Acad Sci U S A.* 2001; 98(2): 676–682.

66. Ishida T, Donishi T, Iwatani J, et al. Interhemispheric disconnectivity in the sensorimotor network in bipolar disorder revealed by functional connectivity and diffusion tensor imaging analysis. *Heliyon.* 2017; 3(6): e00335.

67. Syan SK, Minuzzi L, Smith M, et al. Resting state functional connectivity in women with bipolar disorder during clinical remission. *Bipolar Disord.* 2017; 19(2): 97–106.

68. Lois G, Linke J, Wessa M, Altered functional connectivity between emotional and cognitive resting state networks in euthymic bipolar I disorder patients. *PLoS One.* 2014; 9(10): e107829.

69. Ford KA, Theberge J, Neufeld RJ, Williamson PC, Osuch EA, Correlation of brain default mode network activation with bipolarity index in youth with mood disorders. *J Affect Disord.* 2013; 150(3): 1174–1178.

70. He H, Sui J, Du Y, et al. Co-altered functional networks and brain structure in unmedicated patients with bipolar and major depressive disorders. *Brain Struct Funct.* 2017; 222(9): 4051–4064.

71. Goya-Maldonado R, Brodmann K, Keil M, et al. Differentiating unipolar and bipolar depression by alterations in large-scale brain networks. *Hum Brain Mapp.* 2016; 37(2): 808–818.

72. Bullmore E, Sporns O, Complex brain networks: Graph theoretical analysis of structural and functional systems. *Nat Rev Neurosci.* 2009; 10(3): 186–198.

73. Doucet GE, Bassett DS, Yao N, Glahn DC, Frangou S, The role of intrinsic brain functional connectivity in vulnerability and resilience to bipolar disorder. *Am J Psychiatry.* 2017; 174(12): 1214–1222.

74. Wang Y, Zhong S, Jia Y, et al. Disrupted resting-state functional connectivity in nonmedicated bipolar disorder. *Radiology.* 2016; 280(2): 529–536.

75. Spielberg JM, Beall EB, Hulvershorn LA, et al. Resting state brain network disturbances related to hypomania and depression in medication-free bipolar disorder. *Neuropsychopharmacology.* 2016; 41(13): 3016–3024.

76. He H, Yu Q, Du Y, et al. Resting-state functional network connectivity in prefrontal regions differs between unmedicated patients with bipolar and major depressive disorders. *J Affect Disord.* 2016; 190: 483–493.

77. Wang Y, Wang J, Jia Y, et al. Shared and specific intrinsic functional connectivity patterns in unmedicated bipolar disorder and major depressive disorder. *Sci Rep.* 2017; 7(1): 3570.

78. Wang Y, Wang J, Jia Y, et al. Topologically convergent and divergent functional connectivity patterns in unmedicated unipolar depression and bipolar disorder. *Transl Psychiatry.* 2017; 7(7): e1165.

79. Wiest G. Neural and mental hierarchies. *Front. Psychol.* 2012 November 26; 3(516).

80. Solms L, Gamwell M. (2006). From Neurology to Psychoanalysis: Sigmund Freud's Neurological Drawings and Diagrams of the Mind, Binghamton University Art Museum.

81. Wang F, Kalmar JH, He Y, et al. Functional and structural connectivity between the perigenual anterior cingulate and amygdala in bipolar disorder. *Biol Psychiatry.* 2009; 66(5): 516–521.

82. Almeida JR, Versace A, Mechelli A, et al. Abnormal amygdala-prefrontal effective connectivity to happy faces differentiates bipolar from major depression. *Biol Psychiatry.* 2009; 66 (5): 451–459.

83. Benson BE, Willis MW, Ketter TA, et al. Differential abnormalities of functional connectivity of the amygdala and hippocampus in unipolar and bipolar affective disorders. *J Affect Disord.* 2014; 168: 243–253.

84. Satterthwaite TD, Kable JW, Vandekar L, et al. Common and dissociable dysfunction of the reward system in bipolar and unipolar depression. *Neuropsychopharmacology.* 2015; 40(9): 2258–2268.

85. Pompei F, Dima D, Rubia K, Kumari V, Frangou S, Dissociable functional connectivity changes during the Stroop task relating to risk, resilience and disease expression in bipolar disorder. *Neuroimage.* 2011; 57(2): 576–582.

86. Nguyen TT, Kovacevic S, Dev SI, et al. Dynamic functional connectivity in bipolar disorder is associated with executive function and processing speed: A preliminary study." *Neuropsychology.* 2017; 31(1): 73–83.

87. Brady RO Jr, Tandon N, Masters GA, et al. Differential brain network activity across mood

states in bipolar disorder. *J Affect Disord.* 2017; 207: 367–376.

88. Ellard KK, J. P. Zimmerman JP, N. Kaur N, et al. Functional connectivity between anterior insula and key nodes of frontoparietal executive control and salience networks distinguish bipolar depression from unipolar depression and healthy control subjects. *Biol Psychiatry Cogn Neurosci Neuroimaging.* 2018; 3(5): 473–484.

89. Yip SW, Mackay CE, Goodwin GM, Increased temporo-insular engagement in unmedicated bipolar II disorder: An exploratory resting state study using independent component analysis. *Bipolar Disord.* 2014; 16 (7): 748–755.

90. Ladouceur CD, Diwadkar VA, White R, et al. Fronto-limbic function in unaffected offspring at familial risk for bipolar disorder during an emotional working memory paradigm. *Dev Cogn Neurosci.* 2013; 5: 185–196.

91. Soehner AM, Bertocci MA, Manelis A, et al. Preliminary investigation of the relationships between sleep duration, reward circuitry function, and mood dysregulation in youth offspring of parents with bipolar disorder. *J Affect Disord.* 2016; 205: 144–153.

92. Acuff HE, Versace A, Bertocci MA, et al. Association of neuroimaging measures of emotion processing and regulation neural circuitries with symptoms of bipolar disorder in offspring at risk for bipolar disorder. *JAMA Psychiatry.* 2018; 75(12): 1241–1251.

93. Acuff HE, Versace A, Bertocci MA, et al. Baseline and follow-up activity and functional connectivity in reward neural circuitries in offspring at risk for bipolar disorder. *Neuropsychopharmacology.* 2019 August; 44(9): 1570–1578.

94. Manelis A, Ladouceur CD, Graur S, et al. Altered amygdala-prefrontal response to facial emotion in offspring of parents with bipolar disorder. *Brain.* 2015; 138(Pt 9): 2777–2790.

95. Meluken I, Ottesen NM, Phan KL, et al. Neural response during emotion regulation in monozygotic twins at high familial risk of affective disorders. *Neuroimage Clin.* 2019; 21: 101598.

96. Hafeman DM, Chase HW, Monk K, et al. Intrinsic functional connectivity correlates of person-level risk for bipolar disorder in offspring of affected parents. *Neuropsychopharmacology.* 2019; 44(3): 629–634.

97. Singh MK, Chang KD, Kelley RG, et al. Early signs of anomalous neural functional connectivity in healthy offspring of parents with bipolar disorder. *Bipolar Disord.* 2014; 16(7): 678–689.

98. Singh MK, Leslie SM, Bhattacharjee K, et al. Vulnerabilities in sequencing and task switching in healthy youth offspring of parents with mood disorders. *J Clin Exp Neuropsychol.* 2018; 40(6): 606–618.

99. Sole-Padulles C, Castro-Fornieles J, de la Serna E, et al. Altered cortico-striatal connectivity in offspring of schizophrenia patients relative to offspring of bipolar patients and controls. *PLoS One.* 2016; 11(2): e0148045.

100. Whittaker JR, Foley SF, Ackling E, Murphy K, Caseras X, The functional connectivity between the nucleus accumbens and the ventromedial prefrontal cortex as an endophenotype for bipolar disorder. *Biol Psychiatry.* 2018; 84(11): 803–809.

101. Li CT, Tu PC, Hsieh JC, et al. Functional dysconnection in the prefrontal-amygdala circuitry in unaffected siblings of patients with bipolar I disorder. *Bipolar Disord.* 2015; 17(6): 626–635.

102. Roberts G, Lord A, Frankland A, et al. Functional dysconnection of the inferior frontal gyrus in young people with bipolar disorder or at genetic high risk. *Biol Psychiatry.* 2017; 81 (8): 718–727.

103. Collin G, Scholtens LH, Kahn RS, Hillegers MHJ, van den Heuvel MP, Affected anatomical rich club and structural-functional coupling in young offspring of schizophrenia and bipolar disorder patients. *Biol Psychiatry.* 2017; 82(10): 746–755.

104. Altinay M, Karne H, Anand A, Lithium monotherapy associated clinical improvement effects on amygdala-ventromedial prefrontal cortex resting state connectivity in bipolar disorder. *J Affect Disord.* 2018; 225: 4–12.

105. Spielberg JM, Matyi MA, Karne H, Anand A, Lithium monotherapy associated longitudinal effects on resting state brain networks in clinical treatment of bipolar disorder. *Bipolar Disord.* 2019; 21(4): 361–371.

106. Kazemi R, Rostami R, Khomami S, et al. Bilateral transcranial magnetic stimulation on dlPFC changes resting state networks and cognitive function in patients with bipolar depression. *Front Hum Neurosci.* 2018; 12: 356.

107. Shinn AK, Roh YS, Ravichandran CT, et al. Aberrant cerebellar connectivity in bipolar disorder with psychosis. *Biol Psychiatry Cogn Neurosci Neuroimaging.* 2017; 2(5): 438–448.

108. Samudra N, Ivleva EI, Hubbard NA, et al. Alterations in hippocampal connectivity across the psychosis dimension. *Psychiatry Res.* 2015; 233(2): 148–157.

109. Anticevic A, Savic A, Repovs G, et al. Ventral anterior cingulate connectivity distinguished nonpsychotic bipolar illness from psychotic bipolar disorder and schizophrenia. *Schizophr Bull.* 2015; 41(1): 133–143.

Chapter 8

Magnetic Resonance Spectroscopy Investigations of Bioenergy and Mitochondrial Function in Mood Disorders

Brent M. Kious and Perry F. Renshaw

Abbreviations

AC:	anticonvulsant/mood stabilizer
ACC:	anterior cingulate cortex
adol:	adolescents
ADP:	adenosine diphosphate
AMG:	amygdala
AP:	antipsychotic
ATP:	adenosine triphosphate
B:	bilateral
BD:	bipolar disorder
BD-D;	bipolar, depressed state
BD-E:	bipolar, euthymic state
BDI:	bipolar disorder type I
BDII:	bipolar disorder type II
BD-HM:	bipolar, hypomanic state
BD-M:	bipolar, manic or mixed state
BG:	basal ganglia
β-NTP:	beta nucleotide triphosphate
BZD:	benzodiazepine
CC:	cingulate cortex
Cho:	choline
CK:	creatine kinase
CN:	caudate nucleus
CorCa:	corpus callosum
Cr:	creatine
DACC:	dorsal anterior cingulate cortex
DCC:	dorsal cingulat cortex
DM/DA-PFC:	Dorsomedial-dorsoanterolateral prefrontal cortex
DLPFC:	dorsolateral prefrontal cortex
ECT:	electroconvulsive therapy
FL:	frontal lobes
GABA:	γ-amino butyric acid
Gln:	glutamine

Glu:	glutamate
Glx:	glutamate + glutamine + GABA
GM:	gray matter
HC:	healthy controls
Hippo:	hippocampus
IED:	intermittent explosive disorder
Ins:	insula
L:	Lac: lactate; left
Li:	lithium
M:	medial
MCC:	middle cingulate cortex
MDE:	major depressive episode
MDD:	major depressive disorder
MDD-D:	major depressive disorder, depressed state
MDD-E;	major depressive disorder, euthymic state
mI:	myoinositol
MN:	medication-naïve;
MPFC:	medial prefrontal cortex
NAA:	n-acetyl aspartate
non-resp:	nonresponder
OCC:	occipital cortex
OFC:	orbitofrontal cortex
OL:	occipital lobe
PBO:	placebo
PCC:	posterior cingulate cortex
PCr:	phosphocreatine
PDE:	phosphodiesters
PF:	prefrontal
PGACC:	pregenual anterior cingulate cortex
Pi:	inorganic phosphate
PME:	phosphomonoesters
POC:	parieto-occipital cortex
PPD:	postpartum depression
PS:	photic stimulation
Put:	putamen

(cont.)

R:	right
resp:	responder
rTMS:	repetitive transcranial magnetic stimulation
SGACC:	subgenual anterior cingulate cortex
SSRI:	selective serotonin reuptake inhibitor
TCA:	tricyclic antidepressant
tCr:	total creatine (phosphocreatine + creatine)
Thal:	thalamus;
TP:	total phosphorus
TL:	temporal lobes
T3:	triiodothyronine
UM:	unmedicated
VLPFC:	ventrolateral prefrontal cortex
VOI:	volume of interest
VPFC:	ventral prefrontal cortex
WB:	whole brain
WM:	white matter
↑:	significantly increased/higher
↓:	significantly reduced/lower
−Δ:	no change/not significantly different.

8.1 Introduction

Major depressive disorder (MDD) and bipolar disorder (BD) are likely to be etiologically diverse, resulting from the contributions of multiple pathophysiologic processes present in affected individuals to varying degrees. In MDD, there is abundant evidence that alterations in serotonin and other monoamines (1) and glutamatergic signaling (2) are implicated in its pathogenesis, and most available treatments target these pathways. Likewise, MDD may result from the effects of inflammatory cytokines (3, 4) or oxidative stress (5) on neuronal activity. One set of processes that may bring together these different etiologies, however, is alterations in brain bioenergetics, which can be studied in vivo using magnetic resonance spectroscopy (MRS).

8.2 Magnetic Resonance Spectroscopy and Brain Bioenergetics

Four major spectroscopic techniques have been used to study MDD and BD: proton magnetic resonance spectroscopy (^{1}H-MRS), phosphorus magnetic resonance spectroscopy (^{31}P-MRS), lithium spectroscopy (^{7}Li-MRS), and fluorine magnetic resonance spectroscopy (^{19}F-MRS). The former two methods allow the measurement of metabolites that are directly and indirectly involved in bioenergetic pathways and will be the focus of this chapter.

As noted elsewhere in this volume (CITE), ^{1}H-MRS produces a spectrum that encompasses seven major peaks (though more can be identified with special approaches): choline (Cho), N-acetylaspartate (NAA), total creatine (tCr), myoinositol (mI), the amino acids (AA), lipids, and lactate (Lac) (6). Cho includes a variety of choline-containing compounds with similar resonances: choline, acetylcholine, phosphocholine, cytidine diphosphocholine, and glycerophosphocholine (7). Cho represents membrane biochemistry, as choline is a product of myelin breakdown it is increased by rapid cellular proliferation, as in brain tumors; Cho can also be raised by increases in myelin synthesis and may reflect cellular density (7). Cho indirectly represents brain bioenergetics because it indicates cell growth and proliferation (8, 9), but will not be considered further in this chapter.

The tCr resonance reflects both phosphocreatine (PCr) and creatine (Cr), which are in rapid near-equilibrium because of the creatine kinase (CK) reaction, through which ATP and Cr combine, producing adenosine diphosphate (ADP) and PCr; PCr functions as short-term storage for high-energy phosphate when ATP is generated in excess of energy demands (10). tCr is therefore directly related to brain energy metabolism, though early ^{1}H-MRS studies of MD typically used tCr as a reference, expressing other metabolites as ratios to tCr, on the assumption that tCr levels vary minimally. In fact, tCr can fluctuate under some circumstances, problematizing its use as a reference (11).

The NAA resonance contains N-acetyl aspartate and a small quantity of N-acetyl-aspartyl-glutamate (NAAG) (12). NAA is a direct indicator of mitochondrial activity because it is synthesized in mitochondria (13) by N-acetyltransferase-8 (14) in a fashion correlated with ATP production, oxygen consumption, and glucose utilization (15–17). NAA may serve as a sink for aspartate produced via the mini-citric-acid cycle, which is an alternative pathway for the production of alpha-ketoglutarate for entry into the Krebs cycle (18, 19). NAA is involved in maintaining osmotic homeostasis in cells (20), and is a substrate for the synthesis of NAAG (21). NAAG is a dipeptide composed of NAA and glutamate (22), and may serve as a neurotransmitter (22).

The mI resonance reflects levels of mI, mI–monophosphate, and glycine; mI is the primary constituent of the peak. mI is located primarily in glia such as astrocytes and to be absent from neurons (23), and may be less relevant to the assessment of bioenergetics than other compounds, so will not be further considered.

The AA peak encompasses glutamate (Glu), glutamine (Gln), and gamma aminobutyric acid (GABA) and is designated as "Glx." Increases in Glx indicate increased cellular destruction or neurotransmission, as Glu is an excitatory neurotransmitter active at the N-methyl-D-aspartate receptor, α-amino-3-hydroxy-5-methyl-4-isoxazolepropionic acid receptor, kainite receptor, and metabotropic glutamate receptor (24, 25). Glu is the most abundant neurotransmitter in the brain (26). It is metabolized to Gln, which is stored in astrocytes; astrocytes pass Gln back to neurons where it is converted to Glu (26) (27). Because Glu is an excitatory neurotransmitter, increases in Glx could indicate increased excitatory neurotransmission and thus increased brain energy consumption; increased neurotransmission is linked to increased Krebs cycle activity and glucose consumption (28, 29). Changes in Glu and related metabolites are, however, explored elsewhere in this volume (CITE) and will not be considered here.

The lipid resonance represents brain levels of acetate and macromolecular proteins and is not directly relevant to the assessment of brain bioenergetics. Finally, the Lac resonance measures cellular energy utilization since Lac is a product of glycolysis, which is used by cells whenever the Krebs cycle and oxidative phosphorylation are not sufficient to support energy demands (30, 31).

^{31}P-MRS offers a more direct method of assessing brain bioenergetics because it can measure high-energy phosphate compounds. There are seven chief resonances in the typical ^{31}P-MRS spectrum: phosphomonoesters (PME), inorganic phosphate (Pi), phosphodiesters (PDE), phosphocreatine (PCr), γ-ATP, α-ATP, and β-ATP. Of these, PCr is the dominant and central peak and its relevance to assessing brain bioenergetics has already been mentioned. The ATP resonances α, β, and γ reflect the distinct resonances of the three phosphate groups in the compound. Up to 25% of each ATP signal represents other nucleotide triphosphates, such as guanosine triphosphate (GTP),

uridine triphosphate (UTP), and cytidine triphosphate (CTP). PME and PDE are indirectly related to metabolism because they reflect rates of lipid synthesis and will not be considered further in this review. ^{31}P-MRS also provides an indirect measure of brain pH, which can be estimated from the difference in chemical shift between Pi and PCr (32, 33).

The interpretation of MRS findings in MDD and BD is complicated by multiple factors. We might anticipate that persons with different mood disorders could exhibit different findings even in the same mood state (e.g., depression), that persons with the same disorder might exhibit different findings in different mood states (e.g., mania or depression), and that developmental and degenerative processes associated with age could affect the relative cellular composition and activity of a given brain region, so that adolescents with depression might differ from young adults, who might differ from elderly adults. Similarly, duration of illness and number of mood episodes – both of which affect the clinical manifestations of BD and MDD – could alter metabolite levels, so that persons early in an illness might exhibit different results than persons late in an illness. Women and men may also exhibit different findings because of the effects of sex hormones both concurrently and developmentally. Likewise, medications such as antidepressants (AD), lithium, anticonvulsant (AC) mood stabilizers, and antipsychotics (AP) – many of which have been shown to alter the metabolites studied with both of the major spectroscopic techniques (34) – could alter findings. Moreover, both BD and MDD are likely to result from malfunctions in particular neural circuits, so that abnormalities could exist in brain regions participating in these circuits but not elsewhere. Similarly, tissue type may affect MRS results, as the metabolic activities of gray matter (GM) and white matter (WM) vary widely and are not necessarily coupled. On the other hand, bioenergetic abnormalities might pervade the brain, so that identification of a metabolic abnormality in a given volume of interest (VOI) in persons with a mood disorder does not necessarily show that this region contributes to the condition.

8.3 Major Depressive Disorder

MRS findings in MDD suggest the presence of multiple bioenergetic abnormalities. ^{1}H-MRS studies (Table 8.1) have focused on multiple VOIs in

Table 8.1 ^{1}H-MRS studies in MDD

Publication	Age group	Comparison	VOI	Treatment status	Findings
Charles et al. (68)	Adults ≥63	7 MDD, 10 HC	WM, Thal, and Put	UM ~1 week then nefazodone × 2–3 months	NAA/tCr −Δ in MDD vs. HC, −Δ in MDD pre- and posttreatment; ↓ NAA/Cho in MDD vs. HC and ↑ NAA/Cho with nefazodone
Auer et al. (35)	Adults	19 MDD,18 HC	B ACC, B PL WM	11 SSRI or TCA, 7 UM, 1 other	↓ Glx in MDD vs. HC in ACC; −Δ NAA, tCr
Ende et al. (36)	Adults	17 MDD-D, 24 HC	B Hippo	Pre-/post-ECT	−Δ NAA with ECT; −Δ Lac with ECT
Renshaw et al. (82)	Adults	MDD-D, HC	L CN, L Put	Fluoxetine	−Δ purines in MDD vs. HC; ↓ purines in female fluoxetine resp
Mirza et al. (76)	7–17	18 MDD, 18 HC	B Thal	MN	−Δ tCr in MDD vs. HC
Grachev et al. (65)	Adults	10 MDD + chronic back pain, 10 HC	B DLPFC, B OFC, CC, Thal	Various	↓ NAA in R DLPFC in MDD vs. HC; depression correlated with NAA in R DLPFC.
Michael et al. (74)	Adults	28 MDD-D, 28 HC	L Amg	Pre-/post-ECT. ECT + AD in ECT non-resp	↑ NAA concentrations with ECT or ECT + AD; ↑ Glx in ECT resp; −Δ tCr
Pfleiderer et al. (39)	Adults	17 MDD-D, 17 HC	ACC	Pre-/post-ECT	−Δ tCr, NAA.
Vythilingam et al. (52)	Adults	18 MDD, 20 HC	B CN, B Put	12 SSRI, 1 TCA, 1 nefazodone	↓ NAA/tCr in MDD vs. HC in CN
Gruber et al. (53)	Adults	17 MDD, 17 HC	L PF WM	UM ≥4 weeks	↓ NAA/tCr n MDD vs. HC; ↑ tCr in MDD vs. HC
Gabbay et al. (41)	12–19	14 MDD, 10 HC	B CN, B Put, B Thal	4 MN, 2 UM > 1 year, 8 various	↑ tCr in L CN in MDD vs. HC
Chen et al. (137)	Adults	27 MDD, 19 HC	L F WM, L periventricular WM, L BG	18 UM, 9 AD	↓ NAA/tCr in L F WM
Kaymak et al. (70)	Adults	17 women with first MDE, 13 HC	L DLPFC	UM then AD × 8 weeks	−Δ NAA/tCr, ml/tCr in MDD vs. HC; ↑ ml/tCr with AD

Table 8.1 (cont.)

Publication	Age group	Comparison	VOI	Treatment status	Findings
Nery et al. (77)	Adults	37 MDD, 40 HC	L DLPFC	UM	−Δ between MDD and HC; ↓ tCr in male MDD vs. HC; ↑ tCr in female MDD vs. HC; ↓ NAA in those with longer illness.
Rosa et al. (47)	Adults	36 PPD, 25 HC	B ACC, L DLPFC	UM	↓ NAA in PPD vs. HC; −Δ other metabolites; −Δ in ACC
Huang et al. (69)	Adults	30 poststroke MDD, 20 HC	B Hippo, B Thal	UM, then paroxetine × 6 months	↓ NAA/tCr in MDD vs. HC in Hippo + Thal; ↑ NAA/tCr in L Hippo and B Thal with paroxetine
Portella et al. (61)	Adults	10 first MDE, 16 remitted-recurrent-MDD, 19 chronic-MDD, 15 HC	B VMPFC	AD	↓ NAA in chronic MDD vs. HC vs. first-episode MDD; -Δ tCr
Wang et al. (138)	Adults	24 first MDE, 13 HC	L DLPFC, ACC	MN	↓ NAA/tCr in B DLPFC WM in MDD vs. HC; ↓ Cho/tCr in L DLPFC WM in MDD vs. HC; −Δ in ACC
Wang et al. (67)	Adults	26 first MDE, 13 HC	B Hippo	MN, then duloxetine × 12 weeks	−Δ in MDD vs. HC at baseline; ↑ NAA/tCr in R Hippo with duloxetine
De Diego-Adelino et al. (62)	Adults	52 MDD (20 treatment-resistant, 18 remitted, 14 first-episode), 16 HC	B Hippo	Various	↓ NAA in chronic MDD vs. HC in R Hippo
Tae et al. (63)	Adults	21 women MDD, 26 HC	PGACC	21 UM × 3 months, 11 MN, 21 AD at follow-up	−Δ MDD vs. HC at baseline; ↓ NAA/tCr in MDD vs. HC at follow-up; baseline NAA/tCr inversely correlated with illness duration.
Zhong et al. (98)	Adults	26 MDD, 20 BD-D, 13 HC	PF WM, ACC, Hippo	MN	↓ NAA/tCr in B PF WM in MDD vs. HC; −Δ NAA/Cr in ACC + Hippo

Table 8.1 (cont.)

Publication	Age group	Comparison	VOI	Treatment status	Findings
Jia et al. (139)	Adults	26 first MDE, 13 HC	PF WM, ACC, Hippo	MN	↓ NAA/tCr in MDD vs. HC in L PF WM and R PF WM; -Δ in ACC or Hippo
Zheng et al. (75)	Adults	32 MDD, 28 HC	B ACC	Escitalopram × 2 weeks, then rTMS (18) or sham (14)	↓ NAA in L ACC; NAA normalized in L ACC in rTMS resp
Li et al. (59)	Adults	16 MDD, 10 HC	Ins, ACC, CN, Put, Thal	UM, then 8 weeks cognitive therapy	↓ NAA/tCr in L ACC in MDD vs. HC; ↑ NAA/tCR in L ACC in CBT resp
Li et al. (48)	Adults	20 MDD, 14 BD-D, 20 HC	MPFC, ACC, PCC, PC	UM ≥ 2 weeks	↓ tCr + ↓ NAA in PCC in MDD vs. HC; ↓ Glx in MPFC in MDD vs. HC
Yoon et al. (49)	Adults	34 women MDD, 39 HC	MPFC	Escitalopram at baseline, then Cr or PBO × 8 weeks	↓ NAA in MDD vs. HC; ↓ NAA correlated with ↑ depression; ↑ NAA + ↑ tCr with Cr; −Δ tCr in MDD vs. HC
Cano et al. (73)	Adults	12 MDD, 10 HC	B Hippo	12 AD, 8 AP, 2 Li, 6 BZD, then ECT	−Δ in MDD vs. HC; ↓ NAA/tCr with ECT
Henigsberg et al. (64)	Adults	48 MDD	L DLPFC	AD ≤ 10 years	↓ NAA/tCr in recovery in recurrent depression
Lefebvre et al. (50)	14–22	18 MDD, 15 HC	B Hippo	15 AD, 1 BZD, 1 AC, 2 AP, 1 stimulant	↓ NAA in L Hippo in in MDD vs. HC; NAA inversely correlated with Hippo volume
Njau et al. (51)	Adults	43 MDD, 33 HC	B Hippo, SGACC, D ACC	UM, then ECT	↓ NAA in L Hippo in MDD vs. HC; ↑ tCr + ↓ NAA in dACC, ↑ tCr in sgACC; ↓ NAA in R Hippo with ECT

Please refer to the Abbreviation list on page 83 for more information if needed.

both adults and adolescents. Some studies have not revealed alterations in NAA in MDD (35–46), but many others indicate that NAA measurements are decreased, including in the right dorsolateral prefrontal cortex (DLPFC) (47), posterior cingulate cortex (PCC) (48), medial prefrontal cortex (MPFC) (49), and left Hippo (50, 51). NAA/tCr ratios have been found to be reduced in the basal ganglia (BG) (52), left prefrontal WM (53, 54), bilateral prefrontal WM (55, 56), bilateral Hippo and Thal (57), left DLPFC WM (58), and left ACC (59).

[NAA] or NAA/tCr ratios in the left DLPFC (60), bilateral VMPFC (61), right Hippo (62) and pregenual ACC (63) have been shown to be negatively associated with duration of illness and with illness recurrence (64). Similarly, lower [NAA] in the right DLPFC (65) and MPFC (49) are inversely correlated with MDD severity. The effect of treatment on NAA measurements appears mixed. In one study (66), there were no differences between controls and MDD subjects who were medication-free for at least three months, though the NAA/tCr ratio in the pregenual ACC fell in MDD subjects after they had been taking AD; the authors hypothesized that this was an effect of illness duration, with which NAA/tCr was correlated. In contrast, another study (67) found that there were no differences in NAA/tCr ratios in the bilateral Hippo between treatment-naive depressed subjects and controls, though these ratios increased significantly in the right Hippo after twelve weeks of treatment with duloxetine. Another, early study (68) found that depressed subjects had lower NAA/Cho ratios at baseline compared to HC, and that these levels increased after two to three months of treatment with the AD nefazodone. Similarly, NAA/tCr ratios were lower in the bilateral Hippo and bilateral Thal of depressed subjects compared to controls at baseline, and increased after six months of treatment with the AD paroxetine (69). In contrast, left DLPFC NAA/tCr ratios did not differ between unmedicated MDD subjects and controls, and did not change appreciably after eight weeks of AD treatment (70). Most recently, subjects treated with adjunctive creatine plus escitalopram exhibited increased [NAA] in the MPFC after eight weeks compared to those received placebo plus escitalopram (49).

Neurostimulation techniques such as electroconvulsive therapy (ECT) and repetitive transcranial magnetic stimulation (rTMS) are often effective treatments for depression (71, 72), and appear to affect brain NAA measurements. Two studies (36, 39) found that ECT had no effect on Hippo [NAA], though another showed that NAA/tCr in the bilateral Hippo fell after ECT, with this change correlation with Hippo volume increases (73). Similarly, dorsal ACC and right Hippo [NAA] fell among subjects treated with ECT (51). In contrast, however, [NAA] in the left Amg increased with response to ECT + AD (74).

Similarly, left ACC [NAA] was reduced in MDD subjects taking escitalopram for at least two weeks, though these levels normalized in rTMS responders (75). Psychotherapeutic interventions may affect NAA, as eight weeks of mindfulness-based cognitive therapy was associated with increases in left ACC NAA/tCr ratios (59).

Measures of tCr are less extensively reported in ^{1}H-MRS studies of MDD, and results are mixed. Multiple studies have reported no difference in [tCr] in several brain regions (35, 37–39, 44, 47, 61, 76). Still, [tCr] in inferior prefrontal WM was increased in MDD subjects compared to controls (53), and a similar finding was demonstrated in the left caudate nucleus (CN), though no differences were found in the ipsilateral Put or Thal (41). Studies have also shown reduced [tCr] in MDD in the L DLPFC (77), PCC (48), and Hippo (51). The last of those studies indicated that treatment with ECT was associated with increases in dorsal ACC and subgenual ACC [tCr]. Likewise, oral creatine supplementation in subjects with MDD significantly increases [tCr] (49).

^{31}P-MRS studies in MDD (Table 8.2) provide an additional stream of information about bioenergetically relevant metabolites in MDD. Although some studies have been negative (78, 79), in general there is evidence that MDD is associated with reduced β-NTP. Moore et al. (80) first demonstrated that BG [β-NTP] was reduced in MDD. Later, it was shown that FC (frontal cortex) [β-NTP] was reduced in MDD (81). Renshaw et al. (82) found that although BG [β-NTP] and total purine levels did not differ between MDD and controls, [β-NTP] was 21% lower in fluoxetine responders than nonresponders. In female adolescents with MDD, baseline depression severity is negatively correlated with [β-NTP] (83).

PCr levels have most often been reported to be unchanged in persons with depression, but there are consistent reports that such levels increase with AD treatment. In several studies, [PCr] did not differ in the FC of depressed subjects and controls (81, 84). Still, treatment with acetyl-L-carnitine for twelve weeks was associated with an AD response and [PCr] in the PFC increased in tandem with improvements in depression severity (85). Likewise, Kondo et al. (83) found that adolescent females treated with fluoxetine and adjunctive creatine exhibited increases in [PCr].

A significant barrier to interpreting MRS studies of bioenergetic markers (as well as other

Table 8.2 ^{31}P-MRS studies in MDD

Publication	Age group	Comparison	VOI	Treatment status	Findings
Kato et al. (79)	Adults	12 MDD (MDD-D + MDD-E), 10 BD (BD-D + BD-E), 12 HC	30 mm frontal axial slice	8 TCA, 1 Li	−Δ MDD-D vs. MDD-E; −Δ MDD-D/MDD-E vs. HC
Moore et al. (140)	Adults	35 MDD-D, 18 HC	B BG	UM	↓ β-NTP in MDD vs. HC
Volz et al. (81)	Adults	14 MDD, 8 HC	B FC	UM ≥ 7 days	↓ total ATP + ↓ B-ATP in MDD vs. HC; −Δ PCr or pH
Renshaw et al. (82)	Adults	38 MDD, 22 HC	B BG	MN, then fluoxetine	−Δ purines in MDD vs. HC. ↓ purines in female fluoxetine resp vs. non-resp; ↓ β-NTP in fluoxetine resp vs. non-resp
Pettegrew et al. (85)	Adults >65	2 MDD, 6 HC	PFC	Acetyl-l-carnitine × 12 weeks	↑ PCr in MDD with carnitine correlated with improvement in depression
Iosifescu et al. (84)	Adults	19 MDD, 9 HC	20 mm-thick axial slice	SSRI at baseline, then T3	−Δβ-NTP, tNTP, PCr, pH; ↑ PCr at baseline predicted resp to T3; ↑ tNTP + ↓ PCr in T3 resp correlated with improvement in depression
Forester et al. (86)	Age ≥55	13 MDD, 10 HC	WB GM, WB WM	UM then sertraline × 12 weeks	↓ β-NTP and tNTP in MDD vs. HC; ↓ tNTP with sertraline; ↓ tNTP in WM pre-treatment; ↑ pH in GM pre-treatment, normalized with treatment
Kondo et al. (83)	13–18	5 girls with MDD, 10 female HC	25 mm central axial slice	Fluoxetine + creatine	Baseline depression correlated with pH and negatively correlated with β-NTP; ↑ PCr with creatine
Harper et al. (141)	56–82	10 MDD, 8 HC	WB GM, WB WM	UM ≥1 week	↑ β-NTP in WM correlated with ↑ Stroop; ↑ PCr in GM correlated with ↑ Stroop

Table 8.2 (cont.)

Publication	Age group	Comparison	VOI	Treatment status	Findings
Harper et al. (88)	Adults	50 MDD, 30 HC	WB GM, WB WM	UM	↑ PCr + ↓ Pi in GM + ↓ PCr in WM in MDD vs. HC; depression negatively correlated with Pi in WM but positively correlated with PCr in GM

Please refer to the Abbreviation list on page 83 for more information if needed.

metabolites) is differences in GM and WM composition of VOIs. Forester et al. (86) examined thirteen patients with MDD and ten controls and looked at whole-brain metabolites segmented into GM and WM. They found that total tissue (GM+WM) [β-NTP] and the concentration of total NTP ([tNTP]) were lower in depressed subjects and that [tNTP] decreased after twelve weeks of treatment with sertraline. When the authors looked at the two different tissue types, they found that [tNTP] was reduced in WM but not in GM before treatment. In a study of ten older subjects with MDD, with the whole brain segmented into GM and WM, increased WM [β-NTP] was positively associated with the Stroop score, a measure of executive function, while increased GM [PCr] showed the same association (87). The same group later looked at GM versus WM metabolites in a larger study encompassing fifty subjects with MDD. They found that [PCr] was significantly elevated in GM but reduced in WM, and that depression ratings were correlated with GM [PCr], though not with WM [PCr] (88). One way of interpreting these seemingly inconsistent data, which suggest both that AD response is associated with increasing [PCr] and that higher [PCr] and [tCr] are associated with depression, is that increased GM [PCr] is associated with depression but is also a marker of AD response-readiness, such that persons with depression are less able to respond to ADs if they have lower [PCr]. Indeed, this was the interpretation offered by Iosifescu et al. (84), who found that subjects with MDD who responded to triiodothyronine (T3)

supplementation exhibited increased [tNTP] but reduced [PCr], while elevated baseline [PCr] predicted response to T3.

There is little data regarding alterations in pH in MDD. In one study, pH was increased in whole-brain GM in unmedicated subjects with MDD, and normalized with treatment with sertraline (86); in another study, pH was increased in MDD in female adolescents in a fashion correlated with depression severity (83). Volz et al. (81) found, however, that pH did not differ significantly between subjects with depression and controls. Reports of alterations in Pi are also limited; in their study of GM versus WM segmentation, Harper et al. (88) found that Pi levels were reduced in the GM of depressed subjects but showed a trend toward being increased in the WM of depressed subjects, correlated with depression severity.

8.4 Bipolar Disorder

Spectroscopic investigations of BD are perhaps more extensive than those of MDD, to date, but interpretation of these studies is rendered more difficult than in MDD because of greater differences in medication exposure as well as the larger number of mood states investigated, including mania (BD-M), hypomania (BD-HM), euthymia (BD-E), depression (BD-D), and mixed (BD-Mx). In general, however, spectroscopic findings are similar across mood states, with exceptions noted later.

^{1}H-MRS studies in BD (Table 8.3) evince significant perturbations in multiple bioenergetic markers. Most studies in BD have suggested that [NAA] and NAA/tCr are reduced in brain regions implicated in BD, including in the DLPFC

Table 8.3 ^{1}HMRS studies in BD

Publication	Age group	Comparison	VOI	Treatment status	Findings
Sharma et al. (100)	Adults	4 BD-M, 1 MDD with psychosis, 9 HC	B BG, OCC	Li	$-\Delta$ in OCC in BD vs. HC; ↑ NAA/tCr in BG in BD vs. HC
Ohara et al. (102)	Adults	10 BD, 10 HC	B BG	7 Li	$-\Delta$ NAA/tCr + NAA/Cho in BD vs. HC
Hamakawa et al. (142)	Adults	23 BD-E, 8 BD-D, 20 HC	B FL	13 Li, 7 AD, 3 UM	↓ tCr in L FL in BD-D vs. BD-E; ↑ tCr in R FL in male BD vs. female BD
Moore et al. (143)	Adults	9 BD, 14 HC	B ACC	5 Li, 4 AC, 3 SSRI, 2 TCA, 4 UM	↑ tCr in R ACC in subjects with AD vs. without AD
Winsberg et al. (92)	Adults	10 BDI, 10 BDII (euthymic), 20 HC	B DLPFC	UM ≥2 weeks	↓ NAA/tCr in BDI vs. HC in B DLPFC; ↓ NAA/tCr in BDII vs. HC in R DLPFC
Davanzo et al. (104)	Average 11±3	9 BD-M, 2 BD-HM, 11 HC	ACC	5 AP, 4 stimulant, 1 AC, 2 UM, then all Li	$-\Delta$ NAA/tCr in BD vs. HC at baseline
Deicken et al. (101)	Adults	15 BD-E, 15 HC	B Thal	Various	↑ NAA in BD vs. HC; ↑ NAA in L Thal vs. R Thal in BD; ↑ tCr in BD vs. HC
Cecil et al. (93)	16–35	17 BD-M, 21 HC	MFC GM	Various	↓ NAA in BD-M vs. HC
Bertolino et al. (95)	Adults	7 BD-D, 6 BD-E, 3 BD-HM, 1 BD-M, 17 HC	B Hippo, DLPFC, superior temporal gyrus, inferior frontal gyrus, OC, ACC, PCC, centrum semiovale, PF WM, Thal, Put	6 UM, 6 Li, 1 AP	↓ NAA/tCr in Hippo in BD vs. HC; $-\Delta$ NAA/Cho
Cecil et al. (112)	8–12	7 BD, 2 MDD, 10 HC	FC, F WM, cerebellar vermis	8 UM, 1 AD + AP	↓ NAA + tCr in BD vs. HC in cerebellar vermis
Deicken et al. (96)	Adults	15 BD-E, 20 HC	B Hippo	7 AC, 4 Li, 3 AP, 4 AD, 1 UM	↓ tCr + NAA in BD-E
Dager et al. (114)	Adults	32 BD, 26 HC	M F WM, ACC, Put, CN, Ins, Thal, parietal WM, OCC	UM	$-\Delta$ tCr in GM or WM in BD vs. HC; tCr inversely correlated with depression severity
Brambilla et al. (107)	Adults	10 BD, 32 HC	L DLPFC	6 Li, 4 UM	$-\Delta$ NAA + tCr; ↑ NAA/tCr with Li

Table 8.3 (cont.)

Publication	Age group	Comparison	VOI	Treatment status	Findings
					vs. UM BD vs. HC
DelBello et al. (108)	Adol	20 BD-M, 10 HC	B VPFC	UM, then olanzapine	−Δ NAA in BD overall; ↑ VPFC NAA in olanzapine remitters vs. non-remitters
Sassi et al. (89)	Adol	14 BD, 18 HC	L DLPFC	8 Li, 4 AC, 2 UM	↓ NAA in BD vs. HC
Frye et al. (115)	Adults	23 BD-D, 12 HC	ACC, MCC, MPFC	5 Li at baseline, 18 UM, then lamotrigine × 12 weeks	↑ tCr in BD vs. HC at baseline; tCr normalized w lamotrigine
Kim et al. (131)	Adults	42 BD with rapid cycling	M F GM	UM × 3 days, then quetiapine × 12 weeks	↓ Lac during follow-up, esp. in quetiapine resp; change in Lac correlated with change in mania rating
Olvera et al. (91)	Average 13	23 BDI, 12 BDII, 36 HC	L DLPFC	10 MN, 20 AC, 4 other	↓ NAA in BD vs. HC. −Δ tCr in BD vs. HC; −Δ BDI vs. BDII; NAA inversely correlated with mania severity
Forester et al. (110)	56–85	9 BD	ACC	Li + various	Li levels positively correlated with NAA
Patel et al. (144)	Adol	28 BD-D, 10 HC	ACC, B VLPFC	UM	↑ NAA in BD-D in ACC + B VLPFC; ↑ tCr in B VLPFC
Port et al. (97)	Adults	21 BD, 21 HC	CN, lentiform nucleus, Thal, ACC, DLPFC WM, PC WM, OCC	UM	↓ NAA in B CN + left lentiform nucleus; ↓ tCr in R CN in BD
Ongur et al. (113)	Adults	15 BD-M, 22 HC,	ACC, POC	9 Li, 10 AC, 15 AP, 7 BZD	−Δ tCr BD-M vs. HC
Caetano et al. (90)	Average 13.2 ±2.9	43 BD, 38 HC	MPFC, DLPFC, ACC, PCC, OCC	Various	↓ NAA in MPFC in BD vs. HC. ↓ tCr R MPFC in BD vs. HC. ↓ NAA + ↓ tCr L DLPFC WM in BD vs. HC
Brady et al. (145)	Adults	15 BD-M, 6 HC	ACC, POC	Various	↓ Lac/tCr in BD-E vs. HC; −Δ Lac/tCr BD-M vs. HC; NAA/tCr −Δ
Ozdel et al. (94)	Adults	15 BD-E, 15 HC	B MPFC	6 AC + AP, 5 Li + AP, 2 Li, 1 AC + Li, 1 AC	↓ NAA + tCr in BD vs. HC; -Δ NAA/tCr
Xu et al. (133)	Adults		ACC, PCC, Thal	UM	

Table 8.3 (cont.)

Publication	Age group	Comparison	VOI	Treatment status	Findings
		12 BD-M/BD-HM, 12 BD-D, 20 HC			↑ Lac/tCr in Thal in BD-D vs. HC
Zhong et al et al. (98)	Adults	26 MDD, 20 BD-D, 13 HC	PF WM, ACC, Hippo	MN	↓ L PF WM NAA/Cr in BD vs. HC
Croarkin et al. (99)	Adults	15 BD-D, 9 HC	ACC	UM, then lamotrigine × 12 weeks	↓ NAA BD vs. HC. NAA normalized with lamotrigine. ↓ NAA/Glx in BD vs. HC
Li et al. (48)	Adults	20 MDD, 14 BD-D, 20 HC	mPFC, ACC, PCC, PC	UM ≥2 weeks	↓ tCr + NAA in PCC
Soeiro-de-Souza et al. (134)	Adults	50 BD-E, 38 HC	DACC	23 AC, 29 Li, 23 AP	↑ Lac BD vs. HC
Machado-Vieira et al. (135)	Adults	20 BD-D, 16 HC	DCC	UM ≥6 weeks, then Li × 6 weeks	↑ Lac BD pre-Li, ↓ with Li, correlated with serum lithium levels

Please refer to the Abbreviation list on page 83 for more information if needed.

(89–92), MPFC (90, 93, 94), Hippo (95, 96), BG (97), PF WM (98), ACC (99), and PCC (48). Even so, some studies have found increased NAA in BD, including in the BG (100), ACC and VLPFC (17), and Thal (101). A few studies have also not demonstrated differences in [NAA] or NAA/tCr, including in the BG (102), frontal lobes (FL) (103), ACC (104–106), and left DLPFC (107–109). Given the number of factors that distinguish these studies, it is difficult to determine whether these differences might be explained by differences in mood state, medication exposure, or other variables, though it should be noted that reduced [NAA] or NAA/tCr has been seen in several brain regions in BD-D, BD-E, and BD-M, as well as in medicated and unmedicated subjects. Still, brain lithium levels have been positively correlated with brain [NAA], suggesting that lithium exposure may be an important confound (110).

BD has also been associated with changes in tCr. Overall, studies appear to suggest that [tCr] is reduced in several brain regions in BD, including in the FL (111), cerebellar vermis (112), Hippo (96), CN (97), MPFC (90, 94), DLPFC WM (90), and PCC (48). Several studies have failed to find

alterations in [tCr] in BD, including in the L DLPFC (91, 107, 109) and ACC (105, 113). Dager et al. (114) found that there were no significant differences in [tCr] between unmedicated BD subjects and controls in a variety of GM and WM regions including the MFC, ACC, Put, CN, Ins, Thal, parietal cortex, and OCC. They did, however, show that depression severity in BD was inversely correlated with [tCr]. A few studies have suggested that [tCr] is increased in BD, including in the Thal (114), ACC and MPFC (115), and VLPFC (17). These discrepant findings are not clearly explained by differences in treatment status, mood state, or other factors, suggesting that more research is needed.

PCr constitutes the majority of the tCr signal, so alterations in [tCr] in BD would be expected to coincide with alterations in [PCr]. To date, however, few ^{31}P-MRS studies (Table 8.4) indicate that this is true. In BD-E subjects, Kato et al. (79) found that, in a central 30 mm axial slice, [PCr] trended toward being reduced. In a later study, the same group demonstrated lower [PCr] in subjects with BDII compared to controls, though no difference in [PCr] in subjects with BDI compared to

Table 8.4 3^1P-MRS studies in BD

Publication	Age group	Comparison	VOI	Treatment status	Findings
Kato et al. (79)	Adults	12 MDD (MDD-D + MDD-E), 10 BD (BD-D + BD-E), 12 HC	30 mm frontal axial slice	11 BD-D Li, 3 BD-D Li	↑ pH BD-E vs. BD-D
Kato et al. (127)	Adults	17 BD (BD-M + BD-E)	30 mm frontal axial slice	Li +/- AP	pH ↑ BD-M vs. BD-E; ph ↓ BD-E vs. HC; −Δ pH BD-M vs. HC.
Kato et al. (128)	Adults	31 BDI, 9 BDII, 60 HC	30 mm frontal axial slice	Li	↓ pH BD vs. HC
Kato et al. (116)	Adults	15 BDII, 14 BDI, 29 HC	30 mm frontal axial slice	Various	↓ pH in BDI vs. HC; −Δ PCr in BDI vs. HC; ↓ PCr in BDII vs. HC; −Δ PCr in BDII depressed vs. euthymic
Deicken et al. (146)	Adults	12 BD-E, 14 HC	B TL	UM	PME ↓ BDE vs. HC; otherwise −Δ
Murashita et al. (123)	Adults	19 BD, 25 HC	OCC	Li, then PS	−Δ PCr with PS in Li resp; in Li non-resp; ↓ PCr with PS
Hamakawa et al. (129)	Adults	13 BD-E, 10 HC	B BG	8 Li, 6 AC, 2 AD, 10 AP	pH ↓ BD-E vs. HC; otherwise −Δ
Jensen et al. (122)	Adults	11 BD-D, 9 HC	30 mm axial slice	Various, then triacetyluridine × 6 weeks	−Δ BD vs. HC; ↑ pH triacetyluridine resp vs. non-resp
Brennan et al. (119)	Adults	20 BD-D	WB	Various, then acetyl-L-carnitine or PBO	−Δ pH or other metabolite related to time or treatment arm
Sikoglu et al. (126)	11–20	8 BD, 8 HC	FL	6 Li	pH −Δ BD vs. HC; ↑ pH with age in BD; ↓ Pi in BD vs. HC; −Δ PCr
Weber et al. (117)	11–21	19 BD-M, 14 BD-E, 20 HC	B ACC, L VLPFC	UM ≥2 weeks	↓ pH + ADP in ACC in BD-M vs. HC; ↓ ADP in L VLPFC in BD-E vs. H; ↓ PCr in L VLPFC in BD-E vs. HC.
Shi et al. (124)	Adults	14 BD-E, 11 BD-D, 23 HC	FL, CorCa, Thal, OL	5 UM, 4 Li, 11 AD, 2 AP, 8 AC	Rate constant for CK reaction −Δ; β-NTP/TP correlated with rate constant for CK reaction.
Yuksel et al. (125)	Adults	21 BD-E, 2 BD-D, 22 HC	OCC	Various, then PS	−Δ PCr, ATP, or pH; ↓ ATP in BD with PS but not HC; ↓ PCr in HC

Table 8.4 (cont.)

Publication	Age group	Comparison	VOI	Treatment status	Findings
					but not BD with PS
Dudley et al. (118)	12–21	16 BD-M, 8 BD-E, 19 HC	WB GM vs. WM	UM	↓ PCr in WB and right hemisphere GM in BD; ↓ ATP in WB and right hemisphere WM in BD
Du et al. (121)	Adults	20 BD + psychosis, 28 HC	FL	Various	PCr/ATP −Δ BD vs. HC; rate constant for CK reaction ↓ 13% in BD vs. HC

Please refer to the Abbreviation list on page 83 for more information if needed.

controls (116). They also found that L VLPFC [PCr] was significantly reduced in BD-E subjects compared to controls (117). Dudley et al.(118) also showed that [PCr] was reduced in the whole brain as well as right hemisphere GM in BD irrespective of mood state. Multiple other studies, however, indicate that there are no significant differences between BD subjects' [PCr] and those of healthy controls (119–126). Interpretation of these studies tends, however, to be limited by the fact that they included subjects in different mood states. Several intriguing studies have demonstrated dynamic abnormalities in PCr synthesis in BD. Murashita et al. (123) found that in nineteen subjects with BD, all of whom were treated with lithium, [PCr] fell after photic stimulation (a method of increasing metabolic activity in the visual cortex) in subjects who did not respond to lithium, but remained stable in lithium-responsive subjects and controls. This suggested that subjects with BD have a deficit in PCr production after metabolic stress that is improved by lithium. In a similar study, however, Yuksel et al. (125) compared twenty-three subjects with BD taking various medications to matched controls; they found that [PCr] fell in response to photic stimulation in controls, but not in BD subjects, though PCr/ATP ratios were reduced in BD, and [ATP] fell in BD in response to photic stimulation. Both studies, therefore, suggest some inefficiency in the creatine kinase reaction in BD. Shi et al. (124) used magnetization transfer to estimate the rate constant for the creatine kinase reaction in

BD, however, and found that it did not differ significantly between BD-E, BD-D, and controls. In contrast to this, however, Du et al. (121) studied twenty subjects with a first episode of BD-D or BD-M with psychotic features; they found that although PCr/ATP did not significantly differ between BD subjects and controls, there was a 13% reduction in the rate constant for the creatine kinase reaction. The difference between these two studies may be due to the absence of psychosis among the subjects studied by Shi et al., or to the difference in mood states, as many of the subjects studied by Du and colleagues were manic (as well as psychotic).

Few studies, apart from those examining reaction kinetics mentioned earlier, have reported abnormalities of ATP in BD, though Dudley et al. (118) found that [ATP] was reduced in the whole-brain and right-hemisphere WM in BD-M and BD-E. Similarly, results from studies reporting pH in BD have been mixed. Kato et al. (79) found that pH was elevated in depressed subjects with BD compared to euthymic subjects, while a later study by the same group found that pH was elevated in BD-M compared to BD-E and lower in BD-E than in healthy controls (127). Subsequently, Kato and colleagues found that pH was reduced in BD subjects in a variety of mood states compared to controls (128), and that pH was lower in BD-E than in controls (116). A later study also suggested that pH is reduced in BD-E in the BG (129). Weber et al. (117) identified lower pH in the ACC in BD-M compared to controls, though no such difference in the L VLPFC. In a study of eleven patients with BD treated with various baseline medications, subjects who responded to augmentation with triacetyluridine for six weeks exhibited an increase in pH compared to nonresponders (130).

Together, these studies suggest that subjects with BD may rely on glycolysis more readily than healthy controls; in principle, changes in the CK reaction, suggested by studies described earlier, would reduce the efficiency with which PCr is produced and thus with which it can buffer ATP when bioenergetic demands are increased; this could lead to an increased reliance on glycolysis in those cases. Still, many studies have failed to find variations in pH in BD. Kato et al. (127) found that pH did not differ between BD-M and controls, and Brennan et al. found that pH did not change in response to treatment in twenty subjects with BD-D treated with acetyl-L-carnitine and alpha-lipoic acid compared to those treated with placebo (119). Similarly, pH did not differ in aggregate between subjects in BD-M, BD-E, BD-Mx, BD-D, and healthy controls (126), while there was no difference in pH in the OCC (125).

As noted previously, increases in lactate (Lac) represent a shift toward anaerobic glycolysis and would be expected to be inversely correlated with changes in pH. In BD, reductions in [Lac] have been associated with antimanic response to quetiapine in medial frontal GM (131). Lac/tCr appears to be reduced in BD-E in the ACC but does not differ in BD-M from HC in that region (132), while the ratio is increased in unmedicated subjects with BD-D in the ACC (133). In other studies, Lac is increased in ACC in BD-E (134) and DCC in BD-D, where it appeared to fall with the response to lithium (135).

8.5 Conclusion

Numerous spectroscopic studies suggest that alterations in brain bioenergetics may contribute to the pathogenesis of both MDD and BD. Although the interpretation of these results is still rendered difficult by wide variations in subject populations, mood states, VOIs, and other factors, and though findings are at times contradictory, the weight of evidence indicates that, in MDD, symptom severity is related to reductions in energy utilization, marked by increased [PCr], particularly in GM regions, such as ACC and left DLPFC, that are associated with neural circuits independently implicated in

depression. This reduction in energy utilization may be due to hypoactivity in these regions; antidepressant treatment, by increasing activity in these regions, may increase energy utilization and thereby make use of PCr stores. For subjects with relative depletion of PCr, however, response to treatment is inhibited. In BD, it appears that at least a subset of patients – perhaps those who are responsive to lithium – may suffer from inefficiencies in the CK reaction, oxidative phosphorylation, or the Krebs cycle, which may lead to both reductions in [PCr] as well as inefficient production of ATP under conditions of high energy demand. Clearly, however, more information is needed to complete these emerging stories, suggesting the importance of further research.

References

1. Fakhoury M. Revisiting the serotonin hypothesis: Implications for major depressive disorders. *Mol Neurobiol.* 2016; **53**(5): 2778–2786.

2. Lener MS, Niciu MJ, Ballard ED, et al. Glutamate and gamma-aminobutyric acid systems in the pathophysiology of major depression and antidepressant response to ketamine. *Biological Psychiatry.* 2017; **81**(10): 886–897.

3. Young JJ, Bruno D, Pomara N. A review of the relationship between proinflammatory cytokines and major depressive disorder. *Journal of Affective Disorders.* 2014; **169**: 15–20.

4. Slavich GM, Irwin MR. From stress to inflammation and major depressive disorder: A social signal transduction theory of depression. *Psychological Bulletin.* 2014; **140**(3): 774.

5. Maes M, Galecki P, Chang YS, Berk M. A review on the oxidative and nitrosative stress (O&NS) pathways in major depression and their possible contribution to the (neuro) degenerative processes in that illness. *Progress in Neuro-Psychopharmacology and Biological Psychiatry.* 2011; **35**(3): 676–692.

6. Cecil KM. Proton magnetic resonance spectroscopy: Technique for the neuroradiologist. *Neuroimaging Clinics of North America.* 2013; **23**(3): 381–392.

7. Miller BL, Changl L, Booth R, et al. In vivo 1 H MRS choline: Correlation with in vitro chemistry/ histology. *Life Sciences.* 1996; **58**(22): 1929–1935.

8. Scremin OU, Jenden DJ. Acetylcholine turnover and release: the influence of energy metabolism and systemic choline availability. Progress in Brain Research. **98**: Elsevier; 1993. p. 191–5.

9. Djuricic B, Olson SR, Assaf HM, et al. Formation of free choline in brain tissue during in vitro energy

deprivation. *Journal of Cerebral Blood Flow & Metabolism.* 1991; **11**(2): 308–313.

10. Wallimann T, Wyss M, Brdiczka D, Nicolay K, Eppenberger H. Intracellular compartmentation, structure and function of creatine kinase isoenzymes in tissues with high and fluctuating energy demands: The'phosphocreatine circuit'for cellular energy homeostasis. *Biochemical Journal.* 1992; **281**(Pt 1): 21.

11. Li BSY, Wang H, Gonen O. Metabolite ratios to assumed stable creatine level may confound the quantification of proton brain MR spectroscopy. *Magnetic Resonance Imaging.* 2003 October; **21** (8): 923–928.

12. Choi C, Ghose S, Uh J, et al. Measurement of N-acetylaspartylglutamate in the human frontal brain by 1 H-MRS at 7 T. *Magnetic Resonance in Medicine.* 2010; **64**(5): 1247–1251.

13. Ariyannur PS, Madhavarao CN, Namboodiri AMA. N-acetylaspartate synthesis in the brain: Mitochondria vs. microsomes. *Brain Research.* 2008; **1227**: 34–41.

14. Wiame E, Tyteca D, Pierrot N, et al. Molecular identification of aspartate N-acetyltransferase and its mutation in hypoacetylaspartia. *Biochemical Journal.* 2010; **425**(1): 127–139.

15. Moreno A, Ross BD, Blüml S. Direct determination of the N-acetyl-l-aspartate synthesis rate in the human brain by 13 C MRS and [1-13 C]glucose infusion. *Journal of Neurochemistry.* 2001; **77**(1): 347–350.

16. Choi I-Y, Gruetter R, editors. In vivo 13 C NMR measurement of total brain glycogen concentrations in the conscious rat. *Proc Intl Soc Mag Reson Med;* 2001.

17. Patel TB, Clark JB. Synthesis of N-acetyl-l-aspartate by rat brain mitochondria and its involvement in mitochondrial/cytosolic carbon transport. *Biochemical Journal.* 1979; **184**(3): 539–46.

18. Yudkoff M, Nelson D, Daikhin Y, Erecińska M. Tricarboxylic acid cycle in rat brain synaptosomes. Fluxes and interactions with aspartate aminotransferase and malate/aspartate shuttle. *Journal of Biological Chemistry.* 1994; **269**(44): 27414–27420.

19. Moffett JR, Ross B, Arun P, Madhavarao CN, Namboodiri AMA. N-Acetylaspartate in the CNS: From neurodiagnostics to neurobiology. *Progress in Neurobiology.* 2007; **81**(2): 89–131.

20. Baslow MH. N-Acetylaspartate in the Vertebrate Brain: Metabolism and Function. *Neurochemical Research.* 2003; **28**(6): 941–53.

21. Arun P, Madhavarao CN, Moffett JR, Namboodiri M. Regulation of N-acetylaspartate and N-acetylaspartylglutamate biosynthesis by protein kinase activators. *Journal of Neurochemistry.* 2006; **98**(6): 2034–2042.

22. Neale JH, Bzdega T, Wroblewska B. N-Acetylaspartylglutamate: The most abundant peptide neurotransmitter in the mammalian central nervous system. *J Neurochem.* 2000; **75**(2): 443–452.

23. Brand A, Richter-Landsberg C, Leibfritz D. Multinuclear NMR studies on the energy metabolism of glial and neuronal cells. *Developmental Neuroscience.* 1993; **15**(3–5): 289–298.

24. Moretto E, Murru L, Martano G, Sassone J, Passafaro M. Glutamatergic synapses in neurodevelopmental disorders. *Progress in Neuro-Psychopharmacology and Biological Psychiatry.* 2018; **84**: 328–342.

25. Kew JN, Kemp JA. Ionotropic and metabotropic glutamate receptor structure and pharmacology. *Psychopharmacology.* 2005; **179**(1): 4–29.

26. Anderson CM, Swanson RA. Astrocyte glutamate transport: Review of properties, regulation, and physiological functions. *Glia.* 2000; **32**(1): 1–14.

27. Hertz L, Zielke HR. Astrocytic control of glutamatergic activity: Astrocytes as stars of the show. *Trends in Neurosciences.* 2004; **27**(12): 735–743.

28. Sibson NR, Dhankhar A, Mason GF, et al. Stoichiometric coupling of brain glucose metabolism and glutamatergic neuronal activity. *Proceedings of the National Academy of Sciences.* 1998; **95**(1): 316–321.

29. Chadi G. Abdallah, Lihong Jiang, Henk M. De Feyter, et al. Glutamate metabolism in major depressive disorder. *American Journal of Psychiatry.* 2014; **171**(12): 1320–1327.

30. Sappey-Marinier D, Calabrese G, Fein G, et al. Effect of photic stimulation on human visual cortex lactate and phosphates using 1 H and 31P magnetic resonance spectroscopy. *Journal of Cerebral Blood Flow & Metabolism.* 1992; **12**(4): 584–592.

31. Fox PT, Raichle ME, Mintun MA, Dence C. Nonoxidative glucose consumption during focal physiologic neural activity. *Science (New York, NY).* 1988; **241**(4864): 462–464.

32. Cichocka M, Kozub J, Urbanik A. PH Measurements of the brain using phosphorus magnetic resonance spectroscopy ((31)PMRS) in healthy men – comparison of two analysis methods. *Polish Journal of Radiology.* 2015; **80**: 509–514.

33. Petroff OA, Prichard JW, Behar KL, et al. Cerebral intracellular pH by 31P nuclear magnetic

resonance spectroscopy. *Neurology*. 1985; **35**(6): 781–788.

34. Szulc A, Wiedlocha M, Waszkiewicz N, et al. Proton magnetic resonance spectroscopy changes after lithium treatment. *Systematic Review*. *Psychiatry Research Neuroimaging*. 2018; **273**: 1–8.

35. Auer DP, Pütz B, Kraft E, et al. Reduced glutamate in the anterior cingulate cortex in depression: An in vivo proton magnetic resonance spectroscopy study. *Biological Psychiatry*. 2000; **47**(4): 305–313.

36. Ende G, Braus DF, Walter S, Weber-Fahr W, Henn FA. The hippocampus in patients treated with electroconvulsive therapy: A proton magnetic resonance spectroscopic imaging study. *Archives of General Psychiatry*. 2000; **57**(10): 937–943.

37. Farchione TR, Moore GJ, Rosenberg DR. Proton magnetic resonance spectroscopic imaging in pediatric major depression. *Biological Psychiatry*. 2002; **52**(2): 86–92.

38. Kumar A, Thomas A, Lavretsky H, et al. Frontal white matter biochemical abnormalities in late-life major depression detected with proton magnetic resonance spectroscopy. *American Journal of Psychiatry*. 2002; **159**(4): 630–636.

39. Pfleiderer B, Michael N, Erfurth A, et al. Effective electroconvulsive therapy reverses glutamate/glutamine deficit in the left anterior cingulum of unipolar depressed patients. *Psychiatry Research: Neuroimaging*. 122(3): 185–192.

40. Hasler G, van der Veen J, Tumonis T, et al. Reduced prefrontal glutamate/glutamine and γ-aminobutyric acid levels in major depression determined using proton magnetic resonance spectroscopy. *Archives of General Psychiatry*. 2007; **64**(2): 193–200.

41. Gabbay V, Hess DA, Liu S, et al. Lateralized caudate metabolic abnormalities in adolescent major depressive disorder: A proton MR spectroscopy study. *American Journal of Psychiatry*. 2007; **164**(12): 1881–1889.

42. Glodzik-Sobanska L, Slowik A, McHugh P, et al. Single voxel proton magnetic resonance spectroscopy in post-stroke depression. *Psychiatry Research: Neuroimaging*. 2006; **148**(2): 111–120.

43. Block W, Traber F, von Widdern O, et al. Proton MR spectroscopy of the hippocampus at 3 T in patients with unipolar major depressive disorder: Correlates and predictors of treatment response. *The International Journal of Neuropsychopharmacology / Official Scientific Journal of the Collegium Internationale Neuropsychopharmacologicum*. 2009; **12**(3): 415–422.

44. McEwen AM, Burgess DT, Hanstock CC, et al. Increased glutamate levels in the medial prefrontal cortex in patients with postpartum depression. *Neuropsychopharmacology : Official Publication of the American College of Neuropsychopharmacology*. 2012; **37**(11): 2428–2435.

45. Wang X, Li Y-H, Li M-H, et al. Glutamate level detection by magnetic resonance spectroscopy in patients with post-stroke depression. *European Archives of Psychiatry and Clinical Neuroscience*. 2012; **262**(1): 33–38.

46. Wang Y, Jia Y, Chen X, et al. Hippocampal N-acetylaspartate and morning cortisol levels in drug-naive, first-episode patients with major depressive disorder: Effects of treatment. *Journal of Psychopharmacology*. 2012 November; **26**(11): 1463–1470.

47. Rosa CE, Soares JC, Figueiredo FP, et al. Glutamatergic and neural dysfunction in postpartum depression using magnetic resonance spectroscopy. *Psychiatry Research: Neuroimaging*. 2017; **265**: 18–25.

48. Li H, Xu H, Zhang Y, et al. Differential neurometabolite alterations in brains of medication-free individuals with bipolar disorder and those with unipolar depression: A two-dimensional proton magnetic resonance spectroscopy study. *Bipolar Disorders*. 2016; **18**(7): 583–590.

49. Yoon S, Kim JE, Hwang J, et al. Effects of creatine monohydrate augmentation on brain metabolic and network outcome measures in women with major depressive disorder. *Biological Psychiatry*. 2016; **80**(6): 439–447.

50. Lefebvre D, Langevin LM, Jaworska N, et al. A pilot study of hippocampal N-acetyl-aspartate in youth with treatment resistant major depression. *Journal of Affective Disorders*. 2017; **207**: 110–113.

51. Njau S, Joshi SH, Espinoza R, et al. Neurochemical correlates of rapid treatment response to electroconvulsive therapy in patients with major depression. *J Psychiatry Neurosci*. 2017; **42**(1): 6–16.

52. Vythilingam M, Charles HC, Tupler LA, et al. Focal and lateralized subcortical abnormalities in unipolar major depressive disorder: An automated multivoxel proton magnetic resonance spectroscopy study. *Biological Psychiatry*. 2003 October; **54**(7): 744–750.

53. Gruber S, Frey R, Mlynárik V, et al. Quantification of metabolic differences in the frontal brain of depressive patients and controls obtained by 1 H-MRS at 3 Tesla. *Investigative Radiology*. 2003; **38** (7): 403–408.

54. Chen CS, Chiang IC, Li CW, et al. Proton magnetic resonance spectroscopy of late-life major depressive disorder. *Psychiatry Research*. 2009; **172** (3): 210–214.

55. Zhong S, Wang Y, Zhao G, et al. Similarities of biochemical abnormalities between major depressive disorder and bipolar depression: A proton magnetic resonance spectroscopy study. *Journal of Affective Disorders.* 2014; **168**: 380–386.

56. Jia Y, Zhong S, Wang Y, et al. The correlation between biochemical abnormalities in frontal white matter, hippocampus and serum thyroid hormone levels in first-episode patients with major depressive disorder. *Journal of Affective Disorders.* 2015; **180**: 162–169.

57. Huang Y, Chen W, Li Y, et al. Effects of antidepressant treatment on N-acetyl aspartate and choline levels in the hippocampus and thalami of post-stroke depression patients: A study using (1)H magnetic resonance spectroscopy. *Psychiatry Research.* 2010; **182**(1): 48–52.

58. Wang Y, Jia Y, Xu G, et al. Frontal white matter biochemical abnormalities in first-episode, treatment-naive patients with major depressive disorder: A proton magnetic resonance spectroscopy study. *Journal of Affective Disorders.* 2012; **136**(3): 620–626.

59. Li Y, Jakary A, Gillung E, et al. Evaluating metabolites in patients with major depressive disorder who received mindfulness-based cognitive therapy and healthy controls using short echo MRSI at 7 Tesla. *Magma (New York, Ny).* 2016; **29**: 523–533.

60. Nery FG, Stanley JA, Chen HH, et al. Normal metabolite levels in the left dorsolateral prefrontal cortex of unmedicated major depressive disorder patients: A single voxel (1)H spectroscopy study. *Psychiatry Research.* 2009; **174**(3): 177–183.

61. Portella MJ, de Diego-Adelino J, Gomez-Anson B, et al. Ventromedial prefrontal spectroscopic abnormalities over the course of depression: A comparison among first episode, remitted recurrent and chronic patients. *Journal of Psychiatric Research.* 2011; **45**(4): 427–434.

62. de Diego-Adelino J, Portella MJ, Gomez-Anson B, et al. Hippocampal abnormalities of glutamate/glutamine, N-acetylaspartate and choline in patients with depression are related to past illness burden. *J Psychiatry Neurosci.* 2013; **38**(2): 107–116.

63. Tae WS, Kim SS, Lee KU, Nam EC, Koh SH. Progressive decrease of N-acetylaspartate to total creatine ratio in the pregenual anterior cingulate cortex in patients with major depressive disorder: Longitudinal 1 H-MR spectroscopy study. *Acta Radiologica.* 2014; **55**(5): 594–603.

64. Henigsberg N, Šarac H, Radoš M, et al. Lower choline-containing metabolites/creatine (Cr) rise and failure to sustain NAA/Cr levels in the dorsolateral prefrontal cortex are associated with

depressive episode recurrence under maintenance therapy: A proton magnetic resonance spectroscopy retrospective cohort study. *Frontiers in Psychiatry.* 2017; **8**: 277.

65. Grachev ID, Ramachandran TS, Thomas PS, Szeverenyi NM, Fredrickson BE. Association between dorsolateral prefrontal N-acetyl aspartate and depression in chronic back pain: An in vivo proton magnetic resonance spectroscopy study. *Journal of Neural Transmission.* 2003; **110**(3): 287–312.

66. Woo Suk T, Sam Soo K, Kang Uk L, Eui-Cheol N, Sung Hye K. Progressive decrease of N-acetylaspartate to total creatine ratio in the pregenual anterior cingulate cortex in patients with major depressive disorder: Longitudinal 1H-MR spectroscopy study. *Acta Radiologica.* 2014; **55**(5): 594–603.

67. Wang Y, Jia Y, Chen X, et al. Hippocampal N-acetylaspartate and morning cortisol levels in drug-naive, first-episode patients with major depressive disorder: Effects of treatment. *Journal of Psychopharmacology (Oxford, England).* 2012; **26**(11): 1463–1470.

68. Charles HC, Lazeyras F, Krishnan KRR, Brain choline in depression: In vivo detection of potential pharmacodynamic effects of antidepressant therapy using hydrogen localized spectroscopy. *Progress in Neuro-Psychopharmacology and Biological Psychiatry.* 1994; **18**(7): 1121–1127.

69. Huang Y, Chen W, Li Y, et al. Effects of antidepressant treatment on & N-acetyl aspartate and choline levels in the hippocampus and thalami of post-stroke depression patients: A study using ^{1}H magnetic resonance spectroscopy. *Psychiatry Research: Neuroimaging.* 2010; **182**(1): 48–52.

70. Kaymak SU, Demir B, Oğuz KK, Şentürk S, Uluğ B. Antidepressant effect detected on proton magnetic resonance spectroscopy in drug-naïve female patients with first-episode major depression. *Psychiatry and Clinical Neurosciences.* 2009; **63**(3): 350–356.

71. Lisanby SH. Electroconvulsive therapy for depression. *New England Journal of Medicine.* 2007; **357**(19): 1939–1945.

72. Berlim MT, van den Eynde F, Tovar-Perdomo S, Daskalakis ZJ. Response, remission and drop-out rates following high-frequency repetitive transcranial magnetic stimulation (rTMS) for treating major depression: a systematic review and meta-analysis of randomized, double-blind and sham-controlled trials. *Psychological Medicine.* 2014; **44**(2): 225–239.

73. Cano M, Martínez-Zalacaín I, Bernabéu-Sanz Á, et al. Brain volumetric and metabolic correlates of electroconvulsive therapy for treatment-resistant depression: A longitudinal neuroimaging study. *Translational Psychiatry*. 2017; **7**: e1023.

74. Michael N, Erfurth A, Ohrmann P, et al. Neurotrophic effects of electroconvulsive therapy: A proton magnetic resonance study of the left amygdalar region in patients with treatment-resistant depression. *Neuropsychopharmacology: Official Publication of the American College of Neuropsychopharmacology*. 2003; **28**: 720.

75. Zheng H, Jia F, Guo G, et al. Abnormal anterior cingulate N-acetylaspartate and executive functioning in treatment-resistant depression after rTMS therapy. *The International Journal of Neuropsychopharmacology / Official Scientific Journal of the Collegium Internationale Neuropsychopharmacologicum*. 2015; **18**(11): pyv059.

76. Mirza Y, O'Neill J, Smith EA, et al. Increased medial thalamic creatine-phosphocreatine found by proton magnetic resonance spectroscopy in children with obsessive-compulsive disorder versus major depression and healthy controls. *Journal of Child Neurology*. 2006; **21**(2): 106–111.

77. Nery FG, Stanley JA, Chen H-H, et al. Normal metabolite levels in the left dorsolateral prefrontal cortex of unmedicated major depressive disorder patients: A single voxel 1 H spectroscopy study. *Psychiatry Research: Neuroimaging*. 2009; **174**(3): 177–183.

78. Iosifescu DV, Renshaw PF. 31P-Magnetic resonance spectroscopy and thyroid hormones in major depressive disorder: Toward a bioenergetic mechanism in depression? *Harvard Review of Psychiatry*. 2003; **11**(2): 51–63.

79. Kato T, Takahashi S, Shioiri T, Inubushi T. Brain phosphorous metabolism in depressive disorders detected by phosphorus-31 magnetic resonance spectroscopy. *Journal of Affective Disorders*. 1992; **26**(4): 223–230.

80. Moore CM, Christensen JD, Lafer B, Fava M, Renshaw PF. Lower levels of nucleoside triphosphate in the basal ganglia of depressed subjects: A phosphorous-31 magnetic resonance spectroscopy study. *American Journal of Psychiatry*. 1997; **154**(1): 116–118.

81. Volz HP, Rzanny R, Riehemann S, et al. 31P magnetic resonance spectroscopy in the frontal lobe of major depressed patients. *European Archives of Psychiatry and Clinical Neuroscience*. 1998; **248**(6): 289–295.

82. Renshaw PF, Parow AM, Hirashima F, et al. Multinuclear magnetic resonance spectroscopy studies of brain purines in major depression. *American Journal of Psychiatry*. 2001; **158**(12): 2048–2055.

83. Kondo DG, Sung Y-H, Hellem TL, et al. Open-label adjunctive creatine for female adolescents with SSRI-resistant major depressive disorder: A 31-phosphorus magnetic resonance spectroscopy study. *Journal of Affective Disorders*. 2011; **135**(1): 354–361.

84. Iosifescu DV, Bolo NR, Nierenberg AA, et al. Brain bioenergetics and response to triiodothyronine augmentation in major depressive disorder. *Biological Psychiatry*. 2008; **63** (12): 1127–1134.

85. Pettegrew JW, Levine J, Gershon S, et al. 31P-MRS study of acetyl-L-carnitine treatment in geriatric depression: Preliminary results. *Bipolar Disorders*. 2002; **4**(1): 61–66.

86. Forester BP, Harper DG, Jensen JE, et al. 31Phosphorus magnetic resonance spectroscopy study of tissue specific changes in high energy phosphates before and after sertraline treatment of geriatric depression. *International Journal of Geriatric Psychiatry*. 2009; **24**(8): 788–797.

87. Harper DG, Joe EB, Jensen JE, Ravichandran C, Forester BP. Brain levels of high-energy phosphate metabolites and executive function in geriatric depression. *International Journal of Geriatric Psychiatry*. 2016; **31**(11): 1241–1249.

88. Harper DG, Jensen JE, Ravichandran C, et al. Tissue type-specific bioenergetic abnormalities in adults with major depression. *Neuropsychopharmacology : Official Publication of the American College of Neuropsychopharmacology*. 2017; **42**(4): 876–885.

89. Sassi RB, Stanley JA, Axelson D, et al. Reduced NAA levels in the dorsolateral prefrontal cortex of young bipolar patients. *American Journal of Psychiatry*. 2005; **162**(11): 2109–2115.

90. Caetano SC, Olvera RL, Hatch JP, et al. Lower N-Acetyl-Aspartate levels in prefrontal cortices in pediatric bipolar disorder: A ^{1}H magnetic resonance spectroscopy study. *Journal of the American Academy of Child & Adolescent Psychiatry*. 2011; **50**(1): 85–94.

91. Olvera RL, Caetano SC, Fonseca M, et al. Low levels of N-Acetyl aspartate in the left dorsolateral prefrontal cortex of pediatric bipolar patients. *Journal of Child and Adolescent Psychopharmacology*. 2007; **17**(4): 461–473.

92. Winsberg ME, Sachs N, Tate DL, et al. Decreased dorsolateral prefrontal N-acetyl aspartate in bipolar disorder. *Biological Psychiatry*. 2000; **47**(6): 475–481.

93. Cecil KM, DelBello MP, Morey R, Strakowski SM. Frontal lobe differences in bipolar disorder as determined by proton MR spectroscopy. *Bipolar Disorders*. 2002; 4(6): 357–365.

94. Özdel O, Kalayci D, Sözeri-Varma G, et al. Neurochemical metabolites in the medial prefrontal cortex in bipolar disorder: A proton magnetic resonance spectroscopy study. *Neural Regeneration Research*. 2012; 7(36): 2929–2936.

95. Bertolino A, Frye M, Callicott JH, et al. Neuronal pathology in the hippocampal area of patients with bipolar disorder: A study with proton magnetic resonance spectroscopic imaging. *Biological Psychiatry*. 2003; 53(10): 906–913.

96. Deicken RF, Pegues MP, Anzalone S, Feiwell R, Soher B. Lower concentration of hippocampal N-acetylaspartate in familial bipolar I disorder. *The American Journal of Psychiatry*. 2003; 160(5): 873–882.

97. Port JD, Unal SS, Mrazek DA, Marcus SM. Metabolic alterations in medication-free patients with bipolar disorder: A 3 T CSF-corrected magnetic resonance spectroscopic imaging study. *Psychiatry Research: Neuroimaging*. 2008; 162(2): 113–121.

98. Zhong S, Wang Y, Zhao G, et al. Similarities of biochemical abnormalities between major depressive disorder and bipolar depression: A proton magnetic resonance spectroscopy study. *Journal of Affective Disorders*. 2014; 168: 380–386.

99. Croarkin PE, Thomas MA, Port JD, et al. N-acetylaspartate normalization in bipolar depression after lamotrigine treatment. *Bipolar Disorders*. 2015; 17(4): 450–457.

100. Sharma R, Venkatasubramanian PN, Bárány M, Davis JM. Proton magnetic resonance spectroscopy of the brain in schizophrenic and affective patients. *Schizophrenia Research*. 1992; 8(1): 43–49.

101. Deicken RF, Eliaz Y, Feiwell R, Schuff N. Increased thalamic N-acetylaspartate in male patients with familial bipolar I disorder. *Psychiatry Research: Neuroimaging*. 2001; 106(1): 35–45.

102. Ohara K, Isoda H, Suzuki Y, et al. Proton magnetic resonance spectroscopy of the lenticular nuclei in bipolar I affective disorder. *Psychiatry Research: Neuroimaging*. 1998; 84(2): 55–60.

103. Castillo M, Kwock L, Courvoisie H, Hooper SR. Proton MR spectroscopy in children with bipolar affective disorder: Preliminary observations. *American Journal of Neuroradiology*. 2000; 21(5): 832.

104. Davanzo P, Thomas MA, Yue K, et al. Decreased anterior cingulate myo-inositol/creatine spectroscopy resonance with lithium treatment in children with bipolar disorder. *Neuropsychopharmacology : Official Publication of the American College of Neuropsychopharmacology*. 2001; 24(4): 359–369.

105. Moore CM, Frazier JA, Glod CA, et al. Glutamine and glutamate levels in children and adolescents with bipolar disorder. *J Am Acad Child Adolesc Psychiatry*. 2007 April; 46(4): 524–534.

106. Pablo Davanzo, Kenneth Yue, M. Albert Thomas, et al. Proton magnetic resonance spectroscopy of bipolar disorder versus intermittent explosive disorder in children and adolescents. *American Journal of Psychiatry*. 2003; 160(8): 1442–1452.

107. Brambilla P, Stanley JA, Nicoletti MA, et al. 1 H magnetic resonance spectroscopy investigation of the dorsolateral prefrontal cortex in bipolar disorder patients. *Journal of Affective Disorders*. 2005; 86(1): 61–67.

108. DelBello MP, Cecil KM, Adler CM, Daniels JP, Strakowski SM. Neurochemical effects of olanzapine in first-hospitalization manic adolescents: A proton magnetic resonance spectroscopy study. *Neuropsychopharmacology : Official Publication of the American College of Neuropsychopharmacology*. 2005; 31: 1264.

109. Michael N, Erfurth A, Ohrmann P, et al. Acute mania is accompanied by elevated glutamate/glutamine levels within the left dorsolateral prefrontal cortex. *Psychopharmacology*. 2003; 168(3): 344–346.

110. Forester BP, Finn CT, Berlow YA, et al. Brain lithium, N-acetyl aspartate and myo-inositol levels in older adults with bipolar disorder treated with lithium: A lithium-7 and proton magnetic resonance spectroscopy study. *Bipolar Disorders*. 2008; 10(6): 691–700.

111. Hamakawa H, Kato T, Shioiri T, Inubushi T, Kato N. Quantitative proton magnetic resonance spectroscopy of the bilateral frontal lobes in patients with bipolar disorder. *Psychological Medicine*. 1999; 29(3): 639–644.

112. Cecil KM, DelBello MP, Sellars MC, Strakowski SM. Proton magnetic resonance spectroscopy of the frontal lobe and cerebellar vermis in children with a mood disorder and a familial risk for bipolar disorders. *Journal of Child and Adolescent Psychopharmacology*. 2003; 13(4): 545–555.

113. Öngür D, Prescot AP, Jensen JE, Cohen BM, Renshaw PF. Creatine abnormalities in schizophrenia and bipolar disorder. *Psychiatry Research: Neuroimaging*. 2009; 172(1): 44–48.

114. Dager SR, Friedman SD, Parow A, et al. Brain metabolic alterations in medication-free patients

with bipolardisorder. *Archives of General Psychiatry*. 2004; **61**(5): 450–458.

115. Frye MA, Watzl J, Banakar S, et al. Increased anterior cingulate/medial prefrontal cortical glutamate and creatine in bipolar depression. *Neuropsychopharmacology : Official Publication of the American College of Neuropsychopharmacology*. 2007; **32**: 2490.

116. Kato T, Takahashi S, Shioiri T, et al. Reduction of brain phosphocreatine in bipolar II disorder detected by phosphorus-31 magnetic resonance spectroscopy. *Journal of Affective Disorders*. 1994; **31**(2): 125–133.

117. Weber WA, Dudley J, Lee J-H, et al. A pilot study of alterations in high energy phosphoryl compounds and intracellular pH in unmedicated adolescents with bipolar disorder. *Journal of Affective Disorders*. 2013; **150**(3): 1109–1113.

118. Dudley J, DelBello MP, Weber WA, et al. Tissue-dependent cerebral energy metabolism in adolescents with bipolar disorder. *Journal of Affective Disorders*. 2016; **191**: 248–255.

119. Brennan BP, Jensen JE, Hudson JI, et al. A placebo-controlled trial of acetyl-L-carnitine and alpha-lipoic acid in the treatment of bipolar depression. *J Clin Psychopharmacol*. 2013; **33**(5): 627–635.

120. Deicken RF, Fein G, Weiner MW. Abnormal frontal lobe phosphorous metabolism in bipolar disorder. *American Journal of Psychiatry*. 1995; **152**(6): 915–918.

121. Du F, Yuksel C, Chouinard V-A, et al. Abnormalities in high-energy phosphate metabolism in first-episode bipolar disorder measured using 31P-magnetic resonance spectroscopy. *Biological Psychiatry*. 2018 December 1; **84**(11): 797–802.

122. Jensen JE, Daniels M, Haws C, et al. Triacetyluridine (TAU) decreases depressive symptoms and increases brain pH in bipolar patients. *Experimental and Clinical Psychopharmacology*. 2008; **16**(3): 199–206.

123. Murashita J, Kato T, Shioiri T, Inubushi T, Kato N. Altered brain energy metabolism in lithium-resistant bipolar disorder detected by photic stimulated 31P-MR spectroscopy. *Psychological Medicine*. 2000; **30**(1): 107–115.

124. Shi XF, Carlson PJ, Sung YH, et al. Decreased brain PME/PDE ratio in bipolar disorder: A preliminary 31P magnetic resonance spectroscopy study. *Bipolar Disorders*. 2015; **17**(7): 743–752.

125. Yuksel C, Du F, Ravichandran C, et al. Abnormal high-energy phosphate molecule metabolism

during regional brain activation in patients with bipolar disorder. *Molecular Psychiatry*. 2015; **20**(9): 1079–1084.

126. Sikoglu EM, Jensen JE, Vitaliano G, et al. Bioenergetic measurements in children with bipolar disorder: A pilot 31P magnetic resonance spectroscopy study. *PloS One*. 2013; **8**(1): e54536.

127. Kato T, Takahashi S, Shioiri T, Inubushi T. Alterations in brain phosphorous metabolism in bipolar disorder detected by in vivo 31P and 7Li magnetic resonance spectroscopy. *Journal of Affective Disorders*. 1993; **27**(1): 53–59.

128. Kato T, Shioiri T, Murashita J, et al. Phosphorus-31 magnetic resonance spectroscopy and ventricular enlargement in bipolar disorder. *Psychiatry Research*. 1994; **55**(1): 41–50.

129. Hamakawa H, Murashita J, Yamada N, et al. Reduced intracellular pH in the basal ganglia and whole brain measured by 31P-MRS in bipolar disorder. *Psychiatry and Clinical Neurosciences*. 2004; **58**(1): 82–88.

130. Jensen JE, Daniels M, Haws C, et al. Triacetyluridine (TAU) decreases depressive symptoms and increases brain pH in bipolar patients. *Experimental and Clinical Psychopharmacology*. 2008; **16**(3): 199–206.

131. Kim DJ, Lyoo IK, Yoon SJ, et al. Clinical response of quetiapine in rapid cycling manic bipolar patients and lactate level changes in proton magnetic resonance spectroscopy. *Progress in Neuro-Psychopharmacology and Biological Psychiatry*. 2007; **31**(6): 1182–1188.

132. Bradley EH, Curry L, Horwitz LI, Sipsma H, Thompson JW, Elma M. Contemporary evidence about hospital strategies for reducing 30-day readmissions: a national study. *J Am Coll Cardiol*. 2012; **60**.

133. Xu J, Dydak U, Harezlak J, et al. Neurochemical abnormalities in unmedicated bipolar depression and mania: A 2D 1H MRS investigation. *Psychiatry Research: Neuroimaging*. 2013; **213**(3): 235–241.

134. Soeiro-de-Souza MG, Pastorello BF, Leite CdC, et al. Dorsal anterior cingulate lactate and glutathione levels in euthymic bipolar I disorder: 1 H-MRS study. *International Journal of Neuropsychopharmacology*. 2016; **19**(8): pyw032–pyw.

135. Machado-Vieira R, Zanetti MV, Otaduy MC, et al. Increased brain lactate during depressive episodes and reversal effects by lithium monotherapy in drug-naive bipolar disorder: A 3-T 1 H-MRS study. *Journal of Clinical Psychopharmacology*. 2017; **37**(1): 40–45.

136. Yousha M, Joseph ON, Ethan AS, et al. Increased medial thalamic creatine-phosphocreatine found

by proton magnetic resonance spectroscopy in children with obsessive-compulsive disorder versus major depression and healthy controls. *Journal of Child Neurology.* 2006; **21**(2): 106–111.

137. Chen C-S, Chiang IC, Li C-W, Lin W-C, Lu C-Y, Hsieh T-J, et al. Proton magnetic resonance spectroscopy of late-life major depressive disorder. *Psychiatry Research: Neuroimaging.* 2009; **172**(3): 210–4.

138. Wang Y, Jia Y, Xu G, et al. Frontal white matter biochemical abnormalities in first-episode, treatment-naive patients with major depressive disorder: A proton magnetic resonance spectroscopy study. *Journal of Affective Disorders.* 2012; **136**(3): 620–626.

139. Jia Y, Zhong S, Wang Y, et al. The correlation between biochemical abnormalities in frontal white matter, hippocampus and serum thyroid hormone levels in first-episode patients with major depressive disorder. *Journal of Affective Disorders.* 2015; **180**: 162–169.

140. Moore CM, Christensen JD, Lafer B, Fava M, Renshaw PF. Lower levels of nucleoside triphosphate in the basal ganglia of depressed subjects: A phosphorous-31 magnetic resonance spectroscopy study. *American Journal of Psychiatry.* 1997; **154**(1): 116–118.

141. Harper DG, Jensen JE, Ravichandran C, et al. Tissue type-specific bioenergetic abnormalities in adults with major depression. *Neuropsychopharmacology: Official Publication of the American College of Neuropsychopharmacology.* 2016; **42**: 876.

142. Hamakawa H, Kato T, Shioiri T, Inubushi T, Kato N. Quantitative proton magnetic resonance spectroscopy of the bilateral frontal lobes in patients with bipolar disorder. *Psychological Medicine.* 1999; **29**(3): 639–644.

143. Moore CM, Breeze JL, Gruber SA, et al. Choline, myo-inositol and mood in bipolar disorder: A proton magnetic resonance spectroscopic imaging study of the anterior cingulate cortex. *Bipolar Disorders.* 2000; **2**(3p2): 207–216.

144. Patel NC, Cecil KM, Strakowski SM, Adler CM, DelBello MP. Neurochemical alterations in adolescent bipolar depression: A proton magnetic resonance spectroscopy pilot study of the prefrontal cortex. *Journal of Child and Adolescent Psychopharmacology.* 2008; **18**(6): 623–627.

145. Brady Jr RO, Cooper A, Jensen JE, et al. A longitudinal pilot proton MRS investigation of the manic and euthymic states of bipolar disorder. *Translational Psychiatry.* 2012; **2**: e160.

146. Deicken RF, Weiner MW, Fein G. Decreased temporal lobe phosphomonoesters in bipolar disorder. *Journal of Affective Disorders.* 1995; **33**(3): 195–199.

Imaging Glutamatergic and GABAergic Abnormalities in Mood Disorders

Estêvão Scotti-Muzzi, Maria Concepcion Garcia Otaduy, Márcio
Gerhardt Soeiro-de-Souza, and Rodrigo Machado-Vieira

9.1 Background

Glutamate (Glu) and gamma-aminobutyric acid (GABA) are the main brain excitatory and inhibitory neurotransmitters. These neurotransmitters are involved in neural migration, differentiation, and synaptic plasticity (1–6). There are accumulating evidence in literature that the neurobiology of mood disorders may arise from an imbalance between excitatory Glu (7–11) and inhibitory GABA (12–15) in key brain regions involved in mood regulation, such as the anterior cingulate cortex (ACC). Glu and GABA dysfunctions have been reported in patients with mood disorders based on several lines of evidence, such as abnormalities in cerebrospinal fluid (CSF) (16–21) and postmortem brain tissue (PMBT) (1–6). Additionally, glial cells have been reported to be reduced in many brain (including prefrontal cortex (PFC) and anterior cingulate cortex) areas of subjects with bipolar disorder (BD) according to PMBT studies (9, 22). In major depressive disorder (MDD), Glu levels have been reported to be elevated in plasma (12–15) and PMBT studies (16–21).Thus, evidence has encouraged the development of modern neuroimaging techniques that allow the in vivo measurement of Glu and GABA.

9.2 Glutamate

The Glu hypothesis of depression was proposed in the 1990s, when antagonists of the N-methyl-D-aspartate (NMDA) receptor, an ionotropic glutamate receptor, were found to possess antidepressant-like mechanisms of action in mice (23). More recently, it has been reported and replicated that the infusion of low-dose ketamine, an NMDA receptor antagonist, is associated with robust decreases of depressive symptoms, mainly suicidal thoughts, in depressed patients (24–26). This way, the balance between brain levels of Glu and GABA is hypothesized to be as crucial for achieving and sustaining euthymia in the treatment of mood disorders. However, only recently the development of neuroimaging techniques allowed the precise measurement of these metabolites.

Glu is the most abundant excitatory metabolite in the brain (27), and it is continuously recycled between neurons and glial cells. Excess Glu causes excitotoxicity and apoptosis (28), which is also associated with higher levels of intracellular calcium (Ca^{+2}) and production of mitochondrial reactive species. (29, 30). After neuronal Glu is released into the synapse, it is taken up by astrocytes and converted to glutamine (Gln) by Gln synthase (GS) (31) via ketoglutarate from the tricarboxylic acid (TCA) cycle. Moreover, astrocytes deliver energy sources, including glucose and lactate, based on neuronal energy requirements; thus, there is a close link between the glutamatergic system and brain energy metabolism via astrocytic functions (32). The cycle involving neuronal Glu release from neurons and its resynthesis from Gln inside astrocytes is known as the Glu–Gln cycle (33). Glu does not cross the blood–brain barrier, and its concentration in the cellular and extracellular fluid is maintained at lower levels by the Glu–Gln recycling across neurons and astrocytes (34). Since absolute measures of Glu and Gln do not reflect the constant flux through the Glu–Gln cycle, it has been suggested that the Glu/Gln ratio might be more sensitive to measure changes in the Glu–Gln cycle rather than either metabolite alone (35, 36). Thus, the Glu/Gln ratio may potentially provide insights into glutamatergic activity, and changes in this ratio could be interpreted as a measure of Glu–Gln cycle rate. Some groups have theorized that the Glu/Gln ratio might reflect the flux through the Glu–Gln cycle and can serve as an overall indicator of glutamatergic transmission activity (35–42).

9.3 GABA

GABA is the most abundant inhibitory neurotransmitter in the central nervous system (CNS), and it is synthesized in GABAergic neurons from Glu by the enzyme glutamic acid decarboxylase (GAD) (43, 44). GABA synthesis in the human brain depends greatly on the *GAD1* gene, whose expression and protein levels have been reported to be reduced in different brain regions of BD and schizophrenia patients, including in the ACC (5, 45–48). After its release for neurotransmission, GABA is taken up by both GABAergic neurons and by astrocytes. In neurons, it may be stored in vesicles and reused for neurotransmission or it is degraded by the mitochondrial enzyme GABA transaminase (GABA-T) and enters the TCA cycle, being recycled to glutamate and then GABA again, a process known as the GABA shunt. In astrocytes, the GABA is also converted to glutamate and subsequently to glutamine. Glutamine may enter into the TCA cycle or it may be released to neurons for glutamate synthesis as explained earlier (49). Therefore, in the normal brain, there is a physiological Glu–Gln–GABA cycle associated with neurotransmission and TCA (50).

9.4 Magnetic Resonance Spectroscopy

Proton magnetic resonance spectroscopy (^{1}H-MRS) is a noninvasive technique particularly useful to assess the brain neurometabolic profile by measuring the content of several metabolites including glutamate and GABA (52) (Figure 9.1). Briefly, ^{1}H-MRS relies on the same technique used for magnetic resonance imaging (MRI). MRI signal is based on the magnetic properties of the hydrogen nuclei. In MRI, most of the signal arises from water, which is the most abundant molecule, and the effect of chemical shift can be neglected in most cases. In ^{1}H-MRS, however, this effect is explored in order to distinguish between the different molecules or metabolites. For this purpose, the strong water signal in the brain voxel is first saturated, and the residual signal is then displayed as a spectrum, that is, as a function of frequency, in order to identify all signal frequencies present, which will be then assigned to different metabolites ^{1}H. In ^{1}H-MRS frequency, values are given in *parts per million* (ppm), a unit which is independent of the magnetic field strength of the scanner and makes its interpretation easier.

^{1}H-MRS technique is able to detect nearly 80% of brain Glu, with its most prominent peak at 2.34 ppm in the spectrum that arises from the methylene protons near the carboxy-terminal of Glu (52). Gln concentration is estimated to correspond to 40–60% of Glu, but its separate quantification can be obtained only using special ^{1}H-MRS techniques and/or higher magnetic fields. Glu and Gln are very similar molecules, and for this reason, their ^{1}H-MRS signal, represented by broad and complex peaks, overlaps very

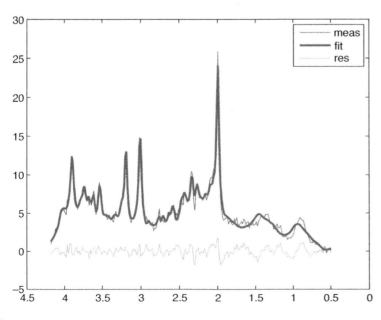

Figure 9.1 One-dimensional projection of the acquired JPRESS spectrum. Measured spectrum in blue, fitted in red, and residual in green. A black and white version of this figure will appear in some formats. For the colour version, refer to the plate section.

strongly. A detailed review of the techniques available to detect Glu and Gln can be found in (49). For this reason, most studies refer to the observed signal as "Glx," which corresponds to a greater proportion of Glu, but also Gln, GABA, and glutathione (GSH). Since Glu and Gln are the major contributions for "Glx," it has been considered a proxy of total glutamatergic neurotransmission (8, 49).

In ^{1}H-MRS spectra, GABA is commonly observed at about 2.28 ppm and is partially overlapped by the Glu peak, being considered nearly 15–20% of Glu concentration (27). Due to such overlapping signals, GABA cannot be quantified with conventional brain ^{1}H-MRS acquisitions, but it is possible to measure it by using magnetic fields with strengths higher than 3.0 T and special pulse sequences such as the J-resolved and J-difference editing sequences (49).

The ACC has been considered a center of integration of cognitive and affective neuronal connections (53). It has been the most studied brain region in affective disorders in ^{1}H-MRS studies. Considering the key role of ACC for affective and cognitive regulations as well as its connective functions between frontolimbic structures (54), there are plenty of studies showing structural and functional abnormalities in the ACC in BD. Reduced ACC gray matter volume has been demonstrated since the work performed by Drevets et al. (55) and then extensively confirmed by several authors (54, 56–58). More recently, Hibar et al. (59) have corroborated this finding in the largest BD sample assessed to date.

9.5 Major Depressive Disorder and Glutamate

Since the first (23) to the most recent studies (24–26), a consistent body of evidence has linked depression physiopathology to Glu as confirmed by a recent meta-analysis (60)(Table 9.1). Most studies have reported a decreased level in MDD patients or no differences in relation to healthy controls (HCs). Recent ^{1}H-MRS meta-analyses that have addressed glutamatergic alterations in MDD across several brain regions have also reported similar results (61, 62). Godfrey et al. (61) investigated Glx data in multiple brain voxels in 520 MDD patients compared to 501 controls across 24 studies, as well as Gln in 444 MDD patients and 420 HCs and found no differences

in either Glx or Gln between MDD and HC. However, when they restricted their analysis to the ACC of 232 MDD patients compared to 226 HCs across 12 studies, Glx was found significantly lower in MDD, although no difference was found for Glu, which remained similar to HC (Table 9.1). Such discrepancies in Glx concentration in whole-brain and specific voxels such as the ACC might be explained by the fact that the former assessment may detect changes in areas not directly related to the etiology of depression. In contrast, changes in neurometabolites in the areas that regulate the cognitive and emotional behaviors such as the ACC (53) are more likely to be implicated in the pathophysiology of MDD. Therefore, more regional and hypothesis-driven ^{1}H-MRS studies assessing Glu are recommended for MDD.

Additionally, Moriguchi et al. (62) performed a meta-analysis of Glx alterations in the medial PFC (mPFC) of 502 MDD as compared to 408 HC subjects and found significantly lower Glx levels, while no changes were observed for Glu or Gln. A subgroup analysis revealed that Glx was decreased in the mPFC of medicated patients with antidepressants compared to controls, and no difference was observed between unmedicated patients and controls (62). Previous meta-analyses have reported decreased Glx, but not Glu, in the PFC of MDD patients as compared to controls (63), and a decrease of both Glx and Glu in the ACC of MDD patients as well as in the whole brain of those under current depressive episodes (64). Overall, there is converging evidence of decreased Glx levels in frontal areas in MDD as compared to controls.

9.6 Bipolar Disorder and Glutamate

^{1}H-MRS studies have documented increased Glx in several brain regions in BD such as: ACC (65–70), dorsolateral PFC (71), basal ganglia (65), hippocampus (40, 65, 66, 72), and occipital cortex (65, 72). Indeed, previous reviews (8, 73) and meta-analyses (74, 75) have confirmed that elevated Glx is likely the most striking neurometabolic abnormality in BD subjects, particularly in frontal areas in all mood states (74, 75). Among these brain regions, the ACC is an important area linked to mood regulation (76, 77) and shows widespread functional and structural abnormalities in patients

Table 9.1 Glutamate ¹H-MRS studies in MDD (ACC voxel)

Study	Disorder	N	Mean age (P/C) (years)	Mood state	Quantified metabolites	Medication	Result	Direction
Auer et al. (2000)	MDD	33	50.2/43.2	Depressed	Glx, Glu	ADP, BZD	S	Decreased
Pfleiderer et al (2003)	MDD	34	61.0/60.1	Depressed	Glx	Medication free	S	Decreased
Mirza et al. (2004)	MDD	26	15.5/15.3	Depressed	Glx	Medication free	S	Decreased
Rosemberg et al. (2005)	MDD	28	15.6/15.4	Depressed	Glu, Gln	Medication free	S	Decreased Glu, no changes in Gln
Bhagwagar et al. (72)	MDD	23	40.6/ 34.3	Euthymic	Glx/Cr	Medication free	NS	Null
Walter et al. (2009)	MDD	43	40/34.6	Depressed	Glu, Gln	Medication free	S	Decreased Gln, no changes in Glu
Taylor et al. (2009)	MDD	30	32.6/31.8	Euthymic	Glx/Cr, Glu/Cr	Medication free	NS	Null
Merkl et al. (2011)	MDD	54	49/36.3	Depressed	Glu	Medication free	S	Decreased
Taylor et al. (2017)	MDD	35	22.5/ 23.9	Depressed	Gln, Gln	Antidepressants	NS	Null
Abdallah et al. (2017)	MDD	39	36.7/35.7	Depressed	Glx, Glu, Gln	Medication free	S	Increased
Gabbay et al. (2017)	MDD	80	16.3/15.8	Depressed	Glx	Medication free	NS	Null
Godlewska et al. (2017)	MDD	105	31.3/31.3	Depressed	Glu, Gln	Medication free	NS	Null
Njau et al. (2017)	MDD	76	43.7/39.3	Depressed	Glx	Medication free	S	Decreased

Glu- glutamate, Gln- glutamine, MDD- unipolar major depressive disorder, ADP- antidepressants, BZD- benzodiazepines, Li- lithium, S- significant, NS- not significant, NM- not mentioned.

with BD (78)(Table 9.2). Most studies have found elevated Glx or Glu levels in BD or no differences in relation to HC. Increased ACC Glu levels seem to be a trait marker intrinsic to BD (79, 80) since several authors have reported this finding in early-onset (81) and medication-free patients (65, 66, 81). Besides, elevated Glu and/or Glx levels have also been reported across different mood states in the ACC but particularly in the depressed (65, 66, 81) and euthymic (67–70) mood states. Indeed, ^{1}H-MRS studies in BD type I euthymic patients indicate Glu cycle metabolite abnormalities and also suggest increased Glx and Glu (67, 68, 72, 82, 83) as well as increased Gln (36, 68, 69) within at least three different brain regions processed with different ^{1}H-MRS sequences (Table 9.2).

Glutamatergic abnormalities in BD also seem to stem from an uncoupled neuron–astrocyte relationship as changes in the Glu–Gln cycle have been documented. Since Glx represents the sum of Glu and Gln signals, studies reporting increased Glx could reflect increased Glu, increased Gln, or even elevated levels of both of these metabolites. Specific ^{1}H-MRS studies reporting Gln measures are scarce in BD. While Ongür et al. (40) reported higher Gln/Glu ratio in the ACC of manic patients, considering it a measure of glutamatergic activity, Moore et al. (84) found that BD children medicated with anticonvulsants, antipsychotics, and antidepressant had higher levels of Gln than medication-naive patients. Similarly, Soeiro-de Souza et al. (36) and Kubo et al. (69) revealed increased levels of Gln in adult euthymic medicated samples treated with combinations of lithium, anticonvulsants, antipsychotics, and antidepressant but the former study revealed higher Gln levels in their subsample under anticonvulsant treatment in relation to the other group class (Table 9.2). Additionally, Frye et al. (66) observed an increase of Gln in response to lamotrigine treatment and Brennan et al. (35) reported an increased Gln/Glu ratio in BD depression after treatment with riluzole, an antagonist of glutamatergic receptors. Although several studies showed that the elevated Glu concentration remained higher in BD patients in relation to controls even when the influence of medication was statistically removed from their analyses (67, 69, 70), anticonvulsants may likely modulate the conversion of Glu into Gln, whatever may underlie their mood stabilizing mechanism of action.

In fact, mood stabilizers have been shown to modulate the Glu concentration in the brain through multiple mechanisms involving the regulation of synaptic Glu uptake, receptor activity, and intracellular signaling cascade functions (85). While anticonvulsants have been shown to decrease the glutamatergic neurotransmission (85), lithium has been reported to both increase (82, 86, 87) and decrease Glx levels (85, 88), whereby this latter finding was corroborated by a recent systematic review(89).

9.7 Major Depressive Disorder and GABA

GABAergic deficit hypothesis (90) has been proposed for MDD based on several lines of evidence indicating that GABA is reduced in plasma (91, 92), CSF (93), and brain tissue (94) of MDD subjects as compared to HC. Similarly, recent meta-analyses on GABA levels in MDD have consistently shown low brain GABA levels relative to HC in several brain regions such as occipital cortex, parieto-occipital (PO) cortex, ventromedial PFC, and ACC (95–97). Importantly, the separate comparison between depressed and remitted MDD subjects showed that the former revealed significantly lower GABA levels than the latter, which achieved similar levels to controls (96). Similarly, Godfrey et al. (61) have assessed in their meta-analysis GABA levels in 356 MDD patients as compared to 366 HC and found significantly lower GABA levels in MDD patients. When the authors restricted their analyses to the ACC (118 MDD patients and 97 HCs), GABA levels remained lower in MDD patients. However, remitted MDD patients showed similar GABA levels to HC. Accordingly, Table 9.3 demonstrates studies that addressed GABA levels in the ACC of MDD in relation to HC.

Changes in GABA levels are implicated not only in the etiology of MDD (90, 98) but also in its recovery; thus, it is considered a state-dependent rather than a trait marker of MDD (61, 95, 97). In fact, normalization of GABA levels in MDD has been reported in response to treatments(61) with selective serotonin reuptake inhibitors (99) and ECT (100). In this way, GABA appears as a promising tool to assess the treatment response in MDD. However, the correlation between lower GABA levels and depressive symptomatology remains poorly understood. It has

Table 9.2 Glutamate ^{1}H-MRS studies in BD (ACC voxel)

Study	Disorder	N	Mean age (P/C) (years)	Mood state	Quantified metabolites	Medication	Result	Direction
Davanzo et al. (2001)	BD I and II	22	11.4/11.4	Manic	Glx/Cr	Li	NS	Null
Davanzo et al.(2003)	BD I	23	9.8/11.7	Manic/DMS	Glx/Cr	ACV, Li, AP	NS	Null
Dager et al. (2004)	BD I and II	58	30.3/31.9	Depressed/DMS	Glx	Medication Free	NS	IndNullç
Frye et al. (2007)	BD I and II	33	37.5/32.9	Manic/hypomanic	Glx/Cr	NM	NS	Null
Frye et al. (2007)B	BD I and II	35	35.6/33	Depressed	Glx/Cr, Glu/Cr Gln/cr	Medication Free	NA	Null
Moore et al. (2007)	BD I	31	12.6 /12.3	DMS	Glu, Gln	ACV, AP, ADP,	NS	Null
Patel et al. (2008)	BD I	38	15.5/14.6	Depressed	Glx	Medication free	S	Increased
Port et al. (2008)	BD I, BD II, and BD-NOS	42	30.8/31.1	DMS	Glx	Medication free	NS	Null
Öngür et al. (2008)	BD I	36	36.3/34.3	Manic	Glu, Gln	Li, ACV, AP	NS	Null
Strawn et al. (2012)	BD I	40	15.4/14.4	Manic /DMS	Glu, Gln	Li, ACV, AP	NS	Null
Xu et al (2013)	BD I and II	44	34/31	DMS	Glx/Cr, Glu/Cr	Medication free	NS	Null
Soeiro-de-Souza et al (2013)	BD I	80	29/29	Euthymic	Glx/Cr, Glu/Cr	ACV, Li, ADP, and AP	S	Increased
Croarkin et al (2015)	BD I and II	24	NM	Depressed	Glx, Glu	ACV	NS	Null
Ehrlich et al (2015)	BD I	63	45.9/39.3	Euthymic	Glu, Gln	ACV, Li, ADP, and AP	S	Increased
Soeiro-de-Souza et al (2015)	BD I	88	31.7/25.7	Euthymic	Glu, Gln	ACV, Li, ADP, and AP	S	Decreased
Cao et al (2016)	BD I	94	35.7/35.4	DMS	Glu	Li, ACV, ADP, and medication-free	NS	Null
Li et al (2016)	NM	33	31/31.7	Depressed	Glx	Medication free	S	Increased
Galińska-Skok (2016)	BD I	37	43/40.2	DMS	Glx/Cr	Li, Ac, Ap, Ad	NS	Null
Kubo et al (2017)	BD I and II	43	45.0/46.4	DMS	Glu, Gln	ACV, Li, and AP	S	Increased
	BD I and II	39	36.8/38.0	NM	Glu	ACV, Li, ADP and AP	NS	Null

Study		N	Age	Mood state	Metabolite	Medication		
Prisciandaro et al. (2017)								
Soeiro-de-Souza et al. (2018)	BD I	208	32.0/28.1	Euthymic	Glu/Cr, Glu/Cr	ACV, Li, and AP	S	Increased
Wise 2018	NM	29	31.44/30	Depressed	Glu/cr	MF	NS	Null

Glu- glutamate, Gln- glutamine, Cr- creatine, BD- Bipolar disorder, NOS- not otherwise specified, DMS- diverse mood states, ACV- anticonvulsants, ADP- antidepressants, AP- antipsychotics, BZD- benzodiazepines, Li- lithium, S- significant, NS- not significant, NM- not mentioned

Table 9.3 GABA ^{1}H-MRS studies in MDD (ACC voxel)

Study	Disorder	N	Mean age (P/C) (years)	Mood state	Quantified metabolite	Medication	Result	Direction
Price et al. (2009)	MDD	57	42.4/37.2	Depressed	GABA	Medication free	NS	Null
Walter et al. (2009)	MDD	43	40/34.6	Depressed	GABA	Medication free	NS	Null
Gabbay et al. (2012)	MDD	41	16.7/16.2	Depressed	GABA/water	Medication free	S	Decreased
Wang et al. (2016)	MDD	32	53.9/ 52.6	Depressed	GABA	Medication free	S	Decreased
Gabbay et al. (2017)	MDD	80	16.3/15.8	Depressed	GABA/water	Medication free	S	Decreased

MDD- unipolar major depressive disorder, S- significant, NS- not significant.

been demonstrated in animal models that chronic stress causes a presynaptic GABA decrease and downregulation of postsynaptic GABA-A receptors (101). Such a GABA decrease in frontal areas might result in a dysregulation of excitatory and inhibitory neurotransmission, leading to alterations in mood and cognition. However, depressive episodes are per se stressful events for those who suffer from MDD and the lower GABA levels might also be a result rather than a cause of the disease. Longitudinal studies assessing GABA levels along several mood episodes would better clarify this issue.

9.8 Bipolar Disorder and GABA

Previous reviews and meta-analyses did not find significant differences in GABA concentration in BD in relation to HC (95, 96). Chiapponi et al. (95) investigated five studies (Table 9.4) about GABA levels in the brain and BD and concluded that given the heterogeneity of the studies it was not possible to state that GABA is different from controls in BD brain. Among these studies, Wang et al. (102) reported higher GABA/Cre ratios in the occipital and PFC regions in a sample of sixteen medicated BD subjects (euthymia, mania, and depression)(102) while Bhagwagar et al. (72) examined the ACC of sixteen unmedicated "recovered" BD patients and eighteen controls and found lower GABA/Cre ratios in the BD group (72). In contrast, Kaufman and colleagues (103) examined the PO and thalamic regions of thirteen BD patients (euthymia, mania, and depression) and eleven controls, reporting no between-group differences (103).

Similarly, among the fewer studies that have examined GABA levels in the ACC of BD patients in relation to HC (Table 9.4), it has been reported increased levels in BD or no significant differences. While Brady and colleagues (13) examined fourteen euthymic BD type I patients and fourteen controls and found higher GABA/Cre ratios in the ACC and also PO cortex of BD patients compared to controls (13), the other studies that measured GABA have reported no differences in these metabolite levels compared to HC in both the basal ganglia (104) and ACC (36, 105). Such contradictory results may be explained by variations in ^{1}H-MRS acquisition methods, brain regions investigated, metabolite quantification and normalization strategies, sample characteristics, and medication status, hampering interpretation of these conflicting findings.

Additionally, there is neither any follow-up study assessing GABA across mood states (hypomania, mania, depression, and euthymia) in BD nor comparing GABA levels between bipolar and unipolar depression (97), which would provide clues on the role of this metabolite in these disorders. However, there are some potential explanations for contrasting between GABA data for MDD and BD. First, there is a larger number of studies that assessed GABA in MDD as compared to BD. Second, it is still a challenge to derive a reliable GABA signal from ^{1}H-MRS spectra and disentangle it from the macromolecular signal, which requires a special ^{1}H-MRS acquisition technique (106). Third, most patients in BD studies were medicated with a combination of lithium, anticonvulsants, antidepressants, and antipsychotics. Since anticonvulsants, benzodiazepines, and antidepressants are known to modulate GABA levels (99, 107), the conflicting findings may likely be influenced by the medication effect. In contrast, as observed for the ACC (Table 9.3), most studies that assessed GABA in MDD, the patients were medication-free, thus providing less biased results.

9.9 Concluding Remarks and Clinical Relevance

There is a considerable body of evidence of glutamatergic and GABAergic abnormalities in mood disorders, likely due to an excitatory/inhibitory imbalance. The Glu and GABA balance in the developing brain is implicated in key processes such as neural migration, differentiation, and synaptic plasticity (2, 4), and consequently the normal adult brain function (108). Thus, it has been proposed that the mood instability and cognitive impairments observed in mood disorders, namely MDD and BD, may result from an excitatory/inhibitory imbalance in cortical regions involved in affect and cognitive regulation as the ACC (109, 110).

Glutamatergic abnormalities have been consistently reported for both BD and MDD. Increased Glu levels have been reported in several cortical regions in BD (8, 73–75), which could be considered a trait marker for this disorder since it has been observed in all mood states. The most accepted theory for the deleterious effects of Glu hyperactivity to cells is based on evidence that a supraphysiological

Table 9.4 GABA ¹H-MRS studies in BD (ACC voxel)

Study	Disorder	N	Mean age (P/C) (years)	Mood state	Quantified metabolite	Medication	Result	Direction
Wang et al. (102)	BD I and BD II	21	34.4/37.2	DMS	GABA/Cr	Li, ACV, AP	S	Increased
Brady et al. (13)	BD I	28	32.6/36.9	Euthymic	GABA/Cr	Li, ACV, ADP, AP, BZD	S	Increased
Soeiro-de-Souza et al. (2015)	BD I	88	31.7/25.7	Euthymic	GABA	Li, ACV, ADP, AP, BZD	NS	Null
Prisciandaro et al. (2017)	BDI and II	39	36.8/38.0	Depressed	GABA/water	Li, ACV,ADP, AP	NS	Null
Huber et al. (2018)	BD I, BD II and BD-NOS	29	17.5/19	Depressed	GABA	NM	NS	Null

Caption: BD- Bipolar disorder, NOS- not otherwise specified, Cr- creatine, DMS – diverse mood states, ACV- anticonvulsants, ADP- antidepressants, AP- antipsychotics, BZD- benzodiazepines, Li- lithium, S- significant, NS- not significant, NM- not mentioned.

activation of the glutamatergic receptors may result in an increased intracellular Ca^{2+} concentration, leading to the activation of Ca^{2+}-dependent enzymes, causing mitochondrial Ca^{2+} overload, oxidative stress and stimulation of apoptotic pathways, resulting, ultimately, in neurotoxicity and neuronal death (74, 111). Therefore, cortical reductions in frontal regions observed in BD (59) may result in part from such hyperglutamatergic state, leading to cognitive and affective dysfunction. Conversely, lower Glu levels have been documented in frontal regions in MDD such as the ACC (61) and mPFC (61, 62), which is considered an indicator of severity and poorer outcome (110). Thus, it has been suggested that successive depressive episodes may result in lower synaptic strength and consequent reduced Glu neurotransmission.

GABAergic abnormalities have also been implicated in mood disorders, particularly in MDD. Reduced GABA levels have been found in several cortical regions in MDD, and its recovery has been associated with the treatment response, thus, it is considered a state-dependent trait marker of MDD (95–97). Such reduced GABA levels observed in MDD has been associated with chronic stress (101) and maybe either a causative factor or a consequence of consecutive depressive episodes. On the other hand, GABA neuroimaging data have provided less positive consistent results for BD than MDD, likely because the positive studies in MDD were executed with medication-free patients, which is harder to achieve in BD than in MDD.

Overall, there is converging evidence of altered Glu levels in both BD and MDD and GABAergic abnormalities only in MDD. Thus, changes in the excitatory/inhibitory neurotransmission, particularly in frontal regions as the ACC, seem to be associated with mood and cognition alterations observed in both disorders. However, the methodological variability across studies (different voxel sizes and locations, acquisition, and post-processing techniques in multiple mood states and BD subtypes in the same sample and possible medication effects) precludes any further conclusions from being drawn. Besides, very few studies have examined simultaneously and longitudinally both neurometabolites Glu and GABA in mood disorders, which would enable us a better understanding of their roles in the neurobiology of BD and MDD and the clinical implications.

Since the frontal areas such as the ACC are associated with cognitive and affective function, and it has been demonstrated reductions of these cortical regions in BD (59), we may infer that the hyperglutamatergic state may underlie the structural and functional changes observed in this region. Additionally, more research is required to understand the longitudinal dynamic changes in Glu levels across the different mood states, would enable us a better understanding of the connections of glutamatergic alterations and BD symptoms. On the other hand, it seems that GABA neuroimage has less positive data in BD than MDD, maybe because the positive studies in MDD were executed with medication-free patients, which is harder to achieve in BD than in MDD.

Further ^{1}H-MRS studies at higher magnetic fields with more sensitive sequences should investigate specific BD subtypes and mood states to increase understanding of the Glu system in BD and help develop novel pharmacological approaches based on the glutamatergic system. Considering that previous studies in patients during mania (40, 112) as well as unipolar and bipolar depressions(65, 66, 110) have indicated altered Glu system metabolites in mood disorders, we may hypothesize that such abnormalities might be a putative neurobiological endophenotype for mood disorders. However, ^{1}H-MRS studies are needed to confirm this hypothesis by comparing not only affected and unaffected subjects but also unaffected first-degree relatives, which so far has not been the case (113).

References

1. Francis PT, Poynton A, Lowe SL, et al. Brain amino acid concentrations and Ca2+-dependent release in intractable depression assessed antemortem. *Brain Res.* 1989; **494**(2): 315–324.

2. Stagg CJ, Bestmann S, Constantinescu AO, et al. Relationship between physiological measures of excitability and levels of glutamate and GABA in the human motor cortex. *J Physiol (Lond).* 2011; **589** (Pt 23): 5845–5855.

3. Eastwood SL, Harrison PJ. Markers of glutamate synaptic transmission and plasticity are increased in the anterior cingulate cortex in bipolar disorder. *Biol Psychiatry.* 2010; **67**(11): 1010–1016.

4. Rossignol E. Genetics and function of neocortical GABAergic interneurons in neurodevelopmental disorders. *Neural Plast*. 2011; **2011**: 649325.

5. Fatemi SH, Hossein Fatemi S, Stary JM, et al. GABAergic dysfunction in schizophrenia and mood disorders as reflected by decreased levels of glutamic acid decarboxylase 65 and 67 kDa and Reelin proteins in cerebellum. *Schizophr Res*. 2005; **72**(2–3): 109–122.

6. Torrey EF, Barci BM, Webster MJ, et al. Neurochemical markers for schizophrenia, bipolar disorder, and major depression in postmortem brains. Biol Psychiatry. 2005; **57**(3): 252–260.

7. Ongür D, Drevets WC, Price JL. Glial reduction in the subgenual prefrontal cortex in mood disorders. *Proc Natl Acad Sci USA*. 1998; **95**(22): 13290–13295.

8. Yüksel C, Ongur D. Magnetic resonance spectroscopy studies of glutamate-related abnormalities in mood disorders. *Biol Psychiatry*. 2010; **68**(9): 785–794.

9. Cotter DR, Pariante CM, Everall IP. Glial cell abnormalities in major psychiatric disorders: the evidence and implications. *Brain Res Bull*. 2001; **55**(5): 585–595.

10. Machado-Vieira R, Salvadore G, Ibrahim LA, Diaz-Granados N, Zarate CA. Targeting glutamatergic signaling for the development of novel therapeutics for mood disorders. *Curr Pharm Des*. 2009; **15**(14): 1595–1611.

11. Machado-Vieira R, Manji HK, Zarate CA. The role of the tripartite glutamatergic synapse in the pathophysiology and therapeutics of mood disorders. *Neuroscientist*. 2009; **15**(5): 525–539.

12. Kim JS, Schmid-Burgk W, Claus D, Kornhuber HH. Increased serum glutamate in depressed patients. *Arch Psychiatr Nervenkr*. 1982; **232**(4): 299–304.

13. Brady RO, McCarthy JM, Prescot AP, et al. Brain gamma-aminobutyric acid (GABA) abnormalities in bipolar disorder. *Bipolar Disord*. 2013; **15**(4): 434–439.

14. Altamura CA, Mauri MC, Ferrara A, et al. Plasma and platelet excitatory amino acids in psychiatric disorders. *Am J Psychiatry*. 1993; **150**(11): 1731–1733.

15. Mauri MC, Ferrara A, Boscati L, et al. Plasma and platelet amino acid concentrations in patients affected by major depression and under fluvoxamine treatment. *Neuropsychobiology*. 1998; **37**(3): 124–129.

16. Rajkowska G. Cell pathology in mood disorders. *Semin Clin Neuropsychiatry*. 2002; **7**(4): 281–292.

17. Levine J, Panchalingam K, Rapoport A et al. Increased cerebrospinal fluid glutamine levels in depressed patients. *Biol Psychiatry*. 2000; **47**(7): 586–593.

18. Hashimoto K, Sawa A, Iyo M. Increased levels of glutamate in brains from patients with mood disorders. *Biol Psychiatry*. 2007; **62**(11): 1310–1316.

19. Frye MA, Tsai GE, Huggins T, Coyle JT, Post RM. Low cerebrospinal fluid glutamate and glycine in refractory affective disorder. *Biol Psychiatry*. 2007; **61**(2): 162–166.

20. Gerner RH, Fairbanks L, Anderson GM, et al. CSF neurochemistry in depressed, manic, and schizophrenic patients compared with that of normal controls. *Am J Psychiatry*. 1984; **141**(12): 1533–1540.

21. Berrettini WH, Nurnberger JI, Hare TA, Simmons-Alling S, Gershon ES. CSF GABA in euthymic manic-depressive patients and controls. *Biol Psychiatry*. 1986; **21**(8–9): 844–846.

22. Rajkowska G. Postmortem studies in mood disorders indicate altered numbers of neurons and glial cells. *Biol Psychiatry*. 2000; **48**(8): 766–777.

23. Trullas R, Skolnick P. Functional antagonists at the NMDA receptor complex exhibit antidepressant actions. *Eur J Pharmacol*. 1990; **185**(1): 1–10.

24. Berman RM, Cappiello A, Anand A, et al. Antidepressant effects of ketamine in depressed patients. *Biol Psychiatry*. 2000; **47**(4): 351–354.

25. Mathew SJ, Shah A, Lapidus K, et al. Ketamine for treatment-resistant unipolar depression: Current evidence. *CNS Drugs*. 2012; **26**(3): 189–204.

26. Zarate CA, Brutsche NE, Ibrahim L, et al. Replication of ketamine's antidepressant efficacy in bipolar depression: A randomized controlled add-on trial. *Biol Psychiatry*. 2012; **71**(11): 939–946.

27. Govindaraju V, Young K, Maudsley AA. Proton NMR chemical shifts and coupling constants for brain metabolites. *NMR Biomed*. 2000; **13**(3): 129–153.

28. Hashimoto R, Hough C, Nakazawa T, Yamamoto T, Chuang D-M. Lithium protection against glutamate excitotoxicity in rat cerebral cortical neurons: Involvement of NMDA receptor inhibition possibly by decreasing NR2B tyrosine phosphorylation. *J Neurochem*. 2002; **80**(4): 589–597.

29. Kumar A, Singh RL, Babu GN. Cell death mechanisms in the early stages of acute glutamate neurotoxicity. *Neurosci Res*. 2010; **66**(3): 271–278.

30. Gigante AD, Young LT, Yatham LN, et al. Morphometric post-mortem studies in bipolar disorder: Possible association with oxidative stress

and apoptosis. *Int J Neuropsychopharmacol.* 2011; **14**(8): 1075–1089.

31. Martinez-Hernandez A, Bell KP, Norenberg MD. Glutamine synthetase: Glial localization in brain. *Science.* 1977; **195**(4284): 1356–1358.

32. Waagepetersen HS, Sonnewald U, Schousboe A. Glutamine, Glutamate, and GABA: metabolic aspects. In: Lajtha A, Oja S, Schousboe A, Saransaari P, editors. *Handbook of Neurochemistry and Molecular Neurobiology: Amino Acids and Peptides in the Nervous System.* New York: Springer; 2007, pp. 1–21.

33. Rothman DL, De Feyter HM, de Graaf RA, Mason GF, Behar KL. 13 C MRS studies of neuroenergetics and neurotransmitter cycling in humans. *NMR Biomed.* 2011; **24**(8): 943–957.

34. Daikhin Y, Yudkoff M. Compartmentation of brain glutamate metabolism in neurons and glia. *J Nutr.* 2000; **130**(4S Suppl): 1026S–1031S.

35. Brennan BP, Hudson JI, Jensen JE, et al. Rapid enhancement of glutamatergic neurotransmission in bipolar depression following treatment with riluzole. *Neuropsychopharmacology.* 2010; **35**(3): 834–846.

36. Soeiro de Souza MG, Henning A, Machado-Vieira R, et al. Anterior cingulate Glutamate-Glutamine cycle metabolites are altered in euthymic bipolar I disorder. *Eur Neuropsychopharmacol.* 2015; **25** (12): 2221–2229.

37. Igarashi H, Kwee IL, Nakada T, Katayama Y, Terashi A. 1 H magnetic resonance spectroscopic imaging of permanent focal cerebral ischemia in rat: Longitudinal metabolic changes in ischemic core and rim. *Brain Res.* 2001; **907**(1–2): 208–221.

38. Iltis I, Koski DM, Eberly LE, et al. Neurochemical changes in the rat prefrontal cortex following acute phencyclidine treatment: An in vivo localized (1)H MRS study. *NMR Biomed.* 2009; **22**(7): 737–744.

39. Mlynárik V, Kohler I, Gambarota G, et al. Quantitative proton spectroscopic imaging of the neurochemical profile in rat brain with microliter resolution at ultra-short echo times. *Magn Reson Med.* 2008; **59**(1): 52–58.

40. Ongur D, Jensen JE, Prescot AP, et al. Abnormal glutamatergic neurotransmission and neuronal-glial interactions in acute mania. *Biol Psychiatry.* 2008; **64**(8): 718–726.

41. Théberge J, Bartha R, Drost DJ, et al. Glutamate and glutamine measured with 4.0 T proton MRS in never-treated patients with schizophrenia and healthy volunteers. *Am J Psychiatry.* 2002; **159**(11): 1944–1946.

42. Théberge J, Al-Semaan Y, Williamson PC, et al. Glutamate and glutamine in the anterior cingulate and thalamus of medicated patients with chronic schizophrenia and healthy comparison subjects measured with 4.0-T proton MRS. *Am J Psychiatry.* 2003; **160**(12): 2231–2233.

43. Erlander MG, Tillakaratne NJ, Feldblum S, Patel N, Tobin AJ. Two genes encode distinct glutamate decarboxylases. *Neuron.* 1991; **7**(1): 91–100.

44. Bu DF, Erlander MG, Hitz BC, et al. Two human glutamate decarboxylases, 65-kDa GAD and 67-kDa GAD, are each encoded by a single gene. *Proc Natl Acad Sci USA.* 1992; **89**(6): 2115–2119.

45. Guidotti A, Auta J, Davis JM, et al. Decrease in reelin and glutamic acid decarboxylase67 (GAD67) expression in schizophrenia and bipolar disorder: a postmortem brain study. *Arch Gen Psychiatry.* 2000; **57**(11): 1061–1069.

46. Heckers S, Stone D, Walsh J, et al. Differential hippocampal expression of glutamic acid decarboxylase 65 and 67 messenger RNA in bipolar disorder and schizophrenia. *Arch Gen Psychiatry.* 2002; **59**(6): 521–529.

47. Woo T-UW, Walsh JP, Benes FM. Density of glutamic acid decarboxylase 67 messenger RNA-containing neurons that express the N-methyl-D aspartate receptor subunit NR2A in the anterior cingulate cortex in schizophrenia and bipolar disorder. *Arch Gen Psychiatry.* 2004; **61**(7): 649–657.

48. Thompson M, Weickert CS, Wyatt E, Webster MJ. Decreased glutamic acid decarboxylase(67) mRNA expression in multiple brain areas of patients with schizophrenia and mood disorders. *J Psychiatr Res.* 2009; **43**(11): 970–977.

49. Maddock RJ, Buonocore MH. MR spectroscopic studies of the brain in psychiatric disorders. *Curr Top Behav Neurosci.* 2012; **11**: 199–251.

50. Cooper AJL, Jeitner TM. Central role of glutamate metabolism in the maintenance of nitrogen homeostasis in normal and hyperammonemic brain. *Biomolecules.* 2016 March 26; **6**(2): 16.

51. Walls AB, Waagepetersen HS, Bak LK, Schousboe A, Sonnewald U. The glutamine-glutamate/GABA cycle: Function, regional differences in glutamate and GABA production and effects of interference with GABA metabolism. *Neurochem Res.* 2015; **40**(2): 402–409.

52. Buonocore MH, Maddock RJ. Magnetic resonance spectroscopy of the brain: A review of physical principles and technical methods. *Rev Neurosci.* 2015; **26**(6): 609–632.

53. Bush G, Luu P, Posner M. Cognitive and emotional influences in anterior cingulate cortex. *Trends Cogn Sci (Regul Ed).* 2000; **4**(6): 215–222.

54. Strakowski SM, Adler CM, Almeida J, et al. The functional neuroanatomy of bipolar disorder: A consensus model. *Bipolar Disord*. 2012 June; **14**(4): 313–325. DOI:10.1111/j.1399-5618.2012.01022.x.

55. Drevets WC, Price JL, Simpson JR, et al. Subgenual prefrontal cortex abnormalities in mood disorders. *Nature*. 1997; **386**(6627): 824–827.

56. Haldane M, Frangou S. New insights help define the pathophysiology of bipolar affective disorder: Neuroimaging and neuropathology findings. *Prog Neuropsychopharmacol Biol Psychiatry*. 2004; **28** (6): 943–960.

57. Savitz JB, Price JL, Drevets WC. Neuropathological and neuromorphometric abnormalities in bipolar disorder: View from the medial prefrontal cortical network. *Neurosci Biobehav Rev*. 2014; **42**: 132–147.

58. Drevets WC, Savitz J, Trimble M. The subgenual anterior cingulate cortex in mood disorders. *CNS Spectr*. 2008; **13**(8): 663–681.

59. Hibar DP, Westlye LT, Doan NT, et al. Cortical abnormalities in bipolar disorder: An MRI analysis of 6503 individuals from the ENIGMA Bipolar Disorder Working Group. *Mol Psychiatry*. 2018 April; **23**(4): 932–942.

60. McGirr A, Berlim MT, Bond DJ, et al. A systematic review and meta-analysis of randomized controlled trials of adjunctive ketamine in electroconvulsive therapy: Efficacy and tolerability. *J Psychiatr Res*. 2015; **62**: 23–30.

61. Godfrey KEM, Gardner AC, Kwon S, Chea W, Muthukumaraswamy SD. Differences in excitatory and inhibitory neurotransmitter levels between depressed patients and healthy controls: A systematic review and meta-analysis. *J Psychiatr Res*. 2018; **105**: 33–44.

62. Moriguchi S, Takamiya A, Noda Y, et al. Glutamatergic neurometabolite levels in major depressive disorder: A systematic review and meta-analysis of proton magnetic resonance spectroscopy studies. *Mol Psychiatry*. 2019; **24**: 952–964.

63. Arnone D, Mumuni AN, Jauhar S, Condon B, Cavanagh J. Indirect evidence of selective glial involvement in glutamate-based mechanisms of mood regulation in depression: Meta-analysis of absolute prefrontal neuro-metabolic concentrations. *Eur Neuropsychopharmacol*. 2015; **25**(8): 1109–1117.

64. Luykx JJ, Laban KG, van den Heuvel MP, et al. Region and state specific glutamate downregulation in major depressive disorder: A meta-analysis of (1)H-MRS findings. *Neurosci Biobehav Rev*. 2012; **36**(1): 198–205.

65. Dager SR, Friedman SD, Parow A, et al. Brain metabolic alterations in medication-free patients with bipolar disorder. *Arch Gen Psychiatry*. 2004; **61**(5): 450–458.

66. Frye MA, Watzl J, Banakar S, et al. Increased anterior cingulate/medial prefrontal cortical glutamate and creatine in bipolar depression. *Neuropsychopharmacology*. 2007; **32**(12): 2490–2499.

67. Soeiro de Souza MG, Salvadore G, Moreno RA, et al. Bcl-2 rs956572 polymorphism is associated with increased anterior cingulate cortical glutamate in euthymic bipolar I disorder. *Neuropsychopharmacology*. 2013; **38**(3): 468–475.

68. Ehrlich A, Schubert F, Pehrs C, Gallinat J. Alterations of cerebral glutamate in the euthymic state of patients with bipolar disorder. *Psychiatry Res*. 2015; **233**(2): 73–80.

69. Kubo H, Nakataki M, Sumitani S, et al. 1 H-magnetic resonance spectroscopy study of glutamate-related abnormality in bipolar disorder. *J Affect Disord*. 2017; **208**: 139–144.

70. Soeiro de Souza MG, Otaduy MCG, Machado-Vieira R, et al. Anterior cingulate cortex glutamatergic metabolites and mood stabilizers in euthymic bipolar I disorder patients: A proton magnetic resonance spectroscopy study. *Biol Psychiatry Cogn Neurosci Neuroimaging*. 2018 December; **3**(12): 985–991.

71. Michael N, Erfurth A, Ohrmann P, et al. Metabolic changes within the left dorsolateral prefrontal cortex occurring with electroconvulsive therapy in patients with treatment resistant unipolar depression. *Psychol Med*. 2003; **33**(7): 1277–1284.

72. Bhagwagar Z, Wylezinska M, Jezzard P, et al. Reduction in occipital cortex gamma-aminobutyric acid concentrations in medication-free recovered unipolar depressed and bipolar subjects. *Biol Psychiatry*. 2007; **61**(6): 806–812.

73. Yildiz-Yesiloglu A, Ankerst DP. Neurochemical alterations of the brain in bipolar disorder and their implications for pathophysiology: A systematic review of the in vivo proton magnetic resonance spectroscopy findings. *Prog Neuropsychopharmacol Biol Psychiatry*. 2006; **30**(6): 969–995.

74. Gigante AD, Bond DJ, Lafer B, et al. Brain glutamate levels measured by magnetic resonance spectroscopy in patients with bipolar disorder: A meta-analysis. *Bipolar Disord*. 2012; **14**(5): 478–487.

75. Chitty KM, Lagopoulos J, Lee RSC, Hickie IB, Hermens DF. A systematic review and meta-analysis of proton magnetic resonance

spectroscopy and mismatch negativity in bipolar disorder. *Eur Neuropsychopharmacol.* 2013; **23**(11): 1348–1363.

76. Drevets WC. Functional anatomical abnormalities in limbic and prefrontal cortical structures in major depression. *Prog Brain Res.* 2000; **126**: 413–431.

77. Phillips ML, Drevets WC, Rauch SL, Lane R. Neurobiology of emotion perception I: The neural basis of normal emotion perception. *Biol Psychiatry.* 2003; **54**(5): 504–514.

78. Anticevic A, Savic A, Repovs G, et al. Ventral anterior cingulate connectivity distinguished nonpsychotic bipolar illness from psychotic bipolar disorder and schizophrenia. Schizophr Bull. 2015; **41**(1): 133–143.

79. Liu J, Blond BN, van Dyck LI, et al. Trait and state corticostriatal dysfunction in bipolar disorder during emotional face processing. *Bipolar Disord.* 2012; **14**(4): 432–441.

80. Foland-Ross LC, Thompson PM, Sugar CA, et al. Investigation of cortical thickness abnormalities in lithium-free adults with bipolar I disorder using cortical pattern matching. *Am J Psychiatry.* 2011; **168**(5): 530–539.

81. Patel NC, DelBello MP, Cecil KM, et al. Temporal change in N-acetyl-aspartate concentrations in adolescents with bipolar depression treated with lithium. *J Child Adolesc Psychopharmacol.* 2008; **18**(2): 132–139.

82. Colla M, Schubert F, Bubner M, et al. Glutamate as a spectroscopic marker of hippocampal structural plasticity is elevated in long-term euthymic bipolar patients on chronic lithium therapy and correlates inversely with diurnal cortisol. *Mol Psychiatry.* 2009; **14**(7): 696–704, 647.

83. Senaratne R, Milne AM, MacQueen GM, Hall GBC. Increased choline-containing compounds in the orbitofrontal cortex and hippocampus in euthymic patients with bipolar disorder: A proton magnetic resonance spectroscopy study. *Psychiatry Res.* 2009; **172**(3): 205–209.

84. Moore CM, Frazier JA, Glod CA, et al. Glutamine and glutamate levels in children and adolescents with bipolar disorder: A 4.0-T proton magnetic resonance spectroscopy study of the anterior cingulate cortex. *J Am Acad Child Adolesc Psychiatry.* 2007; **46**(4): 524–534.

85. Friedman SD, Dager SR, Parow A, et al. Lithium and valproic acid treatment effects on brain chemistry in bipolar disorder. *Biol Psychiatry.* 2004; **56**(5): 340–348.

86. Machado-Vieira R, Gattaz WF, Zanetti MV, et al. A longitudinal (6-week) 3 T (1)H-MRS study on the effects of lithium treatment on anterior cingulate cortex metabolites in bipolar depression. *Eur Neuropsychopharmacol.* 2015; **25**(12): 2311–2317.

87. Zanetti MV, Otaduy MC, de Sousa RT, et al. Bimodal effect of lithium plasma levels on hippocampal glutamate concentrations in bipolar II depression: A pilot study. *Int J Neuropsychopharmacol.* 2014 October 31; **18** (6): pyu058.

88. O'Donnell T, Rotzinger S, Nakashima TT, et al. Chronic lithium and sodium valproate both decrease the concentration of myo-inositol and increase the concentration of inositol monophosphates in rat brain. *Brain Res.* 2000; **880**(1–2): 84–91.

89. Szulc A, Wiedlocha M, Waszkiewicz N, et al. Proton magnetic resonance spectroscopy changes after lithium treatment. *Systematic review.* *Psychiatry Res Neuroimaging.* 2018; **273**: 1–8.

90. Luscher B, Shen Q, Sahir N. The GABAergic deficit hypothesis of major depressive disorder. *Mol Psychiatry.* 2011; **16**(4): 383–406.

91. Petty F, Schlesser MA. Plasma GABA in affective illness. *A Preliminary Investigation. J Affect Disord.* 1981; **3**(4): 339–343.

92. Petty F, Sherman AD. Plasma GABA levels in psychiatric illness. *J Affect Disord.* 1984; **6**(2): 131–138.

93. Gerner RH, Hare TA. CSF GABA in normal subjects and patients with depression, schizophrenia, mania, and anorexia nervosa. *Am J Psychiatry.* 1981; **138**(8): 1098–1101.

94. Honig A, Bartlett JR, Bouras N, Bridges PK. Amino acid levels in depression: A preliminary investigation. *J Psychiatr Res.* 1988; **22**(3): 159–164.

95. Chiapponi C, Piras F, Piras F, Caltagirone C, Spalletta G. GABA system in schizophrenia and mood disorders: A mini review on third-generation imaging studies. *Front Psychiatry.* 2016; **7**: 61.

96. Schür RR, Draisma LWR, Wijnen JP, et al. Brain GABA levels across psychiatric disorders: A systematic literature review and meta-analysis of (1) H-MRS studies. *Hum Brain Mapp.* 2016; **37**(9): 3337–3352.

97. Romeo B, Choucha W, Fossati P, Rotge J-Y. Meta-analysis of central and peripheral γ-aminobutyric acid levels in patients with unipolar and bipolar depression. *J Psychiatry Neurosci.* 2018; **43**(1): 58–66.

98. Kalueff AV, Nutt DJ. Role of GABA in anxiety and depression. *Depress Anxiety.* 2007; **24**(7): 495–517.

99. Sanacora G, Mason GF, Rothman DL, Krystal JH. Increased occipital cortex GABA concentrations in depressed patients after therapy with selective serotonin reuptake inhibitors. *Am J Psychiatry.* 2002; **159**(4): 663–665.

100. Sanacora G, Mason GF, Rothman DL, et al. Increased cortical GABA concentrations in depressed patients receiving ECT. *Am J Psychiatry.* 2003; **160**(3): 577–579.

101. Verkuyl JM, Hemby SE, Joëls M. Chronic stress attenuates GABAergic inhibition and alters gene expression of parvocellular neurons in rat hypothalamus. *Eur J Neurosci.* 2004; **20**(6): 1665–1673.

102. Wang PW, Sailasuta N, Chandler RA, Ketter TA. Magnetic resonance spectroscopy measurement of cerebral gamma-aminobutyric acid concentrations in patients with bipolar disorders. *Acta Neuropsychiatrica.* 2006; **18**: 120–126.

103. Kaufman RE, Ostacher MJ, Marks EH, et al. Brain GABA levels in patients with bipolar disorder. *Prog Neuropsychopharmacol Biol Psychiatry.* 2009; **33**(3): 427–434.

104. Godlewska BR, Yip SW, Near J, Goodwin GM, Cowen PJ. Cortical glutathione levels in young people with bipolar disorder: A pilot study using magnetic resonance spectroscopy. *Psychopharmacology (Berl).* 2014; **231**(2): 327–332.

105. Prisciandaro JJ, Tolliver BK, Prescot AP, et al. Unique prefrontal GABA and glutamate disturbances in co-occurring bipolar disorder and alcohol dependence. *Transl Psychiatry.* 2017; 7(7): e1163.

106. Levy LM, Degnan AJ. GABA-based evaluation of neurologic conditions: MR spectroscopy. *AJNR Am J Neuroradiol.* 2013; **34**(2): 259–265.

107. Mesdjian E, Ciesielski L, Valli M, et al. Sodium valproate: Kinetic profile and effects on GABA levels in various brain areas of the rat. *Prog Neuropsychopharmacol Biol Psychiatry.* 1982; **6**(3): 223–233.

108. Rubenstein JLR, Merzenich MM. Model of autism: Increased ratio of excitation/inhibition in key neural systems. *Genes Brain Behav.* 2003; **2**(5): 255–267.

109. Krystal JH, Sanacora G, Blumberg H, et al. Glutamate and GABA systems as targets for novel antidepressant and mood-stabilizing treatments. *Mol Psychiatry.* 2002; 7(Suppl 1): S71–80.

110. Lener MS, Niciu MJ, Ballard ED, et al. Glutamate and gamma-aminobutyric acid systems in the pathophysiology of major depression and antidepressant response to ketamine. *Biol Psychiatry.* 2017; **81**(10): 886–897.

111. Soeiro de Souza MG, Machado-Vieira R, Soares Bio D, Do Prado CM, Moreno RA. COMT polymorphisms as predictors of cognitive dysfunction during manic and mixed episodes in bipolar I disorder. *Bipolar Disord.* 2012; **14**(5): 554–564.

112. Michael N, Erfurth A, Ohrmann P, et al. Acute mania is accompanied by elevated glutamate/glutamine levels within the left dorsolateral prefrontal cortex. *Psychopharmacology (Berl).* 2003; **168**(3): 344–346.

113. Hajek T, Bernier D, Slaney C, et al. A comparison of affected and unaffected relatives of patients with bipolar disorder using proton magnetic resonance spectroscopy. *J Psychiatry Neurosci.* 2008; **33**(6): 531–540.

Chapter 10

Neuroimaging Brain Inflammation in Mood Disorders

Jeffrey H. Meyer

10.1 Introduction

Neuroimaging with positron emission tomography is increasingly developing radioligands that emulate targets traditionally within the domain of postmortem studies. Consequently, markers indicative of neuroinflammatory processes are advancing and enabling rapid assessment of the neuroinflammatory theory of major depressive disorder (MDD). One marker, translocator protein (TSPO), has now had a significant number of investigations in MDD and it is anticipated that investigations of other neuroinflammatory markers will be extended into mood disorders. Of these measures, neuroimaging of monoamine oxidase B demonstrates promising differences between MDD and health. These investigations offer novel potential to stratify MDD by abnormality of neuroinflammatory markers, investigate neuroprogression and assess effects of therapeutics on neuroinflammation in clinical settings.

10.2 Rationale for Neuroimaging Inflammation in Mood Disorders

A strong argument for neuroinflammation to be present in mood disorders is that greater peripheral inflammation is often associated with symptoms found in mood disorders. For example, by the early 2010s, the majority of investigations of peripheral inflammatory markers reported greater plasma levels of the cytokines IL-6 and TNF-α, and to some extent C-reactive protein during MDD, indicating that excessive peripheral inflammation occurs in at least a subset of MDD (1, 2). Another example is that increasing peripheral inflammation may induce depressive symptoms: Twenty to fifty percent of people receiving chronic interferon (IFN-α) treatment for infections or cancer have major depressive episode

(MDE), anxiety, and anorexia (3, 4). Similarly IFN-α treatment is also associated with depressive behaviors in rodents. Also more broadly, inducing peripheral inflammation (e.g., via vaccinations or lipopolysaccharide administration) elicits depression, anxiety, and decreased food intake in humans (5, 6) and rodents (7, 8). While these examples are compelling, several limitations should be mentioned, including that investigations of peripheral inflammation in MDE during 2000–2010 often did not control for body mass index (1, 2), with some investigations comparing MDE with high BMI to healthy with normative BMI; and that it is not established in humans that peripheral inflammation is fully predictive of brain inflammation.

Even so, it is notable that diseases associated with bodily and brain inflammation are associated with particularly high prevalence of mood disorders. Inflammatory bowel disease, a disease with well-established robust peripheral inflammation, is associated with three to five times the usual prevalence of mood disorders. Traumatic brain injury (TBI), which induces brain inflammation (9–12), is frequently associated with depressed mood (13) with 30–50% prevalence of MDE in the first year after TBI (14, 15). Lifetime rates of MDE in systemic lupus erythematosis and multiple sclerosis, illnesses with brain inflammation, are about 50%, which is, again, much higher than the general population (16–21).

The alternative to neuroimaging inflammation is to investigate with postmortem studies and while each offer complementary information, it is more difficult to recruit mood disorder subjects for postmortem studies than for imaging studies. Consistent with this, the majority of studies of inflammatory markers in the brain of mood disorders are either underpowered for moderate effect sizes in mood disorders or they focused on suicide instead. In a sample of twenty-four teenaged suicide victims (seven with MDE) and twenty-four controls, Pandey et al. (22) reported greater levels of IL-6, TNF-α, and IL-1β in the prefrontal cortex. In a postmortem micro-array study of the prefrontal cortex in fourteen medication-free MDE subjects and fourteen healthy, Shelton et al. found increased transcription of cytokines that influence inflammation (23). The study of Shelton et al. is suggestive rather than definitive since the transcripts detected reflected both stimulatory and inhibitory cytokines. Even so, this was interpreted as reflecting increased inflammatory stress in the prefrontal cortex (23). Another postmortem study applied immunohistochemical staining with HLA-DR, a marker of microglial activation in a sample of nine subjects with a MDE secondary to MDD, five subjects with a MDE secondary to bipolar disorder, sixteen subjects with schizophrenia, and ten healthy. While this study was underpowered to detect an effect of MDE diagnosis, there was increased HLA-DR staining in the prefrontal cortex in those who died of suicide (24). More recently in 2018, in a comparison of twenty-three MDD subjects and twenty-three controls, within the hippocampus, the region sampled, Mahajan et al. reported differential expression of several genes involved in inflammation including upregulation of CCL2/MCP-1 and downregulation of ISG15, IFI44L, IFI6, NR4A1/Nur-77 and GABBR1, further supporting evidence of neuroinflammatory changes (25).

10.3 Translocator Protein Imaging

Translocator protein imaging is mainly associated with microglia in inflammation. Five to ten percent of brain cells are microglia that are important for early immune responses in the central nervous system where they detect stimuli such as damage-associated molecular patterns, pathogen-associated molecular patterns, and cytokines (26). In response to these stimuli, microglia become activated, changing their morphology and function. Morphologically, their dendrites alter from being longer and more slender to being thickened, shorter, and their cell body volume becomes larger, and sometimes they become ameboid (27, 28). When activated, microglial function shifts from a detection state into a response state (26, 29). This response state may vary depending on local conditions and includes roles also implicated in fostering chronic

pathological changes such as increased secretion of IL1β, TNFα, IL-6, prostaglandin E2; diverting tryptophan metabolism toward kyurenine production and away from serotonin synthesis through overexpression of 2,3 indoleamine dioxygenase; and greater production of hydrogen peroxide (30). The response state may also include roles attributed to neuroprotective functions like secretion of IL-4, IL-13, IL-10, and TGFα, and phagocytosis of debris (31).

When microglia become activated, they overexpress TSPO, hence TSPO binding represents an important marker of neuroinflammation (32). There has been some debate regarding whether in pathological conditions, elevated TSPO level represent activated microglia versus astroglia. However, empirically, after exposure to stroke, toxins, and lipopolysaccharide administration, the timing of TSPO elevation closely matches the timing of elevations in markers associated with microglial activation but not such changes in markers associated with astroglial activation (33–35). In pathological conditions, it is believed that TSPO in microglia are the main contributors to the overall TSPO binding, although in healthy conditions, selective knockout of TSPO suggests that binding of TSPO to endothelial cells creates a low baseline signal (36). The question of whether TSPO labels human (versus rodent) microglia has also been raised but it has been demonstrated in postmortem human brain with human immunodeficiency virus that activated human microglia are labeled with TSPO (37).

In the mid 1990s the only high-affinity PET radioligand for the translocator protein was [^{11}C](R)PK11195; however, formal modeling quantification in humans took place later in 2006 (38), which demonstrated, despite a number of previous studies applying reference tissue approaches, that the optimal modeling method was a two-tissue compartment and arterial sampling. In general, reference tissue approaches have been questioned for TSPO imaging, since no brain region with free and non-displaceable binding characteristics representative of gray matter have been shown to be substantially devoid of TSPO receptors. In the mid to late 2000s, a new generation of TSPO binding radiotracers emerged which show greatly improved specific binding to free and non-displaceable binding. There are a number of such radiotracers and a representative sample includes [^{11}C]PBR28, [^{18}F]FEPPA, [^{18}F]PBR111, [^{18}F]DPA714, and [^{11}C]ER176 (see Table 10.1).

Table 10.1 Comparison of PET radiotracers for TSPO

	[¹¹C](R)-PK11195	[¹¹C] PBR28	[¹⁸F]FEPPA	[¹⁸F]PBR111	[¹⁸F]DPA714	[¹¹C]ER176
Selectivity	High (43)	High (39)	Excellent (40)	High (44)	Yes (45)	Yes (46)
Reversibility	Very good (38)	Very good (47)	Good in gray matter (48)	Excellent (49)	Excellent	Yes (41)
Brain uptake	good (50)	Very good (47)	Excellent (48)	Very good (49)	Excellent (51)	Very good (41)
Modeling	Two-tissue compartment (38)	Two-tissue compartment (47)	Two-tissue compartment (48)	Two-tissue compartment (49)	Two-tissue compartment with blood volume (51) or with irreversible compartment (42)	Two-tissue compartment (41)
Specific binding to free and non-specific binding ratio	Modest with arterial sampling Low with reference tissue (38)	Very good (47)	High (48)	Very good (49)	Very good (51)	Very good (41)
Reliability	Good for whole brain; poor for regions (50)	Yes in gray matter (52)	Good (personal communication)	Not yet published	Not yet published	Not yet published
Brain-penetrant radioactive metabolites	Unlikely (53)	Negligible to low (39, 40)	Negligible (40)	Negligible (44)	Low (54)	Not yet published
Measureable in diverse regions	Reliability best for whole-brain regions (50)	Yes	Yes	Yes	Yes	Yes (41)

Adapted from Meyer et al. (55)

While Table 10.1 identifies key issues, there are additional advantages and disadvantages for each. [^{11}C]PBR28 is probably the most widely applied technique in neuropsychiatry but has slightly less stable V_T values over the PET scanning period in humans and there is some, but not completely consistent, report of radioactive, brain-penetrant metabolites in rodent brain (39, 40). The design of [^{18}F]PBR111 trades off some of its ratio of specific binding to free and non-displaceable binding for excellent reversibility of its time activity curve, a particular advantage for imaging white matter; however, it has a lesser number of quantifiable regions due to binding of radioactive metabolite to bone. [^{11}C]ER176 is at an earlier stage of development being newer. It is interesting insofar as its distribution volume measure is much less affected by the homozygous state of single nucleotide polymorphism rs6971(41), found in 1% to 10% of subjects, depending on their ethnicity (for other second-generation radioligands, subjects who are homozygous for this genotype are typically excluded from applied neuroimaging studies). This polymorphism causes a single amino acid substitution that reduces the binding of TSPO to all second-generation radioligands. While reliability of TSPO V_T for most

ligands has not been formally reported, it is common for such data to remain unpublished during the first several years of radiotracer application. There are some reports that for a subset of these radiotracers such as [^{11}C]PBR28 and [^{18}F]DPA714, there is an additional irreversible compartment that improves fitting (42).

TSPO PET imaging has been applied to discover that microglial activation occurs during MDE. In a [^{18}F]FEPPA PET study of twenty unmedicated MDE with no active comorbid psychiatric illnesses and twenty controls, the translocator protein specific distribution volume (TSPO V_T), an index of TSPO density, was significantly elevated in the primary regions of the prefrontal cortex, anterior cingulate cortex, and insular cortex by a substantial magnitude of 30%(56) (see Figure 10.1).

Elevated TSPO V_T may occur during several neuroinflammatory changes including microglial activation, astroglial activation, and activation of peripheral macrophages. However, in brain tissue greater TSPO level is best interpreted as reflecting greater levels of microglial activation because the increased TSPO expression in mammalian brain after diverse paradigms like stroke, neurotoxins, and lipopolysaccharide administration (27, 28)

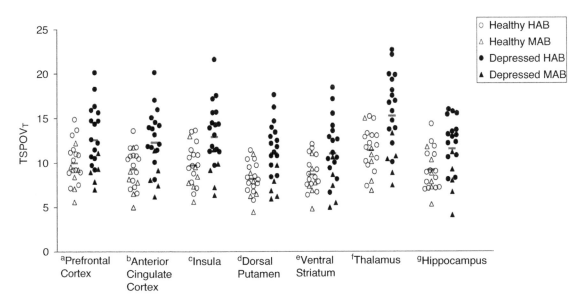

Figure 10.1 Elevated translocator protein density (TSPO V_T) during a major depressive episode (MDE) secondary to major depressive disorder (MDD). TSPO V_T was significantly greater in MDE of MDD (depressed, N = 20, 15 HAB, 5 MAB) compared to controls (healthy, N = 20, 14 HAB, 6 MAB). All second-generation TSPO radioligands, such as [^{18}F]FEPPA, show differential binding according to the SNP rs6971 of the TSPO gene resulting in high-affinity binders (HAB) and mixed-affinity binders (MAB). Red bars indicate means in each group. A black and white version of this figure will appear in some formats. For the colour version, refer to the plate section. Adapted from Setiawan et al. (56)

has a temporal course that closely matches the increased expression of other markers of microglial activation rather than astroglial activation, and peripheral macrophages are typically of low density in human brain. Neuroinflammation, and in particular microglial activation, is a well-established quantitative response to brain injury in neurodegenerative conditions. In addition, induction of microglial activation is implicated in the generation of depressive behaviors in humans and rodents through mechanisms such as the diversion of tryptophan metabolism to kynurenine, stimulation of the hypothalamic–pituitary–adrenal axis and glucocorticoid receptor resistance (29). Thus, given that microglial activation is a marker of advancing disease and is implicated in depressive symptoms it may be advantageous to clinically investigate and categorize chronologically advanced MDD differently.

This has since been demonstrated to be a highly replicable finding, arguably now one of the most replicated findings in mood disorders research (see Table 10.2). Typically across groups, there is 25% to 35% greater TSPO binding in gray matter regions across the brain including prefrontal cortex, anterior cingulate cortex, and insula. However, to date, there have not been studies of TSPO imaging in bipolar disorder or dysthymia.

Elevated TSPO binding also has major implications for neuroprogression, which may be defined as a pathological reorganization of the central nervous system (CNS) along the course of severe mental disorders (4). Chronic microglial activation may become neuroprogressive consequent to its role in responding to accumulating tissue damage and the inherent feed-forward mechanisms from this process (10, 14, 15, 59). Some of these feed-forward mechanisms stem from production of cytokines, complement proteins, reactive oxygen species, and proteinases. The production of cytokines may induce autocrine effects to produce and maintain more activated microglia whereas the latter three processes may lead to cascades of neuronal damage and additional inflammation (15). For example, neuronal damage as secondary to exposure to reactive oxygen species and proteinases may induce microglial activation through microglial detection of damage-associated molecular patterns with upregulation of toll-like receptors (TLR) such as TLR3 and TLR4 receptors, the latter was found in a sample of dorsolateral prefrontal cortex of MDD subjects (16).

In contrast to neuropsychiatric illnesses like Parkinson's disease and Alzheimer's disease in which neuroprogression is firmly established at a neuropathological level, neuroprogression is not well established in MDD, with few investigations demonstrating greater levels of pathology with longer duration of illness (59). While many pathologies have been proposed to be neuroprogressive in MDD, including loss of astroglia and resultant reduced glutamate uptake (5), loss of somatostatin-positive interneurons (6), decreased neurogenesis (7) persistence of elevated MAO-A level (8), hippocampal volume loss (9), and chronic microglial activation (10–12), only hippocampal volume loss has been empirically shown to have greater magnitude of effect with greater duration of MDD, mainly through cross sectional study (9, 13), with mean reductions of 4% overall (9, 13).

Setiawan et al. discovered greater TSPO V_T in the gray matter regions sampled were associated with greater duration of untreated MDD. MDE subjects with history of no antidepressant treatment for ten years or more had 31% to 39% greater TSPO V_T across gray matter regions as compared to healthy subjects, and approximately 30% greater TSPO V_T across these same regions as compared to MDE subjects with short durations of untreated illness (see Figure 10.2 and 10.3). A compelling issue is that there is great potential for pathologically staging MDD, given the increase in TSPO V_T of 14% to 18% per decade. This suggests that duration of untreated MDD may reflect a more precise measure of neuroprogression given its relationship with elevated TSPO V_T, as compared to the current clinical definition of differentiating between single- and multiple-episode MDD.

The second main finding was that total duration of illness predicted greater TSPO V_T and duration of antidepressant exposure was a similar magnitude negative predictor of TSPO V_T throughout the gray matter regions sampled. The yearly increase of TSPO V_T is no longer present when antidepressant treatment occurs since duration of antidepressant exposure is a negative predictor in the model when total duration of MDD is included, and these predictors are of similar magnitude but in the opposite direction. Since most of the antidepressant exposure was selective serotonin reuptake inhibitors or selective serotonin and norepinephrine reuptake

Table 10.2 Comparisons of translocator protein binding between currently depressed and healthy subjects

Study	Diagnosis and number of subjects	Radiotracer	Region	Results
Setiawan et al. (56)	20 Medication-free MDE, MDD, 20 healthy	[¹⁸F]FEPPA	PFC, ACC, insula, 14 gray matter regions	30% elevated in MDE
Li et al. (57)	40 Medication-naïve MDE, MDD, 20 healthy	[¹⁸F]FEPPA	Gray matter, white matter, Frontal Cortex, Temporal Cortex, Hippocampus	~25 to 35% elevated in MDE
Holmes et al. (58)	14 Medication-free MDE, MDD, 13 healthy	[¹¹C](R) PK11195	PFC, ACC, insula	67% elevated in ACC 28% elevated in PFC (n.s.) 24% elevated in ACC (n.s.)
Setiawan et al. (59)	50 MDE (30 new treatment-resistant MDE + previous 20 MDE), 30 healthy	[¹⁸F]FEPPA	PFC, ACC, insula, 14 Gray matter regions	~ 35% elevated in MDE with long history of being untreated
Richards et al. (60)	28 MDE (16 medicated; 12 unmedicated), 20 healthy	[¹¹C]PBR28	sgPFC, ACC	~ 25% elevated in sgPFC ~15% elevated in ACC
Li et al. (61)	50 MDE medication naïve (10 new subjects), 30 healthy (10 new subjects)	[¹⁸F]FEPPA	Gray matter, white matter, frontal cortex, temporal cortex, hippocampus	~25% elevated in MDE

n.s.= non-significant

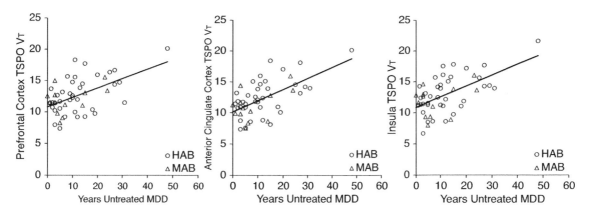

Figure 10.2 Relationship between regional translocator protein distribution volume and duration of untreated major depressive disorder

Analyses of covariance (ANCOVAs) with regional translocator protein distribution volume (TSPO V_T) values as the dependent variable found that the combination of duration of untreated illness and rs6971 genotype, these predictor variables accounted for approximately 50% of the variance in the three prioritized regions. All second-generation TSPO radioligands, such as [^{18}F]FEPPA, show differential binding according to the single-nucleotide polymorphism rs6971 of the TSPO gene resulting in high-affinity binders (HAB) and mixed-affinity binders (MAB).
Adapted from Setiawan et al. (56)

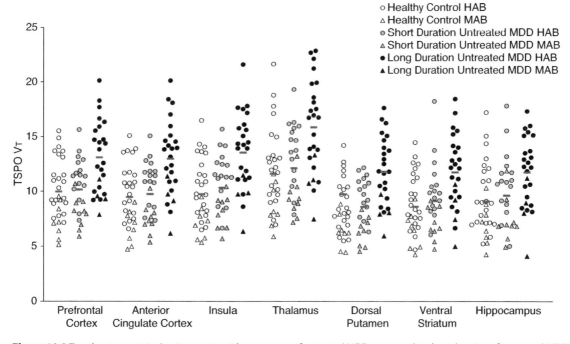

Figure 10.3 Translocator protein density greater with more years of untreated MDD compared to short duration of untreated MDD and healthy controls. A black and white version of this figure will appear in some formats. For the colour version, refer to the plate section.

Group (duration untreated ≥10 years ($N = 25$), duration untreated <10 years ($N = 25$), and healthy ($N = 30$)) and genotype were significant predictor variables in a multivariate analysis of variance with TSPO V_T. Additional comparisons based on the least significant difference test showed significant differences between a long duration of untreated MDD as compared to healthy controls and significant differences between long duration of untreated MDD and short duration of untreated MDD in all of these regions. Second-generation TSPO radioligands, such as [^{18}F]FEPPA, show differential binding according to the single-nucleotide polymorphism rs6971 of the TSPO gene resulting in high-affinity binders (HAB) and mixed-affinity binders (MAB). Red bars indicate means in each group.
Adapted from Setiawan et al. (59)

inhibitors, this provides a context for interpreting literature reports that serotonin reuptake inhibitors reduce induction of microglial activation in cell culture in regards to the brain during clinical treatment in humans (20, 21). The in vitro findings could have been interpreted to indicate that short durations of serotonin reuptake inhibitor treatment strongly reduce microglial activation, but the data of this cross sectional study argue that the yearly accumulation of greater TSPO V_T merely stops. Since inducing microglial activation is associated with concurrent onset of depressed mood and behaviors (29, 30), it may be therapeutically useful to develop superior strategies to modulate and/or reduce microglial activation such as via minocycline administration. Some positive preliminary results of add-on minocycline were shown in a randomized double-blind placebo-controlled trial of MDD (31).

There are several other studies that probed the relationship of TSPO binding to clinical features of

MDE. Richards et al. (60) found that medication-free subjects who also had long histories of MDD have higher levels of TSPO binding. Holmes et al. (58) reported that the presence of current suicidal ideation was associated with greater TSPO binding in the ACC and Li et al. (61) reported that poorer attention performance was associated with greater prefrontal cortex TSPO V_T.

10.4 Novel PET Imaging Probes of Neuroinflammation

In the postmortem field it is common to apply multiple markers to characterize microglial and astroglial activation, whereas this is impractical with PET when arterial sampling is required. However, there will be increasingly greater opportunity to investigate other markers of neuroinflammation in MDE (see Table 10.3). Challenges with these markers are that they are often not specific to individual cell types, and that many of the

Table 10.3 PET imaging of neuroinflammation: molecular targets and potential radiotracers

Molecular target	Cellular expression	Expression in neuroinflammation	Radiotracers investigated
TSPO	Microglia and astrocytes	Upregulated	[11 C]PK11195, [18 F]FEPPA, [18 F]PBR06, [18 F]FEDAA1106, [11 C]PBR28, [11 C]ER176, [18 F]DPA-714
GSK-3	Microglia and astrocytes	Upregulated	[11 C]PF-367, [11 C]SB-216763,
MAO-B	Astrocytes and 5-HT releasing neurons	Upregulated	[11 C]SL25.1188, [11 C]-L-deprenyl, [11 C]-L-deprenyl-D_2, [18 F]fluorodeprenyl-D_2, [18 F]fluororasagiline-D_2,
ROS	Microglia	Upregulated	[11 C]hydromethidine, [11 C]**1**, [18 F]ROStrace, [11 C]ascorbic acid
I_2BS	Astrocytes	Upregulated	[11 C]BU99008
COX-1	Microglia	Upregulated	[11 C]Ketoprofen-methyl ester, [11 C]PS13, [18 F]PS2
COX-2	Microglia	Upregulated	[11 C]MC1
Arachidonic acid	Microglia and astrocytes	Upregulated	[11 C]Arachidonic acid
S1P1	Microglia ≫ astrocytes	Upregulated	[18 F](R)-1-[[3-(6-fluorohexyl)-phenyl]amino-4-oxobutyl]phosphonic acid, [11 C]TZ3321, [18 F]TZ35110, [18 F]TZ43113, [18 F]TZ35104, [18 F]TZ4877, [18 F]TZ4881
CB2	Microglia and astrocytes	Downregulated	[11 C]NE40, [11 C]MA2, [18 F]MA3
Purinergic receptor: P2X$_7$	Microglia ≫ astrocytes	Upregulated	[11 C]A-740003, [11 C]SMW139, [11 C]JNJ-54173717, [11 C]GSK1482160

Adapted from Narayanaswami et al. (62)

radiotracers listed are in development and not yet established for use in humans.

Among these probes, MAO-B imaging has become well advanced for human use, enabling robust quantitation of MAO-B distribution volume (V_T), an index of MAO-B density. [11C] deprenyl was the first radiotracer for MAO-B imaging with PET (63) but it had some limitations of poor reversibility and radioactive metabolites found in both brain and periphery. Subsequently, to improve reversibility, new analogues were created like deuterium-labeled [11C]deprenyl and then deuterium-labeled [18F]deprenyl (64, 65). [18F]deprenyl has been modeled in monkeys, but there is a potential limitation of bias from brain-penetrant metabolites of these compounds (64, 65). Bramoulle et al. (66) discovered a radiotracer with a different structure, [11C] SL25.1188, and the same group modeled it in baboons (67). Unfortunately, the initial production method for [11C]SL25.1188 requires the esoteric carbon-11-labeled phosgene (66) so Vasdev et al. discovered a new synthesis method and then the radiotracer was modeled in humans (68–70). [11C]SL25.1188 has outstanding properties including high reversiblity, brain uptake, and

selectivity for MAO-B; no brain-penetrant meta-bolites; and a very reproducible total V_T measure, which is highly correlated with the known concentration of MAO-B in postmortem human brain ($r^2 > 0.9$) (67–70).

Moriguchi et al. applied [11C]SL25.1188 PET in twenty MDE and twenty healthy and found a 26% greater MAO-B V_T in the prefrontal cortex (71). Interestingly, half of the MDE subjects had MAO-B V_T values exceeding the range in healthy subjects. Differences between MDE and healthy controls were more prominent in PFC regions proximal to the ventrolateral PFC, such as the dorsolateral PFC and orbitofrontal cortex (see Figure 10.4).

In addition, greater duration of MDD illness was associated with greater MAO-B V_T in the PFC (see Figure 10.5), as well as most other cortical regions and the thalamus. The relationship between greater duration of illness and greater regional MAO-B V_T is not accounted for by age because the effect of age on MAO-B V_T is negligible in this sample since age-related effects on MAO-B density do not begin until 55–70 years (72, 73). Greater MAO-B density may occur during reactive astrogliosis and may be associated

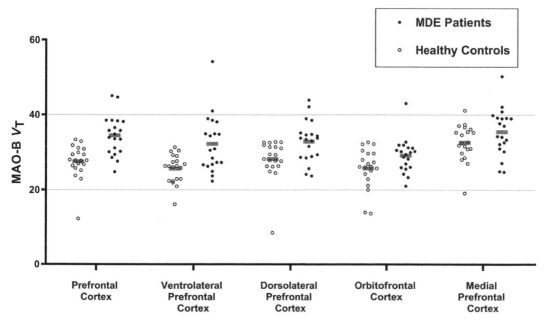

Figure 10.4 Elevated MAO-B distribution volume during MDE in the prefrontal cortex. A black and white version of this figure will appear in some formats. For the colour version, refer to the plate section.

MAO-B V_T was significantly greater in the twenty MDE patients compared with the twenty healthy controls
From Moriguchi et al. (71)

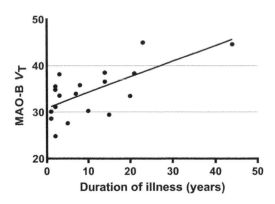

Figure 10.5 Relationship between prefrontal cortex MAO-B distribution volume and duration of illness

Greater MAO-B V_T was significantly associated with longer duration of MDD illness, even after removing highest V_T value in PFC From Moriguchi et al. (71)

with greater duration of untreated illness makes an important empirical case for neuroprogression in MDE. There is a plethora of novel inflammatory markers under development that will aid characterization of neuroinflammation in mood disorders. Among these markers, MAO-B, which may be overexpressed during astroglial activation, is elevated in the PFC, particularly in cases of MDE with longer durations of illness, suggesting further evidence of neuroprogression. Future medication development ideally should target the specific abnormalities of neuroinflammation in mood disorders, a direction increasingly supported by positive results across neuroimaging studies; and future study should investigate other mood disorders in addition to MDD.

with progression of neuropsychiatric diseases such as Alzheimer's disease, amyotrophic lateral sclerosis, multisystem atrophy, and progressive supranuclear palsy (74–76). In these illnesses, GFAP and MAO-B levels are often highly correlated accounting for why greater MAO-B density may be an in vivo marker of reactive astrogliosis (76, 77). Astrogliosis alone would not account for differences between MDD and health, particularly in MDD of shorter duration in younger subjects, since GFAP is reduced in the orbitofrontal, dorsolateral, and subgenual PFC in MDE samples inclusive of younger subjects (78–80). However, these differences are not proven for later stages of MDD as the finding was not present in late-life MDE (81). Furthermore, the two studies that investigated GFAP in relation to age and duration of illness found a much greater rise in GFAP with age in MDD than healthy controls in the region sampled, the dorsolateral prefrontal cortex (82, 83). Hence a reasonable explanation for the association between greater MAO-B with duration of illness is gradually increasing astrogliosis.

10.5 Conclusions

Brain imaging of TSPO has consistently demonstrated elevated binding in MDE subjects, and the best explanation for this is that microglial activation is present when TSPO binding is elevated. Most of the samples investigated were medication free but this was also prominent in cases who have longer histories of medication-free state since onset of the first MDE. The association of greater TSPO binding

References

1. Miller AH, Maletic V, Raison CL. Inflammation and its discontents: The role of cytokines in the pathophysiology of major depression. *Biol Psychiatry*. 2009; **65**(9): 732–741.

2. Dowlati Y, Herrmann N, Swardfager W, et al. A meta-analysis of Cytokines in major depression. *Biol Psychiatry*. 2010 March 1; **67**(5): 446–457.

3. Musselman DL, Lawson DH, Gumnick JF, et al. Paroxetine for the prevention of depression induced by high-dose interferon alfa. *N Engl J Med*. 2001; **344**(13): 961–966.

4. Capuron L, Gumnick JF, Musselman DL, et al. Neurobehavioral effects of interferon-alpha in cancer patients: Phenomenology and paroxetine responsiveness of symptom dimensions. *Neuropsychopharmacology*. 2002; **26**(5): 643–652.

5. Brydon L, Harrison NA, Walker C, Steptoe A, Critchley HD. Peripheral inflammation is associated with altered substantia nigra activity and psychomotor slowing in humans. *Biol Psychiatry*. 2008; **63**(11): 1022–1029.

6. Reichenberg A, Yirmiya R, Schuld A, et al. Cytokine-associated emotional and cognitive disturbances in humans. *Arch Gen Psychiatry*. 2001; **58**(5): 445–452.

7. Salazar A, Gonzalez-Rivera BL, Redus L, Parrott JM, O'Connor JC. Indoleamine 2,3-dioxygenase mediates anhedonia and anxiety-like behaviors caused by peripheral lipopolysaccharide immune challenge. *Horm Behav*. 2012; **62**(3): 202–209.

8. Yang L, Wang M, et al. Systemic inflammation induces anxiety disorder through CXCL12/CXCR4 pathway. *Brain Behav Immun*. 2016; **56**: 352–362.

9. Yu I, Inaji M, Maeda J, et al. Glial cell-mediated deterioration and repair of the nervous system after traumatic brain injury in a rat model as assessed by positron emission tomography. *J Neurotrauma*. 2010; 27(8): 1463–1475.

10. Grossman R, Paden CM, Fry PA, Rhodes RS, Biegon A. Persistent region-dependent neuroinflammation, NMDA receptor loss and atrophy in an animal model of penetrating brain injury. *Future Neurol*. 2012; 7 (3): 329–339.

11. Raghavendra Rao VL, Dogan A, Bowen KK, Dempsey RJ. Traumatic brain injury leads to increased expression of peripheral-type benzodiazepine receptors, neuronal death, and activation of astrocytes and microglia in rat thalamus. *Exp Neurol*. 2000; 161(1): 102–114.

12. Ramlackhansingh AF, Brooks DJ, Greenwood RJ, et al. Inflammation after trauma: Microglial activation and traumatic brain injury. *Ann Neurol*. 2011; 70(3): 374–383.

13. Rapoport MJ. Depression following traumatic brain injury: epidemiology, risk factors and management. *CNS Drugs*. 2012; 26(2): 111–121.

14. Bombardier CH, Fann JR, Temkin NR, Et al. Rates of major depressive disorder and clinical outcomes following traumatic brain injury. *JAMA*. 2010; 303(19): 1938–1945.

15. Jorge RE, Robinson RG, Moser D, et al. Major depression following traumatic brain injury. *Arch Gen Psychiatry*. 2004; 61(1): 42–50.

16. Brey RL, Holliday SL, Saklad AR, et al. Neuropsychiatric syndromes in lupus: prevalence using standardized definitions. *Neurology*. 2002; 58(8): 1214–1220.

17. Nery FG, Borba EF, Viana VS, et al. Prevalence of depressive and anxiety disorders in systemic lupus erythematosus and their association with anti-ribosomal P antibodies. *Prog Neuropsychopharmacol Biol Psychiatry*. 2008; 32 (3): 695–700.

18. Bachen EA, Chesney MA, Criswell LA. Prevalence of mood and anxiety disorders in women with systemic lupus erythematosus. *Arthritis Rheum*. 2009; 61(6): 822–829.

19. Minden SL, Orav J, Reich P. Depression in multiple sclerosis. *Gen Hosp Psychiatry*. 1987; 9(6): 426–434.

20. Sadovnick AD, Eisen K, Ebers GC, Paty DW. Cause of death in patients attending multiple sclerosis clinics. *Neurology*. 1991; 41(8): 1193–1196.

21. Joffe RT, Lippert GP, Gray TA, Sawa G, Horvath Z. Mood disorder and multiple sclerosis. *Arch Neurol*. 1987; 44(4): 376–378.

22. Pandey GN, Rizavi HS, Ren X, et al. Proinflammatory cytokines in the prefrontal cortex of teenage suicide victims. *J Psychiatr Res*. 2012; 46(1): 57–63.

23. Shelton RC, Claiborne J, Sidoryk-Wegrzynowicz M, et al. Altered expression of genes involved in inflammation and apoptosis in frontal cortex in major depression. *Mol Psychiatry*. 2011; 16(7): 751–762.

24. Steiner J, Bielau H, Brisch R, et al. Immunological aspects in the neurobiology of suicide: Elevated microglial density in schizophrenia and depression is associated with suicide. *J Psychiatr Res*. 2008; 42(2): 151–157.

25. Mahajan GJ, Vallender EJ, Garrett MR, et al. Altered neuro-inflammatory gene expression in hippocampus in major depressive disorder. *Prog Neuropsychopharmacol Biol Psychiatry*. 2018; 82: 177–186.

26. Kreutzberg GW. Microglia: A sensor for pathological events in the CNS. *Trends in Neurosciences*. 1996; 19(8): 312–318.

27. Carbonell WS, Murase S, Horwitz AF, Mandell JW. Migration of perilesional microglia after focal brain injury and modulation by CC chemokine receptor 5: An in situ time-lapse confocal imaging study. *J Neurosci*. 2005; 25(30): 7040–7047.

28. Cross AK, Woodroofe MN. Chemokines induce migration and changes in actin polymerization in adult rat brain microglia and a human fetal microglial cell line in vitro. *J Neurosci Res*. 1999; 55(1): 17–23.

29. Gehrmann J, Matsumoto Y, Kreutzberg GW. Microglia: Intrinsic immuneffector cell of the brain. *Brain Research Reviews*. 1995; 20(3): 269–287.

30. Dantzer R, O'Connor JC, Freund GG, Johnson RW, Kelley KW. From inflammation to sickness and depression: When the immune system subjugates the brain. *Nat Rev Neurosci*. 2008; 9(1): 46–56.

31. Wohleb ES, Franklin T, Iwata M, Duman RS. Integrating neuroimmune systems in the neurobiology of depression. *Nat Rev Neurosci*. 2016; 17(8): 497–511.

32. Venneti S, Wiley CA, Kofler J. Imaging microglial activation during neuroinflammation and Alzheimer's disease. *J Neuroimmune Pharmacol*. 2009; 4(2): 227–243.

33. Banati RB, Myers R, Kreutzberg GW. PK ('peripheral benzodiazepine')–binding sites in the CNS indicate early and discrete brain lesions: Microautoradiographic detection of [3 H] PK11195 binding to activated microglia. *J Neurocytol.* 1997; **26**(2): 77–82.

34. Martin A, Boisgard R, Theze B, et al. Evaluation of the PBR/TSPO radioligand [(18)F]DPA-714 in a rat model of focal cerebral ischemia. *J Cereb Blood Flow Metab.* 2010; **30**(1): 230–241.

35. Hannestad J, Dellagioia N, Gallezot JD, et al. The neuroinflammation marker translocator protein is not elevated in individuals with mild-to-moderate depression: A [C]PBR28 PET study. *Brain Behav Immun.* 2013; **33**: 131–138.

36. Betlazar C, Harrison-Brown M, Middleton RJ, Banati R, Liu GJ. Cellular sources and regional variations in the expression of the neuroinflammatory marker translocator protein (TSPO) in the normal brain. *Int J Mol Sci.* 2018 September 11; **19**(9): 2707.

37. Cosenza-Nashat M, Zhao ML, Suh HS, et al. Expression of the translocator protein of 18kDa by microglia, macrophages and astrocytes based on immunohistochemical localization in abnormal human brain. *Neuropathology and Applied Neurobiology.* 2009; **35**(3): 306–328.

38. Kropholler MA, Boellaard R, Schuitemaker A, et al. Evaluation of reference tissue models for the analysis of [11 C](R)-PK11195 studies. *J Cereb Blood Flow Metab.* 2006; **26**(11): 1431–1441.

39. Imaizumi M, Kim HJ, Zoghbi SS, et al. PET imaging with [11 C]PBR28 can localize and quantify upregulated peripheral benzodiazepine receptors associated with cerebral ischemia in rat. *Neurosci Lett.* 2007; **411**(3): 200–205.

40. Wilson AA, Garcia A, Parkes J, et al. Radiosynthesis and initial evaluation of [18 F]-FEPPA for PET imaging of peripheral benzodiazepine receptors. *Nucl Med Biol.* 2008; **35**(3): 305–314.

41. Ikawa M, Lohith TG, Shrestha S, et al. Biomarkers consortium radioligand project T. 11 C-ER176, a radioligand for 18-kDa translocator protein, has adequate sensitivity to robustly image all three affinity genotypes in human brain. *J Nucl Med.* 2017; **58**(2): 320–325.

42. Wimberley C, Lavisse S, Brulon V, et al. Impact of endothelial 18-kDa translocator protein on the quantification of (18)F-DPA-714. *J Nucl Med.* 2018; **59**(2): 307–314.

43. Medran-Navarrete V, Damont A, Peyronneau MA, et al. Preparation and evaluation of novel pyrazolo[1,5-a]pyrimidine acetamides, closely related to DPA-714, as potent ligands for imaging the TSPO 18kDa with PET. *Bioorg Med Chem Lett.* 2014; **24**(6): 1550–1556.

44. Fookes CJ, Pham TQ, Mattner F, et al. Synthesis and biological evaluation of substituted [18 F] imidazo[1,2-a]pyridines and [18 F]pyrazolo[1,5-a] pyrimidines for the study of the peripheral benzodiazepine receptor using positron emission tomography. *J Med Chem.* 2008; **51**(13): 3700–3712.

45. James ML, Fulton RR, Vercoullie J, et al. DPA-714, a new translocator protein-specific ligand: synthesis, radiofluorination, and pharmacologic characterization. *J Nucl Med.* 2008; **49**(5): 814–822.

46. Zanotti-Fregonara P, Zhang Y, Jenko KJ, et al. Synthesis and evaluation of translocator 18 kDa protein (TSPO) positron emission tomography (PET) radioligands with low binding sensitivity to human single nucleotide polymorphism rs6971. *ACS Chem Neurosci.* 2014; **5**(10): 963–971.

47. Fujita M, Imaizumi M, Zoghbi SS, et al. Kinetic analysis in healthy humans of a novel positron emission tomography radioligand to image the peripheral benzodiazepine receptor, a potential biomarker for inflammation. *Neuroimage.* 2008; **40**(1): 43–52.

48. Rusjan P, Wilson AA, Bloomfield PM, et al. Quantification of translocator protein (18kDa) in the human brain with PET and a novel radioligand, [18 F]-FEPPA. *JCBFM.* 2010; **31**(8): 1807–1816.

49. Guo Q, Colasanti A, Owen DR, et al. Quantification of the specific translocator protein signal of 18 F-PBR111 in healthy humans: A genetic polymorphism effect on in vivo binding. *J Nucl Med.* 2013; **54**(11): 1915–1923.

50. Jucaite A, Cselenyi Z, Arvidsson A, et al. Kinetic analysis and test-retest variability of the radioligand [11 C](R)-PK11195 binding to TSPO in the human brain – a PET study in control subjects. *EJNMMI Res.* 2012; **2**: 15.

51. Hagens MHJ, Golla SV, Wijburg MT, et al. In vivo assessment of neuroinflammation in progressive multiple sclerosis: A proof of concept study with [(18)F]DPA714 PET. *J Neuroinflammation.* 2018; **15**(1): 314.

52. Collste K, Forsberg A, Varrone A, et al. Test-retest reproducibility of [(11)C]PBR28 binding to TSPO in healthy control subjects. *Eur J Nucl Med Mol Imaging.* 2016; **43**(1): 173–183.

53. Hashimoto K, Inoue O, Suzuki K, Yamasaki T, Kojima M. Synthesis and evaluation of 11 C-PK 11195 for in vivo study of peripheral-type benzodiazepine receptors using positron

emission tomography. *Ann Nucl Med.* 1989; **3**(2): 63–71.

54. Vicidomini C, Panico M, Greco A, et al. In vivo imaging and characterization of [(18)F]DPA-714, a potential new TSPO ligand, in mouse brain and peripheral tissues using small-animal PET. *Nucl Med Biol.* 2015; **42**(3): 309–316.

55. Meyer J. Novel phenotypes detectable with PET in mood disorders: Elevated monoamine oxidase A and translocator protein level. In: Vasdev N, Alavi A, editors. *PET Clinics: Novel PET Radiotracers with Potential Clinical Applications.* Vol 12. United States: Elsevier; 2017, pp. 361–371.

56. Setiawan E, Wilson AA, Mizrahi R, et al. Role of translocator protein density, a marker of neuroinflammation, in the brain during major depressive episodes. *JAMA Psychiatry.* 2015; **72**(3): 268–275.

57. Li H, Sagar AP, Keri S. Translocator protein (18kDa TSPO) binding, a marker of microglia, is reduced in major depression during cognitive-behavioral therapy. *Prog Neuropsychopharmacol Biol Psychiatry.* 2018; **83**: 1–7.

58. Holmes SE, Hinz R, Conen S, et al. Elevated translocator protein in anterior cingulate in major depression and a role for inflammation in suicidal thinking: A positron emission tomography study. *Biol Psychiatry.* 2018; **83**(1): 61–69.

59. Setiawan E, Attwells S, Wilson AA, et al. Association of translocator protein total distribution volume with duration of untreated major depressive disorder: A cross-sectional study. *Lancet Psychiatry.* 2018; **5**(4): 339–347.

60. Richards EM, Zanotti-Fregonara P, Fujita M, et al. PET radioligand binding to translocator protein (TSPO) is increased in unmedicated depressed subjects. *EJNMMI Res.* 2018; **8**(1): 57.

61. Li H, Sagar AP, Keri S. Microglial markers in the frontal cortex are related to cognitive dysfunctions in major depressive disorder. *J Affect Disord.* 2018; **241**: 305–310.

62. Narayanaswami V, Dahl K, Bernard-Gauthier V, et al. Emerging PET radiotracers and targets for imaging of neuroinflammation in neurodegenerative diseases: Outlook beyond TSPO. *Mol Imaging.* 2018; **17**: 1536012118792317.

63. Fowler JS, MacGregor RR, Wolf AP, et al. Mapping human brain monoamine oxidase A and B with 11 C-labeled suicide inactivators and PET. *Science.* 1987; **235**(4787): 481–485.

64. Fowler JS, Wang GJ, Logan J, et al. Selective reduction of radiotracer trapping by deuterium substitution: Comparison of carbon-11- L-deprenyl and carbon-11-deprenyl-D2 for MAO B mapping. *J Nucl Med.* 1995; **36**(7): 1255–1262.

65. Nag S, Fazio P, Lehmann L, et al. In vivo and in vitro characterization of a novel MAO-B inhibitor radioligand, 18 F-labeled deuterated fluorodeprenyl. *J Nucl Med.* 2016; **57**(2): 315–320.

66. Bramoulle Y, Puech F, Saba W, et al. Radiosynthesis of (S)-5-methoxymethyl-3-[6-(4, 4, 4-trifluorobutoxy) benzo [d] isoxazol-3-yl] oxazolidin-2-[11 C] one ([11 C] SL25. 1188), a novel radioligand for imaging monoamine oxidase-B with PET. *Journal of Labelled Compounds and Radiopharmaceuticals.* 2008; **51**(3): 153–158.

67. Saba W, Valette H, Peyronneau MA, et al. [(11)C] SL25.1188, a new reversible radioligand to study the monoamine oxidase type B with PET: Preclinical characterisation in nonhuman primate. *Synapse.* 2010; **64**(1): 61–69.

68. Vasdev N, Sadovski O, Garcia A, et al. Radiosynthesis of [11 C] SL25. 1188 via [11 C] CO2 fixation for imaging monoamine oxidase B. *Journal of Labelled Compounds and Radiopharmaceuticals.* 2011; **54**(10): 678–680.

69. Vasdev N, Sadovski O, Moran MD, et al. Development of new radiopharmaceuticals for imaging monoamine oxidase B. *Nucl Med Biol.* 2011; **38**(7): 933–943.

70. Rusjan PM, Wilson AA, Miler L, et al. Kinetic modeling of the monoamine oxidase B radioligand [(1)(1)C]SL25.1188 in human brain with high-resolution positron emission tomography. *J Cereb Blood Flow Metab.* 2014; **34** (5): 883–889.

71. Moriguchi S, Wilson AA, Miler L, et al. Monoamine oxidase B total distribution volume in the prefrontal cortex of major depressive disorder: An [11 C]SL25.1188 positron emission tomography study. *JAMA Psychiatry.* 2019 June 1; **6**(6): 634–641.

72. Saura J, Andres N, Andrade C, et al. Biphasic and region-specific MAO-B response to aging in normal human brain. *Neurobiol Aging.* 1997; **18**(5): 497–507.

73. Tong J, Jeffrey H. Meyer, Furukawa Y, Et al. Distribution of monoamine oxidase proteins in human brain: Implications for brain imaging studies. *J Cereb Blood Flow Metab.* 2013; **33**(6): 863–871.

74. Saura J, Luque JM, Cesura AM, et al. Increased monoamine oxidase B activity in plaque-associated astrocytes of Alzheimer brains revealed by quantitative enzyme radioautography. *Neuroscience.* 1994; **62**(1): 15–30.

75. Ekblom J, Jossan SS, Oreland L, Walum E, Aquilonius SM. Reactive gliosis and monoamine

oxidase B. *J Neural Transm Suppl.* 1994; **41**: 253–258.

76. Tong J, Rathitharan G, Jeffrey H. Meyer, et al. Brain monoamine oxidase B and A in human parkinsonian dopamine deficiency disorders. *Brain.* 2017; **140**(9): 2460–2474.

77. Gulyas B, Pavlova E, Kasa P, et al. Activated MAO-B in the brain of Alzheimer patients, demonstrated by [11 C]-L-deprenyl using whole hemisphere autoradiography. *Neurochem Int.* 2011; **58**(1): 60–68.

78. Rajkowska G, Miguel-Hidalgo JJ, Wei J, et al. Morphometric evidence for neuronal and glial prefrontal cell pathology in major depression. *Biol Psychiatry.* 1999; **45**(9): 1085–1098.

79. Ongur D, Drevets WC, Price JL. Glial reduction in the subgenual prefrontal cortex in mood disorders. *Proc Natl Acad Sci U S A.* 1998; **95**(22): 13290–13295.

80. Rajkowska G, Stockmeier CA. Astrocyte pathology in major depressive disorder: Insights from human postmortem brain tissue. *Curr Drug Targets.* 2013; **14**(11): 1225–1236.

81. Khundakar A, Morris C, Oakley A, Thomas AJ. A morphometric examination of neuronal and glial cell pathology in the orbitofrontal cortex in late-life depression. *Int Psychogeriatr.* 2011; **23**(1): 132–140.

82. Si X, Miguel-Hidalgo JJ, O'Dwyer G, Stockmeier CA, Rajkowska G. Age-dependent reductions in the level of glial fibrillary acidic protein in the prefrontal cortex in major depression. *Neuropsychopharmacology.* 2004; **29**(11): 2088–2096.

83. Miguel-Hidalgo JJ, Baucom C, Dilley G, et al. Glial fibrillary acidic protein immunoreactivity in the prefrontal cortex distinguishes younger from older adults in major depressive disorder. *Biol Psychiatry.* 2000; **48**(8): 861–873.

Chapter

11

Imaging Genetic and Epigenetic Markers in Mood Disorders

Sara Poletti, Elena Mazza, Benedetta Vai, and Francesco Benedetti

Genetics explain 60–85% and 31–50% of the risk to develop, respectively, bipolar disorder (BD) (1, 2) and major depressive disorder (MDD) (3, 4). Thus, hereditability has emerged as a crucial factor in the pathophysiology of mood disorders. Early genetics studies focused their attention on specific single-nucleotide polymorphism (SNP), preselected on prior evidence for their functional role in coding products that may influence relevant features of the disorders, also known as candidate gene approach. In these studies, we define risk allele, genetic variants associated with the disorder or worse clinical features such as reduced response to therapeutics, early onset, and higher recurrence. In recent years thanks to the substantial advance in genetic technology, the new cost-effective microarray procedures implemented in genome-wide association studies (GWAS), the list of risk genes associated with mood disorders has rapidly increased (5). However, genetic data explain only a small portion of phenotypical variance of mood disorders (6). In order to fill the gap between genetic asset and phenotype, the focus moved to endophenotypes integrating genetic and neuroimaging data in an imaging genetic perspective (7). This conceptual framework identifies brain function and structure as "intermediate phenotypes" between the genetic vulnerability, such as risk allele, and the disorder, closer to biological pathways than phenotype itself, and thus widely affected by genetic risk variations (8). Insights from meta-analyses and research studies confirm also the hereditability of neuroimaging abnormalities in BD and MDD, as detected in high genetic risk subjects and first-degree relatives of affected patients (9–13).

Parallel to the quest for intermediate phenotypes, a new approach has emerged, which views mood disorders as the result of the modulation of gene expression by environmental stimuli (14) through epigenetic mechanisms. Consequently, epigenetic has also been studied within the imaging genetic approach.

This chapter will address the issue of the identification of imaging genetic and epigenetic biomarkers in MDD and BD, focusing mainly on studies investigating white matter (WM), gray matter (GM), and functional magnetic resonance imaging (fMRI).

11.1 Genome-Wide Association Studies

Recent genetics studies have begun to adopt GWA methods identifying several independent single-nucleotide polymorphisms (SNPs) significantly associated with diagnosis of MDD: OLFM4, TMEM161B-MEF2C, MEIS2-TMCO5A, NEGR1, RSRC1-MLF1, L3MBTL2, VRK2, FHIT, RBFOX1, SORCS3, HACE1-LIN28B, KIAA0020-RFX3, PAX5, RERE, BICC1, PCLO, NCAN, and NETRIN1 (15–17); and BD: TRANK1, ANK3, and ODZ4 genes (18). Only one SNP in the calcium voltage-gated channel subunit alpha1 C (CACNA1C) gene associated with both MDD and BD. Neuroimaging studies explored the effect of the emerged loci from GWAS on both functional and structural brain data in order to elucidate their role in MDD and BD pathophysiology.

Studies in MDD showed that the piccolo presynaptic cytomatrix protein (PCLO), which is involved in establishing active synaptic zones, in synaptic vesicle trafficking, and in monoaminergic neurotransmission, is altered in MDD (19) and is associated with antidepressant treatment response (20). The rs2522833 was associated with a decreased GM in the left temporal pole in drug-naive, first-episode MDD patients carrying C allele (21), whereas A/A, linked to an increased risk of depression, associated with higher GM hippocampal volume and reduced WM lesion volume in patients with late-life MDD (22). fMRI studies showed increased activation in the left amygdala in response to emotional negative stimuli, but no altered prefrontal recruitment on executive function task (23). PCLO*C carriers compared to non-risk 'A' allele carriers showed reduced insula and a trend-wise of anterior cingulate cortex (ACC) and inferior frontal gyrus activation during emotional memory processing (24), and worse memory performance and lower encoding-related hippocampal activation (25). Larger hippocampal volumes (26), only in the absence of early-life adversities (27), and increased activation in brain regions involved in emotion processing have been reported in individuals with the T allele of Bicaudal C homologue 1 (BICC1) gene (27), which has an important role in neuroplasticity. A similar role is played by the NCAN gene, involved in cell adhesion and migration and neurite growth, that impact on subcortical brain structure in healthy and depressed subjects (28). Finally, attention has to be given to (a) the arginine–glutamic acid dipeptide (RE) repeats (RERE) gene, important for normal brain development (29) that was associated with WM alterations in first-episode and drug-naive MDD patients (30); (b) Tescalin gene, involved in neuronal proliferation and differentiation, associated with both WM and GM changes in MDD (31); (c) LHPP gene that encodes an enzyme known as phospholysine phosphohistidine inorganic pyrophosphate phosphatase and influences brain activity in MDD (32).

Studies in BD showed a role of *ANK3* (loci rs10761482, rs10994336, and rs9804190), a gene coding for Ankyrin G, a protein involved in voltage gating in neurotransmission, in neurogenesis and in myelination. Evidences in BD suggest an effect of ANK 3 genes on WM integrity: BD carriers of the risk allele of rs10761482 showed a lower fractional anisotropy (FA), a measure of WM microstructure, in the forceps (33), while rs9804190 risk allele with reduced FA in the uncinate fasciculus and the cingulate gyrus (34). When performing neuropsychological test (N-back test), the rs10994336 SNP risk was associated with hyperactivation of the anterior and posterior cingulate cortex (35). No effect on brain volume and cortical thickness was observed (36). Another SNP involved

in neurotransmission is Neuregulin 1 (NRG1) rs35753505, which affects myelin, neural, and glial cellular growth, differentiation, and death (37). The risk C allele was associated with greater WM volume in the cingulum/parahippocampal gyrus and the callosal body (38) and increased functional response in orbitofrontal cortex (39).

Among the genes related to both MDD and BD, the CACNA1 C gene regulates the L-type voltage-dependent calcium channel 1C subunit, which is involved in mechanisms of neuronal plasticity also indirectly affecting genetic transcription, neuronal signaling, and excitability (40). The rs1006737*A risk allele, possibly linked to a decreased expression of CACNA1C, has been related to MDD and BD (18, 41) with altered functioning of brain regions that have been related to mood disorders (42, 43). In MDD, the A allele associated with an increased activation in the left inferior frontal gyrus and cerebellar areas (44), whereas in BD was associated with greater orbitofrontal thickness (45), reduced GM volume in left putamen, and increased volume in the right amygdala and right hypothalamus (46). Thickness in caudal portion of ACC was also negatively correlated with age only in BD carriers of the risk allele (45). During emotional processing of negative faces, the risk allele associated with higher activation of amygdalae, and lower of ventrolateral prefrontal cortex (47–49). Higher hippocampal functional response has also been detected during emotional tasks (50, 51). During a verbal fluency task, CACNA1C risk allele associated with increased activation in the bilateral prefrontal-temporal and occipital cortex and thalamus (52). Other studies, however, failed in highlighting any significant effect of this gene on brain volume, thickness, WM integrity, and function (36, 53–56).

GWAS studies suggest a detrimental effect of SNPs involved in neurotransmission, neural growth, myelination, and plasticity on brain structure and function both in MDD and BD with a pleiotropic effect on corticolimbic circuitry involved in both affective and cognitive processes, confirming its relevance in mood disorder pathophysiology. It appears that these gene variants can influence brain structure and function, although the mechanism by which this occurs remains to be determined. More research is needed to understand both the function of these genes and their relevance in psychiatric disorders.

11.2 Polygenic Risk Score

Despite these promising results, studying single-risk variants may lead to explain only small effects. In order to evaluate the cumulative effect of multiple risk alleles, a polygenic risk score (PGRS) (also called genetic risk score or genome-wide score) has been developed. PGRS summarises in a single variable the genetic liability to a disorder prompted by GWAS results. For each subject, PGRS is calculated by summing the number of risk alleles, weighted by their effect size emerged from the GWAS study. The role of polygenic risk scoring in mood disorder has been widely investigated (57–59), however, when combining this approach to neuroimaging data in order to identify the influence of genetic factors on brain structure and function, limited and contrasting results emerged.

A higher polygenic risk for MDD and reduced WM integrity and cortical thickness in the medial prefrontal cortex, an area associated with negative affect and poor functioning in social domains, has been highlighted (60, 61). In the only fMRI study performed on MDD-PGRS during a working memory task, a higher PGRS was associated with increased brain activation in right middle frontal gyrus and the right supplementary motor area, whereas a lower PGRS was related to increased activation of the bilateral cerebellum, bilateral middle occipital gyri, bilateral middle frontal gyrus, right precentral gyrus, and left inferior parietal lobule (62).

However, other studies found no evidence for an association between PGRS and either subcortical brain volumes or WM integrity (63, 64) or functional connectivity in MDD (65).

Higher PGRS for BD has been associated with a lower functional response in visual cortex during a face recognition task, whereas signal in ventromedial prefrontal cortex and ACC was higher during working memory, face matching, and verbal fluency tasks (66–68). The volume of amygdala, as well as of globus pallidus, has been previously related to PGRS of BD (69). A resting-state study pointed out significant association between PGRS and functional connectivity between the insula and the bilateral cuneus, precuneus, posterior

cingulate, and midbrain (70). These data suggest a significant effect of the genetic liability for BD of brain functional activity and connectivity in both cognitive and affective processing. On the other side, studies focusing on structural imaging mainly failed in highlighting significant associations between PGRS and WM integrity, subcortical and cortical volumes (71–73). However, a GWAS study investigating average FA, as quantitative phenotype in unaffected relatives of patients with BD and a matched healthy control showed significant associations with SNPs involved in cell adhesion, WM development, and neuronal plasticity (e.g., EPS15L1, ADAM7, LPP, HEPACAM, ROBO4), supporting the role of WM microstructure as endophenotype of BD (74).

11.3 Candidate Gene Studies

Other results for imaging genetics come from the candidate gene approach where SNPs are preselected based on prior evidence for their functional role in coding products that influence relevant neural systems or relevant features previously related to the disorders. Accordingly, SNPs have been selected among genes involved in the activity of neurotransmitters such as serotonin (5-HT), dopamine, and glutamate, growth factors, and response to stress.

The most studied neurotransmitter in depression pathophysiology is 5-HT. Changes in 5-HT synthesis, turnover, and receptor density and structure affect the clinical outcome and pathophysiology of MDD and BD (75, 76), and SNPs involved in serotoninergic transmission have been explored in imaging genetic studies. The s variant of an SNP in the promoter region of the serotonin transporter (5-HTTLPR, SLC6A4 gene) is associated with reduced transcriptional activity (77), leading to lower serotonin transporter (5-HTT) expression and 5-HT reuptake. From a clinical perspective, the 5-HTTLPR*s allele is a risk factor for the development of MDD and in BD was associated with an earlier onset (78) and a worse response to antidepressants (79), whereas l/l showed a worse recurrence of mood episodes (78) and increased hopelessness and suicidal ideation (80, 81). In healthy subjects, 5-HTTLPR*s carriers showed increased amygdala reactivity (82, 83); lower amygdala–ACC functional coupling in response to emotional stimuli, with GM volume reductions in both these regions (84); and concurrent variation in emotional processing performances (85). The long allele of the 5-HTTLPR has been associated with decreased hippocampal GM and WM volumes in patients with MDD (86, 87). These results were confirmed when late-onset patients were considered, whereas a significant association between the 5-HTTLPR*s allele and smaller hippocampal volumes was observed in early-onset (88) and drug naive patients (89).

5-HTTLPR*s allele was also associated with smaller caudate nucleus (90), whereas LA/LA homozygotes (5-HTTLPR tri-allelic) associated with larger left thalamus and putamen volumes (91). However, other studies did not find significant genotype interaction in hippocampal volume (92, 93) and/or amygdala volumes (94), or the orbitofrontal cortex (95). fMRI studies reported (a) no association between 5-HTTLPR gene and amygdala activity or connectivity (96); (b) increased amygdala activation in 5-HTT risk allele carriers to masked emotional faces (97); (c) a lower activation of the medial prefrontal cortex and connectivity with amygdala in MDD (98), confirming an alteration in prefrontal-limbic regulation.

In BD, the 5-HTTLPR*s allele correlated to increased amygdala and reduced dorsolateral prefrontal volume, and WM integrity in several tracts (increased radial diffusivity and mean diffusivity in several brain tracts, including corpus callosum, cingulum bundle, uncinate fasciculus, corona radiata, thalamic radiation, inferior and superior longitudinal fasciculus, and inferior fronto-occipital fasciculus), suggesting demyelination or loss of bundle coherence (99). When considering childhood stress, in a GxE model, researchers found that patients carrying the 5-HTTLPR*s allele showed smaller hippocampal volumes when they had a history of emotional neglect (100). An association between 5-HTTLPR*s allele and alterations in microstructural fronto-limbic WM have been recently reported in depressed elderly patients, who also showed a lower remission rate (101). Related to serotoninergic transmission, an imaging genetic study explored effect of $5-HT_{1A}$ receptor promoter gene polymorphism (rs6295) on functional connectivity during processing of emotional negative stimuli. The risk allele (G/G) associated with worse antidepressant response (102), with a higher risk of committing suicide (103), and a higher coupling between

amygdala and ventrolateral prefrontal cortex for emotional stimuli compared to C carriers, also positively associated with depressive symptoms (104).

Another SNP investigated in mood disorder is the rs4680 on the Catechol-O-methyltransferase (COMT) gene. COMT inactivates extraneuronal dopamine in the brain and a valine (Val) to methionine (Met) transition leads to a decrease of enzymatic activity, resulting in an increased dopamine level (105). This genetic variant affects clinical and prognostic features such as response to antidepressant treatment (106, 107), recurrence of manic or psychotic episodes (108, 109), and rapid-cycling variant of BD (110). Structural studies reported controversial results. Val/Val patients with MDD showed a reduction in FA in several fiber tracts compared to Met carriers (111), suggesting a cortico-limbic network dysfunction in MDD. Conversely, a decreased FA in several fiber tracts (112) and smaller bilateral caudate (113) was reported in Met-carrier MDD patients compared to healthy control but not in Val/Val individuals.

An fMRI emotional processing study showed that activation in the inferior frontal gyrus (IFG), correlated with the number of met-alleles in healthy controls but such correlation was not seen in MDD patients. Moreover, during a working memory task, met-allele was associated with lower activation in the middle frontal gyrus (MFG) in both healthy controls and MDD patients (114). In BD, Val allele compared to Met allele, was associated with enhanced reactivity of the amygdala and reduced activity in ventromedial and lateral prefrontal cortex. Val allele was also associated with higher significant positive functional connectivity between amygdala, dorsolateral prefrontal cortex, and supramarginal gyrus, whereas Met carriers presented a significant negative coupling (115) during processing of negative stimuli. During working memory task, Val/Val displayed decreased activity in the dorsolateral prefrontal cortex (116). Data suggest that COMT affects pleiotropically the reactivity to stimuli in the prefrontal cortex and in amygdala in both healthy controls and BD patients.

Another Val/Met transition has been observed in an SNP (rs6265) in the brain-derived neurotrophic factor (BDNF) gene. The BDNF protein is a neurotrophin affecting cerebral plasticity, neural maturation, survival, and differentiation, and the Met allele may result in reduced transport of BDNF mRNA to dendrites and decreased packaging and secretion of BDNF in neuronal cells (117, 118). Several genetic-neuroimaging studies showed a significant genotype–diagnosis interaction with reduced volume in prefrontal cortex (119), anterior cingulate (120), and hippocampus (121) among MDD Met carriers. When accounting for a history of childhood trauma, Met carriers showed significantly smaller hippocampal volume, outlining the importance of a gene–stress interaction (122).

Met allele and lower BDNF serum levels were reported in ACC and caudal brainstem (pons) in depressed subjects. Additionally, lower BDNF levels in ACC were reported in subjects who had been exposed to early-life adversity and/or committed suicide, shedding light on its possible role in the neurobiology of suicide (123).

BDNF also affects WM microstructure, including the corona radiata, uncinate fasciculus, inferior longitudinal fasciculus, cingulum, and corpus callosum (124, 125), and resulted as a moderator of the association between uncinate fasciculus connectivity and antidepressants treatment response (126) in MDD. Moreover, an interaction effect of both BDNF and 5HTTLPR on the left transverse frontopolar volume was also detected, suggesting their important roles in brain regions involved in emotion processing in MDD (125). fMRI studies found decreased bilateral hippocampal functional connectivity with the temporal cortex and dorsal nexus (127), poorer performance at n-back task associated with hippocampal activation (128) in MDD Met carriers. In contrast with previous results, some studies found no evidence or even reversed data (90, 129, 130), thus, implicating the need to further elucidate these associations.

In BD, the Met allele was associated with reduced volume in hippocampus, in anterior cingulate gyrus, in dorsolateral prefrontal cortex (131, 132), with loss of gyrification, and with GM volume in left hemisphere (133, 134). Effect of rs6265 was not confirmed in pediatric BD patients (135). The abnormalities detected in BD have been suggested as neurobiological underpinning of the cognitive impartments detected in the disorder and associated with Met allele (136) and BDNF peripheral serum level proposed as biomarker for the disorder (137).

Among the neurotransmitters involved in mood disorder, glutamate has a crucial role due to its involvement in both neuronal signaling and neurotoxicity. Some neuroimaging studies focused their attention on D-amino acid oxidase activator (DAOA) and SLC6A15 genes, implicated in the glutamate synthesis and dysfunction. The DAOA rs2391191 was associated with altered region of homogeneity in the cerebellum, right middle frontal gyrus, and left middle temporal gyrus in MDD (138). Moreover, MDD patients with a SLC6A15 risk A-allele showed lower FA than controls with the same genotype in the left parahippocampal cingulum, known to be important in emotional processing (139). An abnormal region of homogeneity of the corpus callosum, cingulum and the frontal, parietal, and temporal lobes was associated with SLC6A15 rs1545843 in MDD patients (140).

After its release, glutamate reuptake is performed by excitatory amino acid transporters (EAATs), involved in maintaining physiological levels of glutamate in the brain. Polymorphisms in genes coding for these transporters affected WM, GM, and functional connectivity, interacting with adverse childhood experience. For EAAT1, rs2731880*T allele leads to reduced EAAT1 expression and glutamate uptake and T/T bipolar patients had a higher significant negative connectivity between the amygdala and ACC and performed better in the face-matching task compared to rs2731880*C carriers (141). For EAAT2-181A > C (rs4354668), when exposed to high stress, the carriers of the C allele showed lower axial diffusivity compared to A/A, whereas when exposed to low stress they showed higher axial diffusivity and higher GM volume (142). Excess of free glutamate may then contribute to vulnerability to stress. Within the Homer family of postsynaptic scaffolding proteins, exerting a crucial role in glutamate-mediated synaptic plasticity affecting synaptic homeostasis, neuroplasticity, the AA genotype of the Homer rs7713917 polymorphism, previously related to mood disorders and suicide (143), associated with lower fractional anisotropy in frontal WM tracts, lower GM, and higher fMRI neural responses to emotional stimuli in medial prefrontal cortex (144).

Other genes involved in the circadian rhythm, myelination, and neuroplasticity have been studied as possible biomarkers of mood disorder. Genes involved in the control system of circadian rhythms, related to core features of BD, such as patterns of sleep, rest, and activity, age at onset of illness, and response to antidepressant treatment (145) have been associated with WM microstructure. Period3 (PER3)$^{4/4}$ homozygotes had increased radial diffusivity and reduced fractional anisotropy, whereas CLOCK 3111 T/C rs1801260*C carriers showed increased mean diffusivity.

The A/A genotype of the transcriptional factor polymorphism of the sterol regulatory element binding protein (SREBF-2, rs1052717), involved in lipid and cholesterol metabolism, associated with increased radial diffusivity and reduced FA in cingulum, corpus callosum, superior and inferior longitudinal fasciculi, and anterior thalamic radiation. These results suggest a role of SREBF-2 in affecting WM integrity possibly related to its effect on myelination processes (146).

Glycogen synthase kinase-3 beta (GSK3β) is involved in the control of gene expression, and affect neurodevelopment and regulation of neuronal polarity, neuronal plasticity, and cell survival (147). Few studies exist in imaging genetics that reported an association of GSK3β rs6438552 and rs12630592 polymorphisms with altered GM volume in the right hippocampus and temporal lobe (148, 149), altered functional brain activity in the thalamus, and parts of the occipital and parietal lobes (150), and an association of GSK3β substrate genes with medial prefrontal cortices (151) in MDD patients.

In BD, a widespread effect on WM integrity and GM volumes was shown in less active glycogen synthase kinase 3-β (GSK3-β) rs334558*C gene-promoter variant. The low-activity C allele was associated with less detrimental clinical features of mood disorders, such as delayed onset and a better clinical response to treatments (152) and higher brain integrity; higher volumes and axial diffusivity were observed in ventral prefrontal cortex and in corpus callosum, forceps major, cingulum bundle, superior and inferior longitudinal fasciculus, fronto-occipital fasciculus, thalamic radiation, corona radiata, and corticospinal tract (153).

Considering the important role that stress seems to play in mood disorder, the glucocorticoid receptor, a mediator of the stress response, has been the focus of several imaging-genetic studies. The gene for the glucocorticoid receptor regulator FK506 binding protein 5 (FKBP5) is a glucocorticoid inducible gene that was found

to be associated with response to antidepressants (154) and the recurrence of depressive episodes (155). In fact alterations of the glucocorticoid system have consistently been reported in MDD (156). Results indicate that the additive effect of connectivity alterations of the right hippocampus and the FKBP5 genotype influence depression risk (157). Moreover, the interaction between the high-risk allele and childhood maltreatment associated with WM changes in the insula and inferior frontal gyrus (158). Other studies showed a volume reduction of portions of the frontal and parietal areas (159) and abnormal functional coupling of regions involved in perception, recognition, and attention allocation (160).

Finally, some study focused on late-onset depression and, as it often precedes the onset of dementia, on the APOE ε4 allele, which is known to be a genetic risk factor for Alzheimer's disease. Geriatric depressed patients with an ApoE ε4-allele showed alteration in hippocampal morphology (161, 162) that seems to be related to cognitive decline (163), smaller right medial frontal gyrus, left middle frontal gyrus and left inferior occipital gyrus (164), abnormal hippocampal functional connectivity (165), and default mode network connectivity (166). An increase in WM hyperintesities has been reported in patients with ApoE ε4-allele (167) who showed chronic course of MDD, a higher number of depressive episodes, and lower age at onset (168).

Although the mechanisms underlying this relationship remain unclear, geriatric depressive patients with the ApoE ε4-allele may be an early manifestation of the AD.

11.4 Epigenetics

Years of research on the genetic basis of several disorders has made clear that genetics is not enough to explain chronic diseases. Besides the DNA sequence inherited from parent to offspring and identical through life and in all the cells and tissues of our body, other information is present in our genome, which is cell and tissue specific and can be modified by the environment especially in critical periods during development but also later in life. This information is epigenetic and epigenetic modifications enable the regulation of gene expression without altering the sequence of the DNA. The most widely studied epigenetic modification is DNA methylation, that refers to the addition of a methyl group onto the 50 carbon of a cytosine ring by DNA methyltransferases (169). When methylation of the gene is done on the promoter region, it interferes with the binding of transcription factors to the promoter region, thereby inhibiting gene expression (170, 171). In this case, a higher degree of methylation is related to decreased gene expression.

As for genetic studies, the exploration of DNA methylation in mood disorders has focused on genes associated with the activity of neurotransmitters involved in the disorder such as serotonin, dopamine, and glutamate but also on glucocorticoid receptor for its role in the response to stress. Indeed, stress is widely considered one of the major factors responsible for the induction of epigenetic changes in mood disorder (172).

DNA methylation in the SLC6A4 promoter has been associated with history of lifetime depression (173), depression severity (174), antidepressant response (175), 5-HTT mRNA levels (176), childhood maltreatment (177), and acute stress (177), whereas hypermethylation was observed in a monozygotic twin with BD but not in controls (178).

Neuroimaging studies investigated SLC6A4 DNA methylation in association with different brain characteristics as WM microstructure, GM volume, and brain function. Medication-naive MDD patients showed elevated SLC6A4 DNA methylation, measured at five cytosine–guanine (CpG) sites of the promoter region, compared to healthy subject. Furthermore, a greater level of methylation was associated with lower fractional anisotropy and axial diffusivity (179), smaller hippocampal volume (CA1, gyrus dentate, and CA2/3) in patients with MDD, and with treatment with SSRI (180). The study of SLC6A4 methylation in an AluJb element in the promoter, a genomic element able to regulate nearby gene expression (181), showed that lower AluJb methylation was lower in MDD patients and associated with decreased amygdala reactivity during an emotional face-matching task. Furthermore, in subject carriers of the 5-HTTLPR/rs25531 risk allele, an increased bilateral amygdala activation was observed (182).

When considering the COMT gene, MDD subjects showed lower methylation at CpG sites 1–5 compared to healthy controls that were associated with lower fractional anisotropy and higher radial diffusivity in the superior longitudinal fasciculus, inferior longitudinal fasciculus, anterior thalamic radiation, and uncinate fasciculus in MDD, whereas the opposite was observed in healthy controls (183).

Two genes involved in the glucocorticoid response to stress have been investigated in epigenetic studies, the glucocorticoid receptor gene NR3CI and the FKBP5 gene. Decreased methylation of FKBP5 was observed in children and adult victims of childhood trauma (184). Also, in MDD, higher childhood trauma predicted lower FKBP5 intron methylation in the carriers of the FKBP5 rs1360780*T allele (185, 186). Lower DNA methylation of intron 7 associated with reduced cortical thickness of the right transverse frontopolar gyrus in the rs1360780*C allele homozygote group (186), reduced GM concentration, and increased hemodynamic response during an emotional recognition task in the inferior frontal orbital gyrus (185).

Methylation in the promoter region of the glucocorticoid receptor NR3C1 gene has been suggested to mediate glucocorticoid resistance by which HPA axis remains activated even after a stressor has ended. Lower methylation at two CpG sites of the NR3C1 promoter has been reported in MDD and associated with lower volume in the cornu ammonis (CA) 2–3 and CA4-dentate gyrus hippocampal subfields whereas, in healthy controls, lower methylations associated with lower volume in the subiculum and presubiculum (187). Greater methylation of exon1D of the NR3C1 gene, which includes a glucocorticoid response element required for transcription factors to bind and trigger autoregulation of the receptor after cortisol release, was associated with increased familial burden of anxious-depressive disorders and reduced resting-state hippocampal connectivity in a monozygotic twin sample (188).

Methylation at the BDNF promoter region has been associated with MDD (189), antidepressant treatment response (190), and suicide (191). Furthermore, in animal models, this methylation associates with BDNF gene expression in neuronal cells (192), suggesting that in regions with greater methylation this might lead to a decreased BDNF release. Indeed, greater BDNF DNA methylation at four CpG sites of the promoter region associates with lower fractional anisotropy in the right anterior corona radiata in MDD (193).

Involved in neuronal proliferation and differentiation, TESC rs7294919 methylation in the CpG pos 2 and pos 3 was greater in MDD, and greater DNA methylation of CpG 3 associated with lower FA and higher RD of the right parahippocampal cingulum (194).

In conclusion, factors affecting core psychopathological features of mood disorders, course and outcome of the illness, and the risk to develop the disorder, do influence brain structure and function, as studied with multimodal brain imaging. In turn, structure and function of the brain, as influenced by genetic variants, have been associated with core characteristics of the illness. This supports imaging genetics as a useful research perspective to investigate the biological underpinnings of mood disorders.

References

1. Barnett JH, Smoller JW. The genetics of bipolar disorder. *Neuroscience.* 2009; **164**(1): 331–343.

2. McGuffin P, Rijsdijk F, Andrew M et al. The heritability of bipolar affective disorder and the genetic relationship to unipolar depression. *Arch Gen Psychiatry.* 2003; **60**(5): 497–502.

3. Jansen R, Penninx BWJH, Madar V, et al. Gene expression in major depressive disorder. *Mol Psychiatr.* 2016; **21**(3): 339–347.

4. Hamet P, Tremblay J. Genetics and genomics of depression. *Metabolism.* 2005; **54** (5 Suppl 1): 10–15.

5. Chen G, Henter ID, Manji HK. Translational research in bipolar disorder: Emerging insights from genetically based models. *Mol Psychiatry.* 2010; **15**(9): 883–895.

6. Goes FS. Genetics of bipolar disorder: Recent update and future directions. *Psychiatr Clin North Am.* 2016; **39**(1): 139–155.

7. Bogdan R, Salmeron BJ, Carey CE, et al. Imaging genetics and genomics in psychiatry: A critical review of progress and potential. *Biological Psychiatry.* 2017; **82**(3): 165–175.

8. Meyer-Lindenberg A, Weinberger DR. Intermediate phenotypes and genetic mechanisms of psychiatric disorders. *Nat Rev Neurosci.* 2006; **7** (10): 818–827.

9. Fusar-Poli P, Howes O, Bechdolf A, Borgwardt S. Mapping vulnerability to bipolar disorder: a systematic review and meta-analysis of neuroimaging studies. *J Psychiatry Neurosci.* 2012; **37**(3): 170–184.

10. Piguet C, Fodoulian L, Aubry JM, Vuilleumier P, Houenou J. Bipolar disorder: Functional

11. Dima D, Roberts RE, Frangou S. Connectomic markers of disease expression, genetic risk and resilience in bipolar disorder. *Transl Psychiatry.* 2016; **6**: e706.

12. Amico F, Meisenzahl E, Koutsouleris N, et al. Structural MRI correlates for vulnerability and resilience to major depressive disorder. *J Psychiatry Neurosci.* 2011; **36**(1): 15–22.

13. Huang H, Fan X, Williamson DE, Rao U. White matter changes in healthy adolescents at familial risk for unipolar depression: A diffusion tensor imaging study. *Neuropsychopharmacology.* 2011; **36**(3): 684–691.

14. Kerner B. Toward a deeper understanding of the genetics of bipolar disorder. *Frontiers in Psychiatry.* 2015; **6**: 105.

15. Sullivan P, Wray N, Consortium PM. Genome-wide association analyses identify 44 risk variants and refine the genetic architecture of major depressive disorder. *Eur Neuropsychopharm.* 2019; **29**: S805.

16. Direk N, Williams S, Smith JA, et al. An analysis of two genome-wide association meta-analyses identifies a new locus for broad depression phenotype. *Biol Psychiat.* 2017; **82**(5): 322–329.

17. Hyde CL, Nagle MW, Tian C, et al. Identification of 15 genetic loci associated with risk of major depression in individuals of European descent. *Nature Genetics.* 2016 September; **48**(9): 1031–1036.

18. Ikeda M, Saito T, Kondo K, Iwata N. Genome-wide association studies of bipolar disorder: A systematic review of recent findings and their clinical implications. *Psychiatry Clin Neurosci.* 2018; **72**(2): 52–63.

19. Leal-Ortiz S, Waites CL, Terry-Lorenzo R, et al. Piccolo modulation of Synapsin1a dynamics regulates synaptic vesicle exocytosis. *Journal of Cell Biology.* 2008; **181**(5): 831–846.

20. Schuhmacher A, Mossner R, Hofels S, et al. PCLO rs2522833 modulates HPA system response to antidepressant treatment in major depressive disorder. *Int J Neuropsychoph.* 2011; **14**(2): 237–245.

21. Igata R, Katsuki A, Kakeda S, et al. PCLO rs2522833-mediated gray matter volume reduction in patients with drug-naive, first-episode major depressive disorder. *Transl Psychiatry.* 2017 May 30; **7**(5): e1140.

22. Ryan J, Artero S, Carriere I, et al. GWAS-identified risk variants for major depressive disorder: Preliminary support for an association with

neuroimaging markers in relatives. *Neurosci Biobehav Rev.* 2015; **57**: 284–296.

late-life depressive symptoms and brain structural alterations. *Eur Neuropsychopharm.* 2016; **26**(1): 113–125.

23. Woudstra S, Bochdanovits Z, van Tol MJ, et al. Piccolo genotype modulates neural correlates of emotion processing but not executive functioning. *Transl Psychiatry.* 2012; **2**: e99.

24. Woudstra S, van Tol MJ, Bochdanovits Z, et al. Modulatory effects of the piccolo genotype on emotional memory in health and depression. *PLoS One.* 2013; **8**(4): e61494.

25. Schott BH, Assmann A, Schmierer P, et al. Epistatic interaction of genetic depression risk variants in the human subgenual cingulate cortex during memory encoding. *Transl Psychiatry.* 2014; **4**: e372.

26. Lewis CM, Ng MY, Butler AW, et al. Genome-wide association study of major recurrent depression in the UK population. *Am J Psychiat.* 2010; **167**(8): 949–957.

27. Bermingham R, Carballedo A, Lisiecka D, et al. Effect of genetic variant in BICC1 on functional and structural brain changes in depression. *Neuropsychopharmacology.* 2012; **37**(13): 2855–2862.

28. Dannlowski U, Kugel H, Grotegerd D, et al. NCAN cross-disorder risk variant is associated with limbic gray matter deficits in healthy subjects and major depression. *Neuropsychopharmacology.* 2015; **40**(11): 2510–2516.

29. Kim BJ, Zaveri HP, Shchelochkov OA, et al. An allelic series of mice reveals a role for RERE in the development of multiple organs affected in chromosome 1p36 deletions. *Plos One.* 2013; **8**(2): e57460.

30. Kakeda S, Watanabe K, Katsuki A, et al. Genetic effects on white matter integrity in drug-naive patients with major depressive disorder: A diffusion tensor imaging study of 17 genetic loci associated with depressive symptoms. *Neuropsych Dis Treat.* 2019; **15**: 375–383.

31. Han KM, Won E, Kang J, et al. TESC gene-regulating genetic variant (rs7294919) affects hippocampal subfield volumes and parahippocampal cingulum white matter integrity in major depressive disorder. *J Psychiat Res.* 2017; **93**: 20–29.

32. Cui LL, Gong XH, Tang YQ, et al. Relationship between the LHPP gene polymorphism and resting-state brain activity in major depressive disorder. *Neural Plasticity.* 2016: 9162590.

33. Ota M, Hori H, Sato N, et al. Effects of ankyrin 3 gene risk variants on brain structures in patients with bipolar disorder and healthy subjects. *Psychiatry Clin Neurosci.* 2016; **70**(11): 498–506.

34. Lippard ETC, Jensen KP, Wang F, et al. Genetic variation of ANK3 is associated with lower white matter structural integrity in bipolar disorder. *Mol Psychiatry.* 2017; **22**(9): 1225.

35. Delvecchio G, Dima D, Frangou S. The effect of ANK3 bipolar-risk polymorphisms on the working memory circuitry differs between loci and according to risk-status for bipolar disorder. *Am J Med Genet B Neuropsychiatr Genet.* 2015; **168B**(3): 188–196.

36. Tesli M, Egeland R, Sonderby IE, et al. No evidence for association between bipolar disorder risk gene variants and brain structural phenotypes. *J Affect Disord.* 2013; **151**(1): 291–297.

37. Falls DL. Neuregulins: Functions, forms, and signaling strategies. *Exp Cell Res.* 2003; **284**(1): 14–30.

38. Cannon DM, Walshe M, Dempster E, et al. The association of white matter volume in psychotic disorders with genotypic variation in NRG1, MOG and CNP: A voxel-based analysis in affected individuals and their unaffected relatives. *Transl Psychiatry.* 2012; **2**: e167.

39. Mechelli A, Prata DP, Fu CH, et al. The effects of neuregulin1 on brain function in controls and patients with schizophrenia and bipolar disorder. *Neuroimage.* 2008; **42**(2): 817–826.

40. Gomez-Ospina N, Tsuruta F, Barreto-Chang O, Hu L, Dolmetsch R. The C terminus of the L-type voltage-gated calcium channel Ca(V)1.2 encodes a transcription factor. *Cell.* 2006; **127**(3): 591–606.

41. Green EK, Grozeva D, Jones I, et al. The bipolar disorder risk allele at CACNA1C also confers risk of recurrent major depression and of schizophrenia. *Mol Psychiatr.* 2010; **15**(10): 1016–1022.

42. Krug A, Nieratschker V, Markov V, et al. Effect of CACNA1C rs1006737 on neural correlates of verbal fluency in healthy individuals. *Neuroimage.* 2010; **49**(2): 1831–1836.

43. Thimm M, Kircher T, Kellermann T, et al. Effects of a CACNA1C genotype on attention networks in healthy individuals. *Psychological Medicine.* 2011; **41**(7): 1551–1561.

44. Backes H, Dietsche B, Nagels A, et al. Genetic variation in CACNA1C affects neural processing in major depression. *J Psychiat Res.* 2014; **53**: 38–46.

45. Soeiro-de-Souza MG, Lafer B, Moreno RA, et al. The CACNA1C risk allele rs1006737 is associated with age-related prefrontal cortical thinning in bipolar I disorder. *Transl Psychiatry.* 2017; **7**(4): e1086.

46. Perrier E, Pompei F, Ruberto G, et al. Initial evidence for the role of CACNA1 C on subcortical

brain morphology in patients with bipolar disorder. *Eur Psychiatry*. 2011; **26**(3): 135–137.

47. Tesli M, Skatun KC, Ousdal OT, et al. CACNA1C risk variant and amygdala activity in bipolar disorder, schizophrenia and healthy controls. *PLoS One*. 2013; **8**(2): e56970.

48. Dima D, Jogia J, Collier D, et al. Independent modulation of engagement and connectivity of the facial network during affect processing by CACNA1C and ANK3 risk genes for bipolar disorder. *JAMA Psychiatry*. 2013; **70**(12): 1303–1311.

49. Jogia J, Ruberto G, Lelli-Chiesa G, et al. The impact of the CACNA1C gene polymorphism on frontolimbic function in bipolar disorder. *Mol Psychiatry*. 2011; **16**(11): 1070–1071.

50. Whalley HC, McKirdy J, Romaniuk L, et al. Functional imaging of emotional memory in bipolar disorder and schizophrenia. *Bipolar Disord*. 2009; **11**(8): 840–856.

51. Bigos KL, Mattay VS, Callicott JH, et al. Genetic variation in CACNA1C affects brain circuitries related to mental illness. *Arch Gen Psychiatry*. 2010; **67**(9): 939–945.

52. Tecelao D, Mendes A, Martins D, et al. The effect of psychosis associated CACNA1C, and its epistasis with ZNF804A, on brain function. *Genes Brain Behav*. 2019; **18**(4): e12510.

53. Mallas E, Carletti F, Chaddock CA, et al. The impact of CACNA1C gene, and its epistasis with ZNF804A, on white matter microstructure in health, schizophrenia and bipolar disorder(1). *Genes Brain Behav*. 2017; **16**(4): 479–488.

54. Soeiro-de-Souza MG, Otaduy MC, Dias CZ, et al. The impact of the CACNA1C risk allele on limbic structures and facial emotions recognition in bipolar disorder subjects and healthy controls. *J Affect Disord*. 2012; **141**(1): 94–101.

55. Wolf C, Mohr H, Schneider-Axmann T, et al. CACNA1 C genotype explains interindividual differences in amygdala volume among patients with schizophrenia. *Eur Arch Psychiatry Clin Neurosci*. 2014; **264**(2): 93–102.

56. Radua J, Surguladze SA, Marshall N, et al. The impact of CACNA1C allelic variation on effective connectivity during emotional processing in bipolar disorder. *Mol Psychiatry*. 2013; **18**(5): 526–527.

57. Byrne EM, Carrillo-Roa T, Penninx BW, et al. Applying polygenic risk scores to postpartum depression. *Arch Womens Ment Health*. 2014; **17**(6): 519–528.

58. Levine ME, Crimmins EM, Prescott CA, et al. A polygenic risk score associated with measures of depressive symptoms among older adults. *Biodemogr Soc Biol*. 2014; **60**(2): 199–211.

59. Mullins N, Power RA, Fisher HL, et al. Polygenic interactions with environmental adversity in the aetiology of major depressive disorder. *Psychological Medicine*. 2016; **46**(4): 759–770.

60. Holmes AJ, Lee PH, Hollinshead MO, et al. Individual differences in amygdala-medial prefrontal anatomy link negative affect, impaired social functioning, and polygenic depression risk. *Journal of Neuroscience*. 2012; **32**(50): 18087–18100.

61. Whalley HC, Sprooten E, Hackett S, et al. Polygenic risk and white matter integrity in individuals at high risk of mood disorder. *Biol Psychiat*. 2013; **74**(4): 280–286.

62. Yuksel D, Dietsche B, Forstner AJ, et al. Polygenic risk for depression and the neural correlates of working memory in healthy subjects. *Prog Neuro-Psychoph*. 2017; **79**: 67–76.

63. Reus LM, Shen X, Gibson J, et al. Association of polygenic risk for major psychiatric illness with subcortical volumes and white matter integrity in UK Biobank. *Sci Rep-Uk*. 2017; **7**: 42140.

64. Wigmore EM, Clarke TK, Howard DM, et al. Do regional brain volumes and major depressive disorder share genetic architecture? A study of Generation Scotland (n=19762), UK Biobank (n=24048) and the English Longitudinal Study of Ageing (n=5766). *Transl Psychiatry*. 2017 August 15; **7**(8): e1205.

65. Wang T, Zhang X, Li A, et al. Polygenic risk for five psychiatric disorders and cross-disorder and disorder-specific neural connectivity in two independent populations. *NeuroImage Clinical*. 2017; **14**: 441–449.

66. Tesli M, Kauppi K, Bettella F, et al. Altered brain activation during emotional face processing in relation to both diagnosis and polygenic risk of bipolar disorder. *PLoS One*. 2015; **10**(7): e0134202.

67. Dima D, Breen G. Polygenic risk scores in imaging genetics: Usefulness and applications. *J Psychopharmacol*. 2015; **29**(8): 867–871.

68. Whalley HC, Papmeyer M, Sprooten E, et al. The influence of polygenic risk for bipolar disorder on neural activation assessed using fMRI. *Transl Psychiatry*. 2012; **2**: e130.

69. Caseras X, Tansey KE, Foley S, Linden D. Association between genetic risk scoring for schizophrenia and bipolar disorder with regional subcortical volumes. *Transl Psychiatry*. 2015; **5**: e692.

70. Wang T, Zhang X, Li A, et al. Polygenic risk for five psychiatric disorders and cross-disorder and

disorder-specific neural connectivity in two independent populations. *Neuroimage Clin.* 2017; **14**: 441–449.

71. Doan NT, Kaufmann T, Bettella F, et al. Distinct multivariate brain morphological patterns and their added predictive value with cognitive and polygenic risk scores in mental disorders. *Neuroimage Clin.* 2017; **15**: 719–731.

72. Whalley HC, Sprooten E, Hackett S, et al. Polygenic risk and white matter integrity in individuals at high risk of mood disorder. *Biol Psychiatry.* 2013; **74**(4): 280–286.

73. Reus LM, Shen X, Gibson J, et al. Association of polygenic risk for major psychiatric illness with subcortical volumes and white matter integrity in UK Biobank. *Sci Rep.* 2017; **7**: 42140.

74. Sprooten E, Fleming KM, Thomson PA, et al. White matter integrity as an intermediate phenotype: Exploratory genome-wide association analysis in individuals at high risk of bipolar disorder. *Psychiatry Res.* 2013; **206**(2–3): 223–231.

75. Serretti A, Cusin C, Benedetti F, et al. Insomnia improvement during antidepressant treatment and CLOCK gene polymorphism. *Am J Med Genet B Neuropsychiatr Genet.* 2005; **137B**(1): 36–39.

76. Zai CC, de Luca V, Strauss J, et al. Genetic factors and suicidal behavior. In: Dwivedi Y, editor. *The Neurobiological Basis of Suicide. Frontiers in Neuroscience.* Boca Raton (FL) Florida, US: CRC Press/Taylor & Francis; 2012, p. 213.

77. Kenna GA, Roder-Hanna N, Leggio L, et al. Association of the 5-HTT gene-linked promoter region (5-HTTLPR) polymorphism with psychiatric disorders: review of psychopathology and pharmacotherapy. *Pharmgenomics Pers Med.* 2012; **5**: 19–35.

78. Smeraldi E, Benedetti F, Zanardi R. Serotonin transporter promoter genotype and illness recurrence in mood disorders. *Eur Neuropsychopharmacol.* 2002; **12**(1): 73–75.

79. Serretti A, Kato M, De Ronchi D, Kinoshita T. Meta-analysis of serotonin transporter gene promoter polymorphism (5-HTTLPR) association with selective serotonin reuptake inhibitor efficacy in depressed patients. *Mol Psychiatry.* 2007; **12**(3): 247–257.

80. Parra-Uribe I, Blasco-Fontecilla H, Garcia-Pares G, et al. Risk of re-attempts and suicide death after a suicide attempt: A survival analysis. *BMC Psychiatry.* 2017; **17**(1): 163.

81. Russ MJ, Lachman HM, Kashdan T, Saito T, Bajmakovic-Kacila S. Analysis of catechol-O-methyltransferase and 5-hydroxytryptamine transporter polymorphisms in patients at risk for suicide. *Psychiatry Res.* 2000; **93**(1): 73–78.

82. Murphy SE, Norbury R, Godlewska BR, et al. The effect of the serotonin transporter polymorphism (5-HTTLPR) on amygdala function: A meta-analysis. *Mol Psychiatry.* 2013; **18**(4): 512–520.

83. Munafo MR, Brown SM, Hariri AR. Serotonin transporter (5-HTTLPR) genotype and amygdala activation: A meta-analysis. *Biol Psychiatry.* 2008; **63**(9): 852–857.

84. Pezawas L, Meyer-Lindenberg A, Drabant EM, et al. 5-HTTLPR polymorphism impacts human cingulate-amygdala interactions: A genetic susceptibility mechanism for depression. *Nat Neurosci.* 2005; **8**(6): 828–834.

85. Jonassen R, Landro NI. Serotonin transporter polymorphisms (5-HTTLPR) in emotion processing: Implications from current neurobiology. *Prog Neurobiol.* 2014; **117**: 41–53.

86. Frodl T, Zill P, Baghai T, et al. Reduced hippocampal volumes associated with the long variant of the tri- and diallelic serotonin transporter polymorphism in major depression. *American Journal of Medical Genetics Part B, Neuropsychiatric Genetics: The Official Publication of the International Society of Psychiatric Genetics.* 2008; **147B**(7): 1003–1007.

87. Frodl T, Meisenzahl EM, Zill P, et al. Reduced hippocampal volumes associated with the long variant of the serotonin transporter polymorphism in major depression. *Arch Gen Psychiat.* 2004; **61**(2): 177–183.

88. Taylor WD, Steffens DC, Payne ME, et al. Influence of serotonin transporter promoter region polymorphisms on hippocampal volumes in late-life depression. *Arch Gen Psychiat.* 2005; **62**(5): 537–544.

89. Eker MC, Kitis O, Okur H, et al. Smaller hippocampus volume is associated with short variant of 5-HTTLPR polymorphism in medication-free major depressive disorder patients. *Neuropsychobiology.* 2011; **63**(1): 22–28.

90. Hickie IB, Naismith SL, Ward PB, et al. Serotonin transporter gene status predicts caudate nucleus but not amygdala or hippocampal volumes in older persons with major depression. *J Affect Disord.* 2007; **98**(1–2): 137–142.

91. Jaworska N, MacMaster FP, Foster J, Ramasubbu R. The influence of 5-HTTLPR and Val66 Met polymorphisms on cortical thickness and volume in limbic and paralimbic regions in depression: A preliminary study. *BMC Psychiatry.* 2016; **16**: 61.

92. Ahdidan J, Foldager L, Rosenberg R, et al. Hippocampal volume and serotonin transporter

polymorphism in major depressive disorder. *Acta Neuropsychiatr.* 2013; **25**(4): 206–214.

93. Cole J, Weinberger DR, Mattay VS, et al. No effect of 5HTTLPR or BDNF Val66 Met polymorphism on hippocampal morphology in major depression. *Genes, Brain, and Behavior.* 2011; **10**(7): 756–764.

94. Hickie IB, Naismith SL, Ward PB, et al. Serotonin transporter gene status predicts caudate nucleus but not amygdala or hippocampal volumes in older persons with major depression. *J Affect Disorders.* 2007; **98**(1–2): 137–142.

95. Taylor WD, Macfall JR, Payne ME, et al. Orbitofrontal cortex volume in late life depression: Influence of hyperintense lesions and genetic polymorphisms. *Psychological Medicine.* 2007; **37**(12): 1763–1773.

96. Costafreda SG, McCann P, Saker P, et al. Modulation of amygdala response and connectivity in depression by serotonin transporter polymorphism and diagnosis. *J Affect Disorders.* 2013; **150**(1): 96–103.

97. Dannlowski U, Ohrmann P, Bauer J, et al. 5-HTTLPR biases amygdala activity in response to masked facial expressions in major depression. *Neuropsychopharmacology: Official Publication of the American College of Neuropsychopharmacology.* 2008; **33**(2): 418–424.

98. Friedel E, Schlagenhauf F, Sterzer P, et al. 5-HTT genotype effect on prefrontal-amygdala coupling differs between major depression and controls. *Psychopharmacology.* 2009; **205**(2): 261–271.

99. Benedetti F, Bollettini I, Poletti S, et al. White matter microstructure in bipolar disorder is influenced by the serotonin transporter gene polymorphism 5-HTTLPR. *Genes Brain Behav.* 2015; **14**(3): 238–250.

100. Frodl T, Reinhold E, Koutsouleris N, et al. Childhood stress, serotonin transporter gene and brain structures in major depression. *Neuropsychopharmacology: Official publication of the American College of Neuropsychopharmacology.* 2010; **35**(6): 1383–1390.

101. Alexopoulos GS, Murphy CF, Gunning-Dixon FM, et al. Serotonin transporter polymorphisms, microstructural white matter abnormalities and remission of geriatric depression. *J Affect Disorders.* 2009; **119**(1–3): 132–141.

102. Parsey RV, Olvet DM, Oquendo MA, et al. Higher 5-HT1A receptor binding potential during a major depressive episode predicts poor treatment response: Preliminary data from a naturalistic study. *Neuropsychopharmacology.* 2006; **31**(8): 1745–1749.

103. Lemonde S, Turecki G, Bakish D, et al. Impaired repression at a 5-hydroxytryptamine 1A receptor gene polymorphism associated with major depression and suicide. *The Journal of Neuroscience.* 2003; **23**(25): 8788–8799.

104. Vai B, Riberto M, Ghiglino D, et al. A 5-HT1A receptor promoter polymorphism influences fronto-limbic functional connectivity and depression severity in bipolar disorder. *Psychiatry Res Neuroimaging.* 2017; **270**: 1–7.

105. Bilder RM, Volavka J, Lachman HM, Grace AA. The catechol-O-methyltransferase polymorphism: Relations to the tonic-phasic dopamine hypothesis and neuropsychiatric phenotypes. *Neuropsychopharmacology.* 2004; **29**(11): 1943–1961.

106. Benedetti F, Dallaspezia S, Colombo C, et al. Effect of catechol-O-methyltransferase Val(108/158)Met polymorphism on antidepressant efficacy of fluvoxamine. *Eur Psychiatry.* 2010; **25**(8): 476–478.

107. Benedetti F, Barbini B, Bernasconi A, et al. Acute antidepressant response to sleep deprivation combined with light therapy is influenced by the catechol-O-methyltransferase Val(108/158)Met polymorphism. *J Affect Disord.* 2010; **121**(1–2): 68–72.

108. Benedetti F, Dallaspezia S, Locatelli C, et al. Recurrence of bipolar mania is associated with catechol-O-methyltransferase Val(108/158)Met polymorphism. *J Affect Disord.* 2011; **132**(1–2): 293–296.

109. Benedetti F, Dallaspezia S, Colombo C, et al. Association between catechol-O-methyltransferase Val(108/158)Met polymorphism and psychotic features of bipolar disorder. *J Affect Disord.* 2010; **125**(1–3): 341–344.

110. Papolos DF, Veit S, Faedda GL, Saito T, Lachman HM. Ultra-ultra rapid cycling bipolar disorder is associated with the low activity catecholamine-O-methyltransferase allele. *Mol Psychiatry.* 1998; **3**(4): 346–349.

111. Seok JH, Choi S, Lim HK, et al. Effect of the COMT val158 met polymorphism on white matter connectivity in patients with major depressive disorder. *Neurosci Lett.* 2013; **545**: 35–39.

112. Hayashi K, Yoshimura R, Kakeda S, et al. COMT Val158 Met, but not BDNF Val66 Met, is associated with white matter abnormalities of the temporal lobe in patients with first-episode, treatment-naive major depressive disorder: A diffusion tensor imaging study. *Neuropsych Dis Treat.* 2014; **10**: 1183–1190.

113. Watanabe K, Kakeda S, Yoshimura R, et al. Relationship between the catechol-O-methyl

transferase Va1108/158 Met genotype and brain volume in treatment-naive major depressive disorder: Voxel-based morphometry analysis. *Psychiat Res-Neuroim.* 2015; **233**(3): 481–487.

114. Opmeer EM, Kortekaas R, van Tol MJ, et al. Influence of COMT val158 met genotype on the depressed brain during emotional processing and working memory. *PLoS One.* 2013; **8**(9): e73290.

115. Vai B, Riberto M, Poletti S, et al. Catechol-O-methyltransferase Val (108/158) Met polymorphism affects fronto-limbic connectivity during emotional processing in bipolar disorder. *European Psychiatry.* 2017; **41**: 53–59.

116. Miskowiak KW, Kjaerstad HL, Stottrup MM, et al. The catechol-O-methyltransferase (COMT) Val158 Met genotype modulates working memory-related dorsolateral prefrontal response and performance in bipolar disorder. *Bipolar Disord.* 2017; **19**(3): 214–224.

117. Hempstead BL. Brain-derived neurotrophic factor: Three ligands, many actions. *Trans Am Clin Climatol Assoc.* 2015; **126**: 9–19.

118. Notaras M, Hill R, van den Buuse M. The BDNF gene Val66 Met polymorphism as a modifier of psychiatric disorder susceptibility: Progress and controversy. *Mol Psychiatry.* 2015; **20**(8): 916–930.

119. Ide S, Kakeda S, Watanabe K, et al. Relationship between a BDNF gene polymorphism and the brain volume in treatment-naive patients with major depressive disorder: A VBM analysis of brain MRI. *Psychiatry Res.* 2015; **233**(2): 120–124.

120. Legge RM, Sendi S, Cole JH, et al. Modulatory effects of brain-derived neurotrophic factor Val66 Met polymorphism on prefrontal regions in major depressive disorder. *Br J Psychiatry.* 2015; **206**(5): 379–384.

121. Frodl T, Schule C, Schmitt G, et al. Association of the brain-derived neurotrophic factor Val66 Met polymorphism with reduced hippocampal volumes in major depression. *Arch Gen Psychiatry.* 2007; **64**(4): 410–416.

122. Carballedo A, Morris D, Zill P, et al. Brain-derived neurotrophic factor Val66 Met polymorphism and early life adversity affect hippocampal volume. *Am J Med Genet B Neuropsychiatr Genet.* 2013; **162B**(2): 183–190.

123. Youssef MM, Underwood MD, Huang YY, et al. Association of BDNF Val66 Met polymorphism and brain BDNF levels with major depression and suicide. *Int J Neuropsychopharmacol.* 2018; **21**(6): 528–538.

124. Alexopoulos GS, Glatt CE, Hoptman MJ, et al. BDNF val66 met polymorphism, white matter abnormalities and remission of geriatric depression. *J Affect Disord.* 2010; **125**(1–3): 262–268.

125. Han KM, Choi S, Kim A, et al. The effects of 5-HTTLPR and BDNF Val66 Met polymorphisms on neurostructural changes in major depressive disorder. *Psychiatry Res Neuroimaging.* 2018; **273**: 25–34.

126. Tatham EL, Hall GBC, Clark D, Foster J, Ramasubbu R. The 5-HTTLPR and BDNF polymorphisms moderate the association between uncinate fasciculus connectivity and antidepressants treatment response in major depression. *European Archives of Psychiatry and Clinical Neuroscience.* 2017; **267**(2): 135–147.

127. Yin YY, Hou ZH, Wang XQ, Sui YX, Yuan YG. The BDNF Val66 Met polymorphism, resting-state hippocampal functional connectivity and cognitive deficits in acute late-onset depression. *J Affect Disorders.* 2015; **183**: 22–30.

128. Opmeer EM, Kortekaas R, van Tol MJ, et al. Influence of COMT val158 met genotype on the depressed brain during emotional processing and working memory. *Plos One.* 2013 September 12; **8** (9): e73290.

129. Gonul AS, Kitis O, Eker MC, et al. Association of the brain-derived neurotrophic factor Val66 Met polymorphism with hippocampus volumes in drug-free depressed patients. *World J Biol Psychia.* 2011; **12**(2): 110–118.

130. Kanellopoulos D, Gunning FM, Morimoto SS, et al. Hippocampal volumes and the brain-derived neurotrophic factor val66 met polymorphism in geriatric major depression. *Am J Geriatr Psychiatry.* 2011; **19**(1): 13–22.

131. Cao B, Bauer IE, Sharma AN, et al. Reduced hippocampus volume and memory performance in bipolar disorder patients carrying the BDNF val66 met met allele. *J Affect Disord.* 2016; **198**: 198–205.

132. Chepenik LG, Fredericks C, Papademetris X, et al. Effects of the brain-derived neurotrophic growth factor val66 met variation on hippocampus morphology in bipolar disorder. *Neuropsychopharmacology.* 2009; **34**(4): 944–951.

133. Matsuo K, Walss-Bass C, Nery FG, et al. Neuronal correlates of brain-derived neurotrophic factor Val66 Met polymorphism and morphometric abnormalities in bipolar disorder. *Neuropsychopharmacology.* 2009; **34**(8): 1904–1913.

134. Mirakhur A, Moorhead TW, Stanfield AC, et al. Changes in gyrification over 4 years in bipolar disorder and their association with the brain-derived neurotrophic factor valine(66) methionine variant. *Biol Psychiatry.* 2009; **66**(3): 293–297.

135. Zeni CP, Mwangi B, Cao B, et al. Interaction between BDNF rs6265 Met allele and low family cohesion is associated with smaller left hippocampal volume in pediatric bipolar disorder. *J Affect Disord.* 2016; **189**: 94–97.

136. Mandolini GM, Lazzaretti M, Pigoni A, et al. The impact of BDNF Val66 Met polymorphism on cognition in bipolar disorder: A review: Special section on "translational and neuroscience studies in affective disorders" section editor, Maria Nobile MD, PhD. This section of JAD focuses on the relevance of translational and neuroscience studies in providing a better understanding of the neural basis of affective disorders. The main aim is to briefly summaries relevant research findings in clinical neuroscience with particular regards to specific innovative topics in mood and anxiety disorders. *J Affect Disord.* 2019; **243**: 552–558.

137. Fernandes BS, Molendijk ML, Kohler CA, et al. Peripheral brain-derived neurotrophic factor (BDNF) as a biomarker in bipolar disorder: a meta-analysis of 52 studies. *BMC Med.* 2015; **13**: 289.

138. Chen J, Xu Y, Zhang J, et al. Genotypic association of the DAOA gene with resting-state brain activity in major depression. *Mol Neurobiol.* 2012; **46**(2): 361–373.

139. Choi S, Han KM, Kang J, et al. Effects of a polymorphism of the neuronal amino acid transporter SLC6A15 gene on structural integrity of white matter tracts in major depressive disorder. *Plos One.* 2016 October 10; **11**(10): e0164301.

140. Wang LJ, Liu ZF, Cao XH, et al. A combined study of SLC6A15 gene polymorphism and the resting-state functional magnetic resonance imaging in first-episode drug-naive major depressive disorder. *Genet Test Mol Bioma.* 2017; **21**(9): 523–530.

141. Poletti S, Riberto M, Vai B, et al. A glutamate transporter EAAT1 gene variant influences amygdala functional connectivity in bipolar disorder. *Journal of Molecular Neuroscience.* 2018; **65**(4): 536–545.

142. Poletti S, Bollettini I, Lorenzi C, et al. White matter microstructure in bipolar disorder is influenced by the interaction between a glutamate transporter EAAT1 gene variant and early stress. *Molecular Neurobiology.* 2018: 1–9.

143. Benedetti F, Poletti S, Locatelli C, et al. A Homer 1 gene variant influences brain structure and function, lithium effects on white matter, and antidepressant response in bipolar disorder: A multimodal genetic imaging study. *Progress in Neuro-Psychopharmacology and Biological Psychiatry.* 2018; **81**: 88–95.

144. Benedetti F, Poletti S, Locatelli C, et al. A Homer 1 gene variant influences brain structure and function, lithium effects on white matter, and antidepressant response in bipolar disorder: A multimodal genetic imaging study. *Prog Neuropsychopharmacol Biol Psychiatry.* 2018; **81**: 88–95.

145. Bollettini I, Melloni EMT, Aggio V, et al. Clock genes associate with white matter integrity in depressed bipolar patients. *Chronobiology International.* 2017; **34**(2): 212–224.

146. Poletti S, Aggio V, Bollettini I, et al. SREBF-2 polymorphism influences white matter microstructure in bipolar disorder. *Psychiatry Research: Neuroimaging.* 2016; **257**: 39–46.

147. Grimes CA, Jope RS. CREB DNA binding activity is inhibited by glycogen synthase kinase-3 beta and facilitated by lithium. *J Neurochem.* 2001; **78**(6): 1219–1232.

148. Inkster B, Nichols TE, Saemann PG, et al. Association of GSK3beta polymorphisms with brain structural changes in major depressive disorder. *Arch Gen Psychiatry.* 2009; **66**(7): 721–728.

149. Inkster B, Simmons A, Cole JH, et al. Unravelling the GSK3 beta-related genotypic interaction network influencing hippocampal volume in recurrent major depressive disorder. *Psychiatric Genetics.* 2018; **28**(5): 77–84.

150. Liu Z, Guo H, Cao XH, et al. A combined study of GSK3 beta polymorphisms and brain network topological metrics in major depressive disorder. *Psychiat Res-Neuroim.* 2014; **223**(3): 210–217.

151. Inkster B, Nichols TE, Saemann PG, et al. Pathway-based approaches to imaging genetics association studies: Wnt signaling, GSK3beta substrates and major depression. *Neuroimage.* 2010; **53**(3): 908–917.

152. Benedetti F, Serretti A, Colombo C, et al. A glycogen synthase kinase 3-beta promoter gene single nucleotide polymorphism is associated with age at onset and response to total sleep deprivation in bipolar depression. *Neurosci Lett.* 2004; **368**(2): 123–126.

153. Benedetti F, Bollettini I, Barberi I, et al. Lithium and GSK3-β promoter gene variants influence white matter microstructure in bipolar disorder. *Neuropsychopharmacology.* 2013; **38**(2): 313.

154. Horstmann S, Lucae S, Menke A, et al. Polymorphisms in GRIK4, HTR2A, and FKBP5 show interactive effects in predicting remission to antidepressant treatment. *Neuropsychopharmacology.* 2010; **35**(3): 727–740.

155. Binder EB, Salyakina D, Lichtner P, et al. Polymorphisms in FKBP5 are associated with

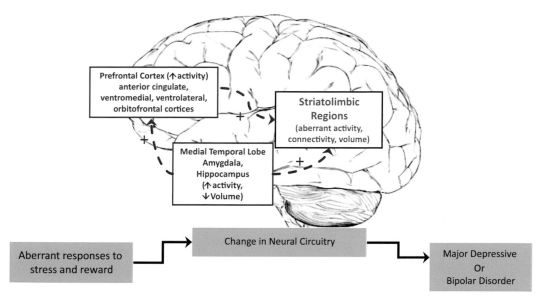

Figure 4.1 Candidate brain regions and circuits associated with aberrant responses to stress and reward in youth with or at risk for a major mood disorder. A black and white version of this figure will appear in some formats.

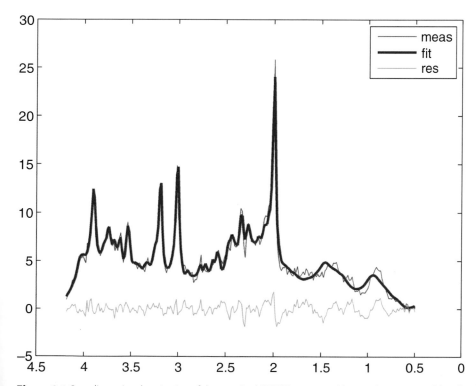

Figure 9.1 One-dimensional projection of the acquired JPRESS spectrum. Measured spectrum in blue, fitted in red, and residual in green. A black and white version of this figure will appear in some formats.

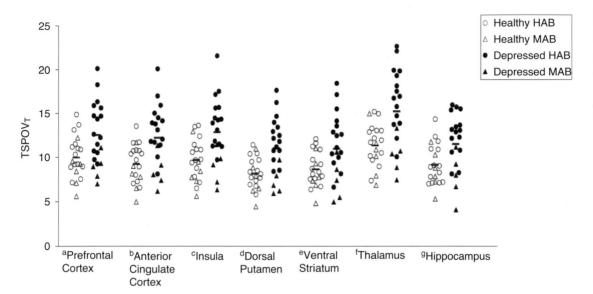

Figure 10.1 Elevated translocator protein density (TSPO V_T) during a major depressive episode (MDE) secondary to major depressive disorder (MDD). TSPO V_T was significantly greater in MDE of MDD (depressed, $N = 20$, 15 HAB, 5 MAB) compared to controls (healthy, $N = 20$, 14 HAB, 6 MAB). All second-generation TSPO radioligands, such as [^{18}F]FEPPA, show differential binding according to the SNP rs6971 of the TSPO gene resulting in high-affinity binders (HAB) and mixed-affinity binders (MAB). Red bars indicate means in each group. A black and white version of this figure will appear in some formats.

Adapted from Setiawan et al. (56)

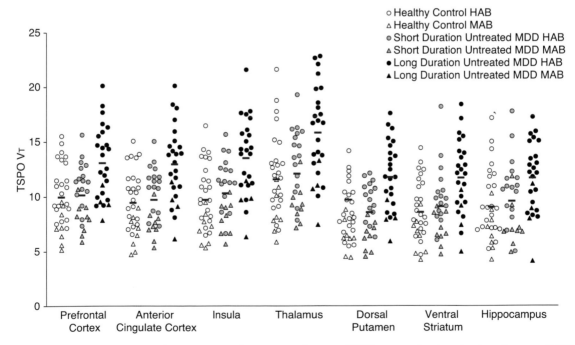

Figure 10.3 Translocator protein density greater with more years of untreated MDD compared to short duration of untreated MDD and healthy controls. A black and white version of this figure will appear in some formats.

Adapted from Setiawan et al. (59)
Group (duration untreated ≥10 years ($N = 25$), duration untreated <10 years ($N = 25$), and healthy ($N = 30$)) and genotype were significant predictor variables in a multivariate analysis of variance with TSPO V_T. Additional comparisons based on the least significant difference test showed significant differences between a long duration of untreated MDD as compared to healthy controls and significant differences between long duration of untreated MDD and short duration of untreated MDD in all of these regions. Second-generation TSPO radioligands, such as [^{18}F]FEPPA, show differential binding according to the single-nucleotide polymorphism rs6971 of the TSPO gene resulting in high-affinity binders (HAB) and mixed-affinity binders (MAB). Red bars indicate means in each group.

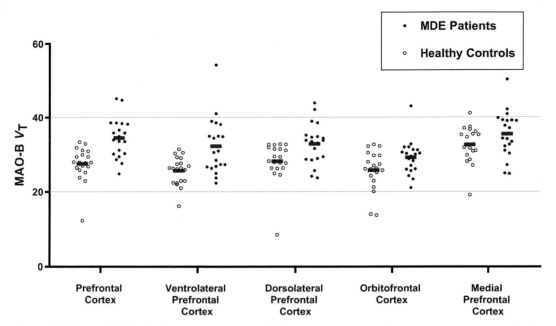

Figure 10.4 Elevated MAO-B distribution volume during MDE in the prefrontal cortex. A black and white version of this figure will appear in some formats.

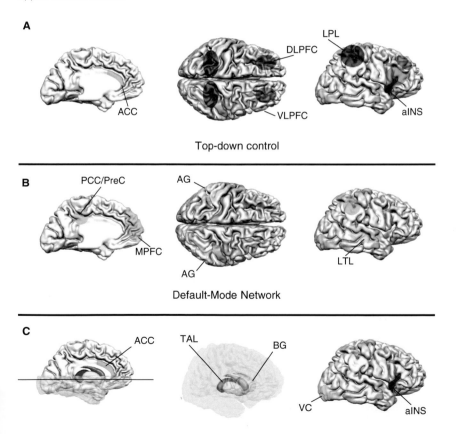

Figure 12.1 Regions recruited during neurofeedback guided self-regulation. A. A distributed network of regions implicated in cognitive control is activated during neurofeedback including lateral parietal and medial as well as lateral prefrontal areas. B. The default mode network shows modulations during neurofeedback that are likely due to the task demand and shifts in internally and externally directed attention, also reflected by deactivation of auditory areas in the lateral temporal lobe. C. Regions implicated in reward learning and visual processing are reliably recruited, including the visual cortex, the anterior cingulate cortex, the anterior insula, the basal ganglia and the thalamus. Abbreviations: ACC: Anterior cingulate cortex; DLPFC: dorsolateral prefrontal cortex; VLPFC: ventrolateral PFC; LPL: lateral parietal lobe; aINS: Anterior insula; PCC/PreC: posterior cingulate cortex / precuneus; MPFC: Medial prefrontal cortex; AG: Angular gyrus; LTL: lateral temporal lobe; TAL: Thalamus; BG: basal ganglia; VC: visual cortex. A black and white version of this figure will appear in some formats.

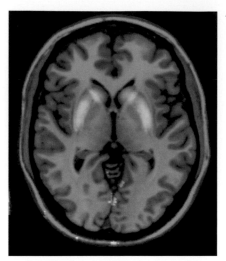

Dopamine Synthesis Capacity

Ki^cer (1/min)

0.00   0.03

Figure 18.3 A normative map of dopamine synthesis capacity as measured with FDOPA PET.
A black and white version of this figure will appear in some formats.

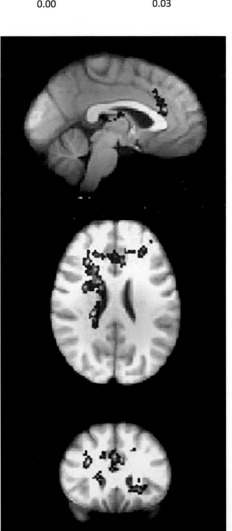

Figure 19.1 This picture illustrates the use of fMRI as a tool in research on treatment response biomarkers. Ths picture presents results of the whole-brain level analysis of response to masked sad vs happy facial expressions (thresholded at Z=2.3 and cluster-corrected with a family wise error (FWE) P<.05). Responders to escitalopram showed increased pre-treatment activation across a number of structures including anterior cingulate cortex, paracingulate gyrus, thalamus and putamen, as compared to non-responders to treatment. For details of the study see Godlewska et al., 2016. A black and white version of this figure will appear in some formats.

increased recurrence of depressive episodes and rapid response to antidepressant treatment. *Nat Genet.* 2004; **36**(12): 1319–1325.

156. Pace TW, Miller AH. Cytokines and glucocorticoid receptor signaling. Relevance to major depression. *Ann N Y Acad Sci.* 2009; **1179**: 86–105.

157. Cordova-Palomera A, de Reus MA, Fatjo-Vilas M, et al. FKBP5 modulates the hippocampal connectivity deficits in depression: A study in twins. *Brain Imaging Behav.* 2017; **11**(1): 62–75.

158. Tozzi L, Carballedo A, Wetterling F, et al. Single-nucleotide polymorphism of the FKBP5 gene and childhood maltreatment as predictors of structural changes in brain areas involved in emotional processing in depression. *Neuropsychopharmacology.* 2016; **41**(2): 487–497.

159. Han KM, Won E, Sim Y, et al. Influence of FKBP5 polymorphism and DNA methylation on structural changes of the brain in major depressive disorder. *Sci Rep-Uk.* 2017; **7**.

160. Tozzi L, Doolin K, Farrel C, et al. Functional magnetic resonance imaging correlates of emotion recognition and voluntary attentional regulation in depression: A generalized psycho-physiological interaction study. *J Affect Disorders.* 2017; **208**: 535–544.

161. Qiu AQ, Taylor WD, Zhao Z, et al. APOE related hippocampal shape alteration in geriatric depression. *Neuroimage.* 2009; **44**(3): 620–626.

162. Kim DH, Payne ME, Levy RM, MacFall JR, Steffens DC. APOE genotype and hippocampal volume change in geriatric depression. *Biol Psychiat.* 2002; **51**(5): 426–429.

163. Sachs-Ericsson N, Sawyer K, Corsentino E, Collins N, Steffens DC. The moderating effect of the APOE epsilon 4 allele on the relationship between hippocampal volume and cognitive decline in older depressed patients. *Am J Geriat Psychiat.* 2011; **19**(1): 23–32.

164. Yuan YG, Zhang ZJ, Bai F, et al. Genetic variation in apolipoprotein E alters regional gray matter volumes in remitted late-onset depression. *J Affect Disorders.* 2010; **121**(3): 273–277.

165. Shu H, Yuan YG, Xie CM, et al. Imbalanced hippocampal functional networks associated with remitted geriatric depression and apolipoprotein E epsilon 4 allele in nondemented elderly: A preliminary study. *J Affect Disorders.* 2014; **164**: 5–13.

166. Wu D, Yuan YG, Ba F, et al. Abnormal functional connectivity of the default mode network in remitted late-onset depression. *J Affect Disorders.* 2013; **147**(1–3): 277–287.

167. Chang KJ, Hong CH, Lee KS, et al. Differential effects of white matter hyperintensity on geriatric depressive symptoms according to APOE-epsilon 4 status. *J Affect Disorders.* 2015; **188**: 28–34.

168. Lavretsky H, Lesser IM, Wohl M, et al. Apolipoprotein-E and white matter hyperintensities in late-life depression. *Am J Geriat Psychiat.* 2000; **8**(3): 257–261.

169. Turecki G, Ota VK, Belangero SI, Jackowski A, Kaufman J. Early life adversity, genomic plasticity, and psychopathology. *Lancet Psychiatry.* 2014; **1**(6): 461–466.

170. Lutz PE, Turecki G. DNA methylation and childhood maltreatment: From animal models to human studies. *Neuroscience.* 2014; **264**: 142–156.

171. Szyf M. The early life social environment and DNA methylation: DNA methylation mediating the long-term impact of social environments early in life. *Epigenetics.* 2011; **6**(8): 971–978.

172. Caspi A, Hariri AR, Holmes A, Uher R, Moffitt TE. Genetic sensitivity to the environment: The case of the serotonin transporter gene and its implications for studying complex diseases and traits. *Am J Psychiatry.* 2010; **167**(5): 509–527.

173. Philibert RA, Sandhu H, Hollenbeck N, et al. The relationship of 5HTT (SLC6A4) methylation and genotype on mRNA expression and liability to major depression and alcohol dependence in subjects from the Iowa adoption studies. *Am J Med Genet B Neuropsychiatr Genet.* 2008; **147B**(5): 543–549.

174. Okada S, Morinobu S, Fuchikami M, et al. The potential of SLC6A4 gene methylation analysis for the diagnosis and treatment of major depression. *J Psychiatr Res.* 2014; **53**: 47–53.

175. Domschke K, Tidow N, Schwarte K, et al. Serotonin transporter gene hypomethylation predicts impaired antidepressant treatment response. *Int J Neuropsychopharmacol.* 2014; **17**(8): 1167–1176.

176. Olsson CA, Foley DL, Parkinson-Bates M, et al. Prospects for epigenetic research within cohort studies of psychological disorder: A pilot investigation of a peripheral cell marker of epigenetic risk for depression. *Biol Psychol.* 2010; **83**(2): 159–165.

177. Kang HJ, Kim JM, Stewart R, et al. Association of SLC6A4 methylation with early adversity, characteristics and outcomes in depression. *Prog Neuropsychopharmacol Biol Psychiatry.* 2013; **44**: 23–28.

178. Sugawara H, Iwamoto K, Bundo M, et al. Hypermethylation of serotonin transporter gene in bipolar disorder detected by epigenome analysis of discordant monozygotic twins. *Transl Psychiatry*. 2011; **1**: e24.

179. Won E, Choi S, Kang J, et al. Association between reduced white matter integrity in the corpus callosum and serotonin transporter gene DNA methylation in medication-naive patients with major depressive disorder. *Transl Psychiatry*. 2016; **6**(8): e866.

180. Booij L, Szyf M, Carballedo A, et al. DNA methylation of the serotonin transporter gene in peripheral cells and stress-related changes in hippocampal volume: A study in depressed patients and healthy controls. *PLoS One*. 2015; **10**(3): e0119061.

181. Kaer K, Speek M. Retroelements in human disease. *Gene*. 2013; **518**(2): 231–241.

182. Schneider I, Kugel H, Redlich R, et al. Association of serotonin transporter gene AluJb methylation with major depression, amygdala responsiveness, 5-HTTLPR/rs25531 polymorphism, and stress. *Neuropsychopharmacology*. 2018; **43**(6): 1308–1316.

183. Na KS, Won E, Kang J, et al. Differential effect of COMT gene methylation on the prefrontal connectivity in subjects with depression versus healthy subjects. *Neuropharmacology*. 2018; **137**: 59–70.

184. Tyrka AR, Ridout KK, Parade SH. Childhood adversity and epigenetic regulation of glucocorticoid signaling genes: Associations in children and adults. *Dev Psychopathol*. 2016; **28**(4pt2): 1319–1331.

185. Tozzi L, Farrell C, Booij L, et al. Epigenetic changes of FKBP5 as a link connecting genetic and environmental risk factors with structural and functional brain changes in major depression. *Neuropsychopharmacology*. 2018; **43**(5): 1138–1145.

186. Han KM, Won E, Sim Y, et al. Influence of FKBP5 polymorphism and DNA methylation on structural changes of the brain in major depressive disorder. *Sci Rep*. 2017; **7**: 42621.

187. Na KS, Chang HS, Won E, et al. Association between glucocorticoid receptor methylation and hippocampal subfields in major depressive disorder. *PLoS One*. 2014; **9**(1): e85425.

188. Palma-Gudiel H, Cordova-Palomera A, Tornador C, et al. Increased methylation at an unexplored glucocorticoid responsive element within exon 1D of NR3C1 gene is related to anxious-depressive disorders and decreased hippocampal connectivity. *Eur Neuropsychopharmacol*. 2018; **28**(5): 579–588.

189. Fuchikami M, Morinobu S, Segawa M, et al. DNA methylation profiles of the brain-derived neurotrophic factor (BDNF) gene as a potent diagnostic biomarker in major depression. *PLoS One*. 2011; **6**(8): e23881.

190. Tadic A, Muller-Engling L, Schlicht KF, et al. Methylation of the promoter of brain-derived neurotrophic factor exon IV and antidepressant response in major depression. *Mol Psychiatry*. 2014; **19**(3): 281–283.

191. Kang HJ, Kim JM, Lee JY, et al. BDNF promoter methylation and suicidal behavior in depressive patients. *J Affect Disord*. 2013; **151**(2): 679–685.

192. Martinowich K, Hattori D, Wu H, et al. DNA methylation-related chromatin remodeling in activity-dependent BDNF gene regulation. *Science*. 2003; **302**(5646): 890–893.

193. Choi S, Han KM, Won E, et al. Association of brain-derived neurotrophic factor DNA methylation and reduced white matter integrity in the anterior corona radiata in major depression. *J Affect Disord*. 2015; **172**: 74–80.

194. Han KM, Won E, Kang J, et al. TESC gene-regulating genetic variant (rs7294919) affects hippocampal subfield volumes and parahippocampal cingulum white matter integrity in major depressive disorder. *J Psychiatr Res*. 2017; **93**: 20–29.

Chapter 12

fMRI Neurofeedback as Treatment for Depression

Leon Skottnik and David E.J. Linden

12.1 Introduction

We urgently need new therapeutic strategies for depression (1). Depression is one of the top three causes of disability in the global disease burden statistic, affecting up to 15% of the population of high-income countries and with increasing prevalence also in low- and middle-income countries. This comes at huge socioeconomic and healthcare costs, especially because a large number of patients develop chronic illness, regardless of the available treatments that are effective for the majority of patients. The mainstay of current management are pharmacological and psychological/psychosocial interventions, and recent innovation has been particularly active in the field of physical interventions, adding transcranial magnetic stimulation (TMS) to the repertoire. Limitations of current treatment options include medication side effects, nonresponse, and frequent relapse. The scale of the public health problem and the limitations of existing treatments underscore the need for better, and more effective, treatment and relapse prevention options. In our opinion, interventions that involve the active collaboration of the patient are particularly promising, which is why the neurofeedback approach that has seen a resurgence in recent years is conceptually rather attractive.

Since its invention over twenty-five years ago, functional magnetic resonance imaging (fMRI) has become one of the most widely used and publicly visible noninvasive techniques to measure brain activation. fMRI-based neurofeedback (fMRI-NF) has the potential to open up new paths to translation. During fMRI-NF training, participants receive feedback on their brain activity in real-time and are instructed to change this activation, for example, by engaging in specific mental imagery. One attractive feature of neurofeedback is that it enables patients to control their own brain activity and thus contributes to their experience of self-efficacy, which is an important therapeutic factor in many neuropsychiatric disorders.

Recent advances in affective neuroscience in general and its application to depression, reviewed in Chapters 7 and 8 of this book, have paved the ground for the identification of neurofeedback targets (2). Modulation of prefrontal cortex and limbic areas could be used to improve emotion regulation, modulation of amygdala, insula and other parts of the salience network to normalize emotional reactivity, modulation of frontoparietal circuits or the default mode network (DMN) to attenuate rumination and tackle cognitive symptoms of depression, and modulation of the reward system to address anhedonia and the amotivational syndrome. The syndromal, multifaceted nature of depression poses a challenge to any unified treatment approach, but also plenty of opportunities to target specific neural substrates with neurofeedback. It is thus perhaps not surprising that depression is one of the clinical areas where fMRI-NF research has advanced most.

12.2 The Neural Basis of Neurofeedback

Although neurofeedback, particularly with EEG, has been applied for decades in research and in clinical settings (3), relatively little is known about the neural effects of neurofeedback. For neurofeedback guided self-regulation, previous research suggests an interplay of reward processing, self-regulation, and learning mechanisms in interaction with brain networks involved in the specific mental task driving the feedback (13). However, studies that investigated the general neural mechanisms of neurofeedback on the whole-brain level are sparse.

Notably, a recent meta-analysis compared whole-brain activation across different neurofeedback tasks, and thereby revealed extensive overlap in brain activation across neurofeedback studies in

151

prefrontal, parietal, occipital as well as subcortical areas and deactivation of the DMN (4). The observed network appeared to be congruent with the main theorized psychological components of neurofeedback interventions (Figure 12.1) and included regions recruited in self-regulation and executive control, particularly the ventrolateral and dorsolateral prefrontal cortex (vlPFC and dlPFC), the anterior cingulate cortex (ACC), the anterior insula (aINS), and clusters in the parietal cortex. Furthermore, it involved activation in regions involved in visual feedback processing and learning, such as the occipital cortex, the basal ganglia

(notably the dorsal and ventral striatum), and the thalamus. In addition, deactivation was observed for main hubs of the DMN, precuneus, posterior cingulate cortex, and lateral parietal cortex, as well as deactivation in Heschl's gyrus, potentially reflecting attention shifts away from auditory processing of scanner noise.

By comparing activation across different (affective as well as non-affective) neurofeedback tasks, the study by Emmert et al. (4) revealed a network of regions that is generally recruited during neurofeedback, but not necessarily specific for neurofeedback. Increases in the implicated parietal-

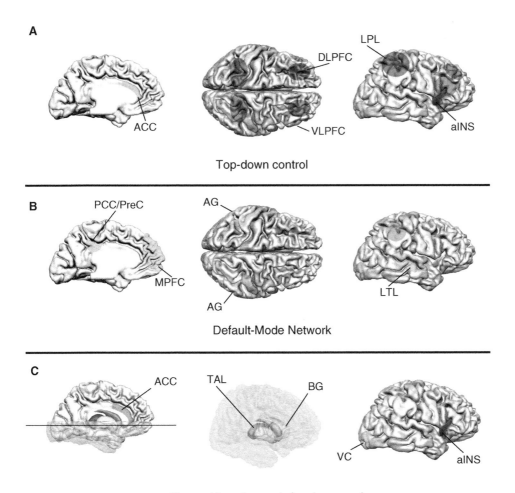

A

LPL

DLPFC

ACC

VLPFC

aINS

Top-down control

B

PCC/PreC

MPFC

AG

AG

LTL

Default-Mode Network

C

ACC

TAL

BG

VC

aINS

Reward learning and visual processing

Figure 12.1 Regions recruited during neurofeedback guided self-regulation. A. A distributed network of regions implicated in cognitive control is activated during neurofeedback including lateral parietal and medial as well as lateral prefrontal areas. B. The default mode network shows modulations during neurofeedback that are likely due to the task demand and shifts in internally and externally directed attention, also reflected by deactivation of auditory areas in the lateral temporal lobe. C. Regions implicated in reward learning and visual processing are reliably recruited, including the visual cortex, the anterior cingulate cortex, the anterior insula, the basal ganglia and the thalamus. Abbreviations: ACC: Anterior cingulate cortex; DLPFC: dorsolateral prefrontal cortex; VLPFC: ventrolateral PFC; LPL: lateral parietal lobe; aINS: Anterior insula; PCC/PreC: posterior cingulate cortex / precuneus; MPFC: Medial prefrontal cortex; AG: Angular gyrus; LTL: lateral temporal lobe; TAL: Thalamus; BG: basal ganglia; VC: visual cortex. A black and white version of this figure will appear in some formats. For the colour version, refer to the plate section.

prefrontal regions are also observed during various self-regulation tasks without neurofeedback (5–7), and deactivation of the DMN is reliably associated with attention-demanding tasks (8–10).

In addition to these shared neural components across neurofeedback tasks, distinct mental tasks and neural targets affect distinguishable, task-specific networks (11). Yet so far, no large-scale comparisons of multiple neurofeedback paradigms have been made, so it is not clear whether certain subgroups of neurofeedback approaches share an even more pronounced neural basis.

In addition to the scarceness of comprehensive whole-brain analysis on neurofeedback, the field also lacks evidence on the temporal properties of the neural processes occurring within involved networks. Taking into account how crucial timing is in operant conditioning (95, 96), these questions appear to be fundamental for the understanding how neurofeedback training can induce learning and reshape the brain. In one of our recent studies, we aimed to contribute to this issue by analyzing brain action across different self-regulation tasks, with and without providing neurofeedback (12). Self-regulation with feedback was accompanied by stronger activation in the striatum, and additional time-resolved analysis revealed that neurofeedback performance was positively correlated with a delayed brain response in the striatum that reflected the accuracy of self-regulation.

Overall, the current state of research suggests that, during neurofeedback interventions, task-general self-regulation processes execute control on mental task-specific areas beyond the neurofeedback target region. During this process, successful self-regulation performance is reinforced through positive feedback. For neurofeedback as a clinical tool, it remains to be specified to what extent processes specific to a given neurofeedback intervention and unspecific effects, such as reinforcement of general self-regulation abilities or improved self-efficacy, differentially contribute to treatment outcomes.

12.3 fMRI-NF Neurofeedback Treatments for Depression

While neurofeedback approaches differ with regard to the neural target that participants train to control, as well as the mental processes used to control the neurofeedback signal, previous theoretical accounts of neurofeedback have argued that neurofeedback-guided self-regulation generally implicates three main components (13): general self-regulation, reward learning, and processes specific to the self-regulation task.

12.3.1 Mechanisms Shared across fMRI-NF Neurofeedback Treatments for Depression

12.3.1.1 Self-regulation

The network recruited during neurofeedback across neurofeedback tasks includes areas implicated in self-regulation across various cognitive and affective tasks (4, 12). Of the recruited regions, especially the aINS, vlPFC, dlPFC, and ACC have previously also been related to different forms of top-down control in emotion regulation: particularly the aINS, vlPFC, dlPFC, and ACC have been shown to contribute to the endogenous generation of emotional states of positive as well as of negative valence, across different self-regulation modalities (5). Additionally, they are recruited during down-regulation of negative emotions across various emotion regulation strategies (6),

The task-unspecific recruitment of these areas in self-regulation suggests that a self-regulation network that contributes to cognitive control in various mental domains is reinforced across different neurofeedback approaches. Our recent neurofeedback study (14) supports this notion also in depression: a neurofeedback control group that performed primarily non-affective self-regulation (visual scenes imagery) showed significant improvements in clinical symptoms that were comparable to improvements of the (emotion-regulation) intervention group. These effects exceeded the expected improvements of placebo effects of other high-tech interventions in depression significantly. Notably, placebo-controlled neurofeedback trials on depression, in which self-regulation performance was not matched between intervention and control group, did not show corresponding improvements for the control group (15). Taken together, these results suggest that neurofeedback regulation alters symptoms of depression across specific neurofeedback tasks, but it is not clear what causes such general effects of neurofeedback. On the one hand, they could be related to improvements in general self-regulation abilities, but on the other hand they could also be related to unspecific effects of positive feedback or increases in self-efficacy.

In addition to top-down control, self-observation constitutes an intrinsic feature of mental self-regulation tasks that supports successful self-regulation (16, 17). It is therefore likely that introspective abilities contribute to such domain-general effects. Of the regions recruited during neurofeedback, especially the anterior insula and the ACC have been shown to play a selective role in introspection (18). Additionally, several studies support a link between altered insula and ACC functioning and alexithymia (19–22).

In the presence of pronounced deficits of subjective experience of internal states, the neurofeedback signal could constitute an external information source on ongoing mental activity. Notably, Zotev et al. (23) were able to show that neurofeedback performance during emotional memory recall was negatively correlated with alexithymia ratings in healthy participants, suggesting a relationship between perception of internal states and neurofeedback performance.

A recent neurofeedback approach motivated by this property of neurofeedback has provided depressed patients with neurofeedback on the effectiveness of mental strategies to control ACC reactivity to negative affective content in depression (24). Neurofeedback performance could predict whether strategies were experienced as being difficult to perform and efficient for controlling negative mood during the neurofeedback training, but were unrelated to ratings acquired before the training, suggesting that the information provided by neurofeedback was indeed used to evaluate subjective experiences. After a one-month follow-up, neurofeedback performance remained predictive of efficacy ratings and predicted how often patients would use certain self-regulation strategies in daily life.

Self-efficacy could be another crucial factor contributing to task-general effects, as perceived self-efficacy shows a negative correlation with subclinical depressive symptoms (25). Additionally, Kavanagh and Wilson (26) showed that improvements in depression correlated with self-efficacy of mood regulation in cognitive therapy and could be used to identify patients who showed remission

over the following twelve months (see also Maddux and Meier (27)).

12.3.1.2 Reinforcement and Regulation of Neural States

When providing feedback on self-regulation performance, successful self-regulation is accompanied by increased activation in the striatum (12), a key region of reward learning (28, 29). It has been shown that neurofeedback with patients with depression can lead to increased coupling between the neurofeedback target area and the dorsal and ventral striatum (30), suggesting that self-regulation reinforcement takes place during depression treatment with neurofeedback.

Besides reinforcing top-down self-regulation, another property of neurofeedback is its association with a decreased activation in the DMN (4, 12). Notably, it has been shown that hyperactivity of the DMN contributes to impaired self-regulation in depression (31) and modulations in DMN connectivity have been related to increased rumination in depression (32, 33). Taking into account the well-observed anticorrelation between attention networks and the DMN, reinforcing an upstate in executive networks as well as a downstate of the DMN could help to reduce the distorting influence of the DMN on ongoing processing in depression (34, 35).

In addition to being associated with a general decrease in DMN activation, neurofeedback provides the possibility to alter specific configurations of DMN connectivity: Young et al. (30) showed that neurofeedback-guided self-regulation with autobiographical memories altered connectivity between the amygdala and various nodes of the DMN. Connectivity changes were associated with memory recall and translated to post-scan resting-state measures. As DMN connectivity has repeatedly been related to alterations in self-referential thought in depression (31–33), Young and colleagues argued that neurofeedback could help to modulate distorted connectivity pattern related to negative self-referential rumination.

Besides its relationship to the DMN, rumination in depression has been repeatedly related to alterations in limbic activity (36–39). Previous neurofeedback approaches have used limbic regions as neurofeedback targets, either for modulating activation in relation to positive (15, 40, 41) or to negative valence (24, 42). The results of

Young et al. (15) revealed that neurofeedback can alter memory recall of autobiographical affective content, a crucial factor contributing to excessive rumination in depression (43, 44).

Overall, reinforcement learning thereby suggests the strong possibility of neurofeedback to modulate automatic neural processes in depression that are not directly accessible for cognitive control. While other forms of self-regulation, such as cognitive reappraisal or meditation, rely on voluntary self-regulation, neurofeedback can even reinforce neural target states when participants are unaware of receiving neurofeedback (45). However, the exact effects of this reinforcement learning likely differ between different neurofeedback target and self-regulation strategies.

12.3.2 Different fMRI-NF Neurofeedback Approaches in Depression

While different neurofeedback approaches share basic mechanisms of self-regulation and reinforcement learning, existing fMRI-NF neurofeedback approaches show considerable variance in methodology (for a recent overview see Thibault et al. (46)). In depression, basic differences between neurofeedback approaches exist with regard to the targeted psychological mechanisms, as well with regard to which neural markers were selected to create the neurofeedback signal (see Tables 12.1 and 12.2)

12.3.2.1 Emotion Regulation: Positive Affect
General Positive Affect

Our first fMRI-NF neurofeedback study performed with depressed patients focused on increasing activation in regions related to positive reactivity, without selecting neurofeedback target regions a priori (40). Individualized target regions were instead selected based on activation in response to positive images during a functional localizer scan. Taking into account that affective states show considerable interindividual variability with regard to associated brain activation (47), this approach ensured that regions were selected that were maximally responsive to positive experience in each participant. Concerning the content of self-regulation strategies, participants were free to modulate activation using individual emotion regulation strategies related to positive affect.

Thereby this neurofeedback procedure aimed at training individually sensitive aspects of positive affect, without restricting self-regulation a priori to an affective subcomponent such as salience or hedonistic value. Results indicated that participants were able to increase activation in the individual regions of interest (ROIs) using positive emotion regulation. In comparison to a control group that performed emotion regulation without receiving neurofeedback, depressive symptoms significantly improved.

While these findings provided first evidence for the clinical relevance of fMRI-NF neurofeedback in depression, they were obtained through a small, non-randomized study and not controlled for unspecific effects of neurofeedback, for example, the placebo effect caused by exposure to a high-technology treatment environment (as has been described in response to sham TMS in depression, see Berlim et al. (48), Berlim et al. (49)). Recently, our group addressed this issue in a randomized clinical trial (14). This trial compared the approach described by Linden et al. (40) to a neurofeedback control protocol that trained patients to increase activation in a non-affective, visual imagery task, using the parahippocampal place area as target region. Although no significant difference between groups was found, there was significant pre–post improvement in depression scores for both groups beyond expected placebo effects, suggesting that a clinically relevant mechanism may have been modulated in both neurofeedback groups (see Section 12.3.1).

Saliency of Positive Affective Experiences

Instead of aiming at generally increasing positive affect, the neurofeedback approach by Young et al. (50) focused on modulating a specific subcomponent of positive affect, that is, the salience of positive affective experience. In depression, salience responses to stimuli with positive valence are significantly impaired (51). In order to improve saliency of positive information in depressed patients, Young et al. (50) provided participants with amygdala neurofeedback that they trained to increase by contemplating positive autobiographical memories. The choice of the amygdala as neurofeedback target was motivated by its multifaceted relevance in depression: in comparison to healthy individuals, patients with depression show increased reactivity to negative stimuli (52–54) and attenuated reactivity to

Table 12.1 Studies applying fMRI-NF in depression

Year Published	Authors	Target process	Neural target	Group design	n	Neurofeedback regulation			Clinical improvements		Transfer	Follow-up	Neural outcome measure
						Baseline	Time	Group	Time	Group			
2012	Linden et al.	Positive affect: upregulation	Individual areas responsive to positive affect	NFI, SR	[8 8]	Y	N	-	Y	Y	-	-	NFP
2014	Young et al.	Positive memories: upregulation	Amygdala	NFI, OB	[14 7]	Y	Y	Y	-	-	Y	-	NFP
2014	Yuan et al.	Positive memories: upregulation	Amygdala	NFI, OB, H	[14 13 27]	-	-	-	Y	N	Y	Y	Connectivity
2016	Zotev et al.	Positive memories: upregulation	Amygdala	NFI, OB	[13 11]	-	-	-	-	-	Y	-	Correlation with EEG
2016	Hamilton et al.	Salience of negative stimuli: downregulation	Individual salience network region	NFI, Sham	[10 10]	-	-	N	-	-	Y	-	Negative reactivity
2017	Yamada et al.	-	FC (increase) between left DLPFC and left precuneus/PCC	-	[3]	-	(Y)	-	(N)	-	-	-	NFP
2017a	Young et al.	Positive memories: upregulation	Amygdala	NFI, OB	[19 17]	Y	Y	Y	Y	Y	-	Y	NFP
2017b	Young et al.	Positive memories: upregulation	Amygdala	NFI, OB	[18 16]	-	-	-	-	-	Y	Y	ROI activation

2018	Young et al.	Positive memories: upregulation	Amygdala	NFI, OB	[18, 16]	-	-	-	-	-	Y	Y	Connectivity
2018	MacDuffie	Reactivity to negative stimuli: downregulation	ACC	NFI	[13]	-	-	-	-	-	-	Y	Correlation with NFP
2018	Mehler et al.	Positive affect: upregulation	Individual areas responsive to positive affect	NFI, OB	[16, 16]	Y	Y	Y	Y	N	N	Y	NFP

Abbreviations: Y = yes, N = no; NFI = neurofeedback intervention, OB = other brain region, H = healthy participants, SR = self-regulation without NF; NFP = neurofeedback performance; WBA = whole-brain activation.

Table 12.2 Registered clinical trials applying fMRI-NF in depression

Year registered	Initiator	Target process	Neural target	Group design	Transfer	Follow-up	Main neural outcome measure	Identifier
2013	Moll	Blame related memories	Connecivity: anterior temporal lobe with septal/subgenual cingulate	NFI, OC	-	-	Connectivity/NFP	NCT01920490
2016	Young	Positive memories: upregulation	Amygdala	NFI, OB	-	Y	-	NCT02709161
2016	Peciña	Positive mood induction	rACC	Placebo, Medicated	-	-	NFP	NCT02674529
2017	Scharnowski	Not defined	Not defined	NFI [Depression, Schizophrenia, Nicotine Dependent], Sham	-	Y	WBA	NCT03165578
2017	Mathiak	Self-regulation abilities	PFC	NFI, OB [Depression Schizophrenia]; H	-	Y	NFP	NCT03183947
2018	Young	Positive memories: upregulation	Amygdala	NFI, OB	-	-	NFP	NCT03428828

Abbreviations: Y = yes; N = no; NFI = neurofeedback intervention, OB = other brain region, H = healthy participants, SR = self-regulation without NF, OC =other connectivity marker; NFP = neurofeedback performance; WBA = whole-brain activation. Retrieved from ClinicalTrials.gov.

positive stimuli (55, 56). Furthermore, it has been shown that the amygdala is a central node of the salience network (57, 58) and modulates the memory system based on affective arousal (59).

Upregulation of amygdala activity using positive autobiographical memories appeared to be effective for reducing clinical symptoms of depression in comparison to a control group receiving neurofeedback from a task-unrelated brain region. Whole-brain activation during a transfer run indicated increased activation in the temporal pole, superior temporal gyrus, and the thalamus for the experimental group in comparison to the control group. These structures have shown to be crucially involved in autobiographical memory (60–62), suggesting connectivity alterations specific to the trained mental task.

The training effects appeared to extend to post intervention mood ratings, with amygdala neurofeedback being associated with improved mood in indices of positive as well as to negative valence (50), supporting the effectiveness of amygdala-focused treatments for emotional states with positive as well as negative valence. A second clinical trial replicated the clinical improvements of this neurofeedback approach with higher sample size (15) and, currently, two ongoing clinical trials further test clinical efficacy of this approach by examining whether neurofeedback can support cognitive-behavioral therapy (63) and by targeting treatment-unresponsive patients (64), see Table 12.2.

In addition to outcomes in primary clinical measures, more general (neural) intervention effects were further investigated by Yuan et al. (41): comparison between pre- and post-training resting-state scans revealed elevated hypoconnectivity of the amygdala after the training, which predicted decreases in depression severity for the intervention group. Specifically, alterations in connectivity between the amygdala, temporal regions, and the hippocampus were observed, supporting mental task-specific alterations in the memory system. Connectivity analysis of the second trial data set (30) underlined the relationship between alterations in amygdala connectivity with training outcomes: Amygdala connectivity to the precuneus and the inferior frontal gyrus during neurofeedback predicted symptom improvements, suggesting clinically relevant alterations in processing of self-referential information and emotion regulation (for self-referential processing related to the precuneus, see Zhu et al. (32), Hamilton et al. (33), Sheline et al. (31) and for IFG (inferior frontal gyrus) involvement in positive emotion-regulation, see Engen et al. (5), Engen et al. (65)).

Notably, Young et al. (66) additionally demonstrated that effects of this neurofeedback approach could transfer to amygdala reactivity beyond the neurofeedback training. Increased amygdala activation during neurofeedback was associated with increased amygdala reactivity to happy faces and decreased reactivity to sad faces, as well as improved processing of positive stimuli in a behavioral test battery. Such transfer from neurofeedback training runs to markers of emotional reactivity provides a promising outlook for neurofeedback as a therapeutic tool, as this suggests that neurofeedback can induce changes in bottom-up-driven processes in depression.

12.3.2.2 Emotion Regulation: Negative Affect
General Negative Affect

So far, extensive research that focuses on self-regulation of general negative affect with fMRI-NF neurofeedback is lacking for depression. A previous paradigm developed by MacDuffie et al. (24) has, however, used neurofeedback to evaluate effectiveness of CBT strategies to down-regulate ACC activation in response to negative autobiographical content. As self-regulation behavior was significantly predicted by neurofeedback performance even one month after the neurofeedback intervention, results demonstrate the strong relevance of self-regulation of brain activation related to negative affective states for the treatment of depression. However, despite applying a functional localizer, target areas for this study were restricted to the ACC and results thereby likely reflect a preselection of affective processing that involves the ACC. Additionally, a currently running clinical trial (Mathiak (67), see Table 12.2) aims to train participants to regulate PFC activation using emotional reappraisal, a commonly used, effective strategy for regulation of negative affect (6). However, results from studies that apply an individualized approach equivalent to Linden et al. (40) to negative affect are still pending at this point.

Saliency of Negative Affective Experiences

Taking into account the meta-analytic finding that depression is associated with altered activation in the saliency network in response to negative affective content (68), Hamilton et al. (42) demonstrated that neurofeedback from subject-specific ROIs in the saliency network can reduce reactivity in the ROIs to negative images. These training effects were additionally reflected in decreased ratings of negative affect in response to the images.

While this study focused on reducing the salience response to negative affective images in a non-neurofeedback transfer task, it did not provide evidence for increased self-regulation performance through neurofeedback. Notably, an early study by Caria et al. (69) showed that healthy participants were able to upregulate aINS activation (a key hub of the salience network), which correlated with increased negative emotion ratings to subsequently presented negative images. Recently, a study by Herwig et al. (70) showed that amygdala reactivity to negative affective images can be downregulated. While these studies suggest that neurofeedback can indeed modulate negative salience responses, future clinical trials are necessary in order to determine whether patients with depression can gain reliable control over their hyperactive salience response through neurofeedback.

12.3.2.3 Connectivity Neurofeedback

Instead of providing feedback from mean activation in ROIs, connectivity neurofeedback approaches provide participants with feedback on how far activation between different regions becomes (de)synchronized. The distributed alterations in connectivity that accompany neurofeedback interventions in depression (30, 41), as well as the importance of interregional connectivity for emotion regulation (71, 72) and emotion processing (72, 73) suggest that a large number of clinically relevant processes are manifested at the level of interregional connectivity.

While connectivity alterations in response to neurofeedback procedures that target the average activation in a ROI (see Sections 12.3.2.1 and 12.3.2.2) demonstrate that these approaches, too, modulate interregional connectivity, patients are not aware of alterations in brain connectivity in these scenarios. It remains an open question at this point whether connectivity neurofeedback can provide additional therapeutic value compared to regional neurofeedback in depression because no head-to-head comparisons have been performed.

So far, evidence for the efficacy of connectivity neurofeedback in depression is sparse. One recent clinical trial on depression tests the possibility of modulating connectivity between the anterior temporal lobe and the septal/subgenual cingulate with neurofeedback, in relation to subjective experience of self-blame. Initial results indicated that participants are able to modulate connectivity in relation to feelings of guilt (74), but results on the clinical efficacy of this approach are still pending.

While this approach aimed to modulate functional coupling related to defined mental processes, depression is also associated with alterations in large-scale connectivity pattern at rest for which underlying psychological mechanisms are not clear (75–77). Remarkably, connectivity patterns during resting state have been shown to function as sensitive biomarkers for depression (Drysdale et al. (78), but also see Dinga et al. (79)).

Taking this into account, Yamada et al. (80) extracted neurofeedback information based on resting-state connectivity biomarkers for depression diagnosis and severity of symptoms, instead of focusing on altering connectivity specific to a certain psychological process. Preliminary results indicated that participants were able to control the provided connectivity marker, and showed a trend toward improvement of depressive symptoms. While these early results are preliminary and based on a small sample, this approach has potential for clinical applications due to its data-driven nature.

Another approach that captures distributed information from fMRI signals relies on the multivariate decoding of brain activation, for example, in relation to specific emotional states. Pilot work has demonstrated that participants can increase activation patterns related to specific emotions (81). It remains to be tested in clinical trials whether this methodology can also be used to reinforce desirable emotional states in patients with depression with clinical benefits.

12.4 Discussion

The research discussed in this chapter provides evidence across various studies that fMRI-NF constitutes a promising treatment option for depression. While fMRI-NF carries the potential to influence a multitude of functional mechanisms, the existing evidence is largely unstructured, due to the lack of standardized treatment designs and the variability in applied neurofeedback approaches.

The clinical potential of fMRI-NF for depression is therefore far from being fully exploited.

While this chapter focused on the functional mechanisms and the efficacy of fMRI-NF treatments for treating depression, extensive research is also needed to understand how neurofeedback would interact with other forms of treatment, and, under which circumstances certain types of neurofeedback treatments are preferable and which treatment combinations result in optimal effects. Important steps toward creating standard neurofeedback treatments will be to examine which neurofeedback approaches are most effective or whether different approaches are particularly effective for certain subgroups of patients. At this moment, direct comparisons between different fMRI-NF treatments for depression have not been performed. Likewise, it is not clear whether effects of neurofeedback are modulated by psychotherapy or pharmacological treatments. With regard to such interactions with other treatment options, especially combinations between brain stimulation techniques such as TMS, could provide novel treatment options and insights into the neural basis of depression, as both approaches offer flexible control over neural treatment effects. While first closed-loop neurofeedback-TMS systems have been implemented (82, 83), the applicability of this approach for depression remains an open question.

Another group of treatments that shows potential for being combined with neurofeedback are biofeedback trainings that take respiratory or cardiac activity as feedback rather than brain activation. Such biofeedback approaches, such as heart rate variability biofeedback, also have been shown to reduce symptoms of depression (see Siepmann et al. (84); Karavidas et al. (85)), and could contribute to the training of self-regulation strategies, interoceptive abilities, as well as self-efficacy in patients with depression (see Gevirtz (86)). In addition, meditation-based treatments share several psychological core aspects with biofeedback interventions, for example, training of self-regulation skills and introspection (87–89), and can reduce depressive symptoms (90). Because these approaches are not as costly and resource-intensive as fMRI-NF approaches, but potentially require more training sessions, combining such interventions with neurofeedback could provide a possibility to allow for continuous self-regulation training, while reducing treatment costs.

Furthermore, due to the necessity for neurofeedback setups to acquire brain data, neurofeedback can be utilized as a research/diagnostic tool at the same time as it is applied for treatment purposes. Ongoing clinical trials exploit this feature of neurofeedback, by using neurofeedback performance as a marker to evaluate responsiveness to pharmacological treatments (91) or by treating patients with different mental disorders within the same neurofeedback trial (92), allowing for structured comparisons of self-regulation and reward-learning deficits across psychopathologies.

Overall, the review of the evidence for fMRI-NF in depression has shown that, regardless of the range of activities and paradigms tested in the field, only a small number of studies have applied rigorous trials methodology, and no definitive information about its efficacy (let alone the differential efficacy of different protocols) is available. One of the main challenges of the field is the definition of appropriate control conditions for randomized trials (see Sorger et al. (93)). Another is the need for standardization, both of outcome measures and of intervention protocols, to allow for meta-analysis (94). The feasibility demonstrated by the early clinical trials, as well as the very good safety record of fMRI-neurofeedback, makes this an attractive line to pursue further, both for refinement of interventional protocols (especially regarding combination with psychological and other neuromodulation interventions) and for testing in larger efficacy trials. One critique that is often raised concerns the high costs of fMRI scanning compared to EEG neurofeedback or psychological interventions, but if similar effects can be obtained with a smaller number of sessions, an fMRI-based methodology can still be cost-effective.

References

1. Linden DE. Neurofeedback and networks of depression. *Dialogues Clin Neurosci*. 2014; **16**(1): 103–112.

2. Esmail S, Linden DE. Emotion regulation networks and neurofeedback in depression. *Cognitive Sciences*. 2011; **6**(2): 101.

3. Linden DE. *Brain Control: Developments in Therapy and Implications for Society*. Springer; 2014.

4. Emmert K, Kopel R, Sulzer J, et al. Meta-analysis of real-time fMRI neurofeedback studies using individual participant data: How is brain regulation mediated? *Neuroimage*. 2016; **124**: 806–812.

5. Engen HG, Kanske P, Singer T. The neural component-process architecture of endogenously generated emotion. *Social Cognitive and Affective Neuroscience*. 2016; **12**(2): 197–211.

6. Dörfel D, Lamke J-P, Hummel F, et al. Common and differential neural networks of emotion regulation by detachment, reinterpretation, distraction, and expressive suppression: a comparative fMRI investigation. *Neuroimage*. 2014; **101**: 298–309.

7. Cohen JR, Berkman ET, Lieberman MD. Intentional and incidental self-control in ventrolateral PFC. In: Donald T. Stuss and Robert T. Knight. editors. *Principles of Frontal Lobe Function*. 2nd edition. Oxford University Press; 2013, pp. 417–40.

8. Anderson JS, Ferguson MA, Lopez-Larson M, Yurgelun-Todd D. Connectivity gradients between the default mode and attention control networks. *Brain Connectivity*. 2011; **1**(2): 147–157.

9. Singh KD, Fawcett I. Transient and linearly graded deactivation of the human default-mode network by a visual detection task. *Neuroimage*. 2008; **41**(1): 100–112.

10. Sridharan D, Levitin DJ, Menon V. A critical role for the right fronto-insular cortex in switching between central-executive and default-mode networks. *Proceedings of the National Academy of Sciences*. 2008; **105**(34): 12569–12574.

11. Scharnowski F, Veit R, Zopf R, et al. Manipulating motor performance and memory through real-time fMRI neurofeedback. *Biological Psychology*. 2015; **108**: 85–97.

12. Skottnik L, Sorger B, Kamp T, Linden D, Goebel R. Success and failure of controlling the real-time functional magnetic resonance imaging neurofeedback signal are reflected in the striatum. *Brain and Behavior*. 2019 March; **9**(3): e01240.

13. Sitaram R, Ros T, Stoeckel L, et al. Closed-loop brain training: The science of neurofeedback. *Nature Reviews Neuroscience*. 2017; **18**(2): 86.

14. Mehler DM, Sokunbi MO, Habes I, et al. Targeting the affective brain—a randomized controlled trial of real-time fMRI neurofeedback in patients with depression. *Neuropsychopharmacology*. 2018; **43**(13): 2578.

15. Young KD, Siegle GJ, Zotev V, et al. Randomized clinical trial of real-time fMRI amygdala neurofeedback for major depressive disorder: Effects on symptoms and autobiographical memory recall. *American Journal of Psychiatry*. 2017 August 1; **174**(8): 748–755.

16. Herwig U, Kaffenberger T, Jäncke L, Brühl AB. Self-related awareness and emotion regulation. *NeuroImage*. 2010; **50**(2): 734–741.

17. Beer JS, Heerey EA, Keltner D, Scabini D, Knight RT. The regulatory function of self-conscious emotion: Insights from patients with orbitofrontal damage. *Journal of Personality and Social Psychology*. 2003; **85**(4): 594.

18. Schooler JW, Smallwood J, Christoff K, et al. Meta-awareness, perceptual decoupling and the wandering mind. *Trends in Cognitive Sciences*. 2011; **15**(7): 319–326.

19. Ernst J, Böker H, Hättenschwiler J, et al. The association of interoceptive awareness and alexithymia with neurotransmitter concentrations in insula and anterior cingulate. *Social Cognitive and Affective Neuroscience*. 2013; **9**(6): 857–863.

20. Deng Y, Ma X, Tang Q. Brain response during visual emotional processing: An fMRI study of alexithymia. *Psychiatry Research: Neuroimaging*. 2013; **213**(3): 225–229.

21. Goerlich-Dobre KS, Bruce L, Martens S, Aleman A, Hooker CI. Distinct associations of insula and cingulate volume with the cognitive and affective dimensions of alexithymia. *Neuropsychologia*. 2014; **53**: 284–292.

22. Hogeveen J, Bird G, Chau A, Krueger F, Grafman J. Acquired alexithymia following damage to the anterior insula. *Neuropsychologia*. 2016; **82**: 142–148.

23. Zotev V, Krueger F, Phillips R, et al. Self-regulation of amygdala activation using real-time fMRI neurofeedback. *PloS One*. 2011; **6**(9): e24522.

24. MacDuffie KE, MacInnes J, Dickerson KC, et al. Single session real-time fMRI neurofeedback has a lasting impact on cognitive behavioral therapy strategies. *NeuroImage: Clinical*. 2018; **19**: 868–875.

25. Muris P. Relationships between self-efficacy and symptoms of anxiety disorders and depression in a normal adolescent sample. *Personality and Individual Differences*. 2002; **32**(2): 337–348.

26. Kavanagh DJ, Wilson PH. Prediction of outcome with group cognitive therapy for depression. *Behaviour Research and Therapy*. 1989; **27**(4): 333–343.

27. Maddux JE, Meier LJ. Self-Efficacy and Depression. Self-Efficacy, Adaptation, and Adjustment. Springer; 1995. 143–169.

28. Bartra O, McGuire JT, Kable JW. The valuation system: A coordinate-based meta-analysis of BOLD fMRI experiments examining neural correlates of subjective value. *Neuroimage*. 2013; **76**: 412–427.

29. Balleine BW, Delgado MR, Hikosaka O. The role of the dorsal striatum in reward and

decision-making. *Journal of Neuroscience*. 2007; **27**(31): 8161–8165.

30. Young KD, Siegle GJ, Misaki M, et al. Altered task-based and resting-state amygdala functional connectivity following real-time fMRI amygdala neurofeedback training in major depressive disorder. *NeuroImage: Clinical*. 2018; **17**: 691–703.

31. Sheline YI, Barch DM, Price JL, et al. The default mode network and self-referential processes in depression. *Proceedings of the National Academy of Sciences*. 2009; **106**(6): 1942–1947.

32. Zhu X, Wang X, Xiao J, et al. Evidence of a dissociation pattern in resting-state default mode network connectivity in first-episode, treatment-naive major depression patients. *Biological Psychiatry*. 2012; **71**(7): 611–617.

33. Hamilton JP, Furman DJ, Chang C, et al. Default-mode and task-positive network activity in major depressive disorder: Implications for adaptive and maladaptive rumination. *Biological Psychiatry*. 2011; **70**(4): 327–333.

34. Marchetti I, Koster EH, Sonuga-Barke EJ, De Raedt R. The default mode network and recurrent depression: A neurobiological model of cognitive risk factors. *Neuropsychology Review*. 2012; **22**(3): 229–251.

35. Belleau EL, Taubitz LE, Larson CL. Imbalance of default mode and regulatory networks during externally focused processing in depression. *Social Cognitive and Affective Neuroscience*. 2014; **10**(5): 744–751.

36. Burkhouse KL, Jacobs RH, Peters AT, et al. Neural correlates of rumination in adolescents with remitted major depressive disorder and healthy controls. *Cognitive, Affective, & Behavioral Neuroscience*. 2017; **17**(2): 394–405.

37. Mandell D, Siegle GJ, Shutt L, Feldmiller J, Thase ME. Neural substrates of trait ruminations in depression. *Journal of Abnormal Psychology*. 2014; **123**(1): 35.

38. Siegle GJ, Steinhauer SR, Thase ME, Stenger VA, Carter CS. Can't shake that feeling: event-related fMRI assessment of sustained amygdala activity in response to emotional information in depressed individuals. *Biological Psychiatry*. 2002; **51**(9): 693–707.

39. Siegle GJ, Carter CS, Thase ME. Use of fMRI to predict recovery from unipolar depression with cognitive behavior therapy. *American Journal of Psychiatry*. 2006; **163**(4): 735–738.

40. Linden DE, Habes I, Johnston SJ, et al. Real-time self-regulation of emotion networks in patients with depression. *PloS One*. 2012; **7**(6): e38115.

41. Yuan H, Young KD, Phillips R, et al. Resting-state functional connectivity modulation and sustained changes after real-time functional magnetic resonance imaging neurofeedback training in depression. *Brain Connectivity*. 2014; **4**(9): 690–701.

42. Hamilton JP, Glover GH, Bagarinao E, et al. Effects of salience-network-node neurofeedback training on affective biases in major depressive disorder. *Psychiatry Research: Neuroimaging*. 2016; **249**: 91–96.

43. Teasdale JD, Green HA. Ruminative self-focus and autobiographical memory. *Personality and Individual Differences*. 2004; **36**(8): 1933–1943.

44. Sutherland K, Bryant RA. Rumination and overgeneral autobiographical memory. *Behaviour Research and Therapy*. 2007; **45**(10): 2407–2416.

45. Ramot M, Grossman S, Friedman D, Malach R. Covert neurofeedback without awareness shapes cortical network spontaneous connectivity. *Proceedings of the National Academy of Sciences*. 2016; **113**(17): E2413–E20.

46. Thibault RT, MacPherson A, Lifshitz M, Roth RR, Raz A. Neurofeedback with fMRI: A critical systematic review. *Neuroimage*. 2018; **172**: 786–807.

47. Hamann S, Canli T. Individual differences in emotion processing. *Current Opinion in Neurobiology*. 2004; **14**(2): 233–238.

48. Berlim MT, Van den Eynde F, Daskalakis ZJ. Clinically meaningful efficacy and acceptability of low-frequency repetitive transcranial magnetic stimulation (rTMS) for treating primary major depression: a meta-analysis of randomized, double-blind and sham-controlled trials. *Neuropsychopharmacology*. 2013; **38**(4): 543.

49. Berlim M, Van den Eynde F, Tovar-Perdomo S, Daskalakis Z. Response, remission and drop-out rates following high-frequency repetitive transcranial magnetic stimulation (rTMS) for treating major depression: A systematic review and meta-analysis of randomized, double-blind and sham-controlled trials. *Psychological Medicine*. 2014; **44**(2): 225–239.

50. Young KD, Zotev V, Phillips R, Misaki M, Yuan H, Drevets WC, et al. Real-time fMRI neurofeedback training of amygdala activity in patients with major depressive disorder. *PloS One*. 2014; **9**(2): e88785.

51. Yang Y, Zhong N, Imamura K, et al. Task and resting-state fMRI reveal altered salience responses to positive stimuli in patients with major depressive disorder. *PLOS ONE*. 2016; **11**(5): e0155092.

163

52. Sheline YI, Barch DM, Donnelly JM, et al. Increased amygdala response to masked emotional faces in depressed subjects resolves with antidepressant treatment: An fMRI study. *Biological Psychiatry.* 2001; **50**(9): 651–658.

53. Drevets WC, Price JL, Bardgett ME, et al. Glucose metabolism in the amygdala in depression: Relationship to diagnostic subtype and plasma cortisol levels. *Pharmacology Biochemistry and Behavior.* 2002; **71**(3): 431–447.

54. Drevets WC. Neuroimaging abnormalities in the amygdala in mood disorders. *Annals of the New York Academy of Sciences.* 2003; **985**(1): 420–444.

55. Victor TA, Furey ML, Fromm SJ, Öhman A, Drevets WC. Relationship between amygdala responses to masked faces and mood state and treatment in major depressive disorder. *Archives of General Psychiatry.* 2010; **67**(11): 1128–1138.

56. Suslow T, Konrad C, Kugel H, et al. Automatic mood-congruent amygdala responses to masked facial expressions in major depression. *Biological Psychiatry.* 2010; **67**(2): 155–160.

57. Seeley WW, Menon V, Schatzberg AF, Keller J, Glover GH, Kenna H, et al. Dissociable intrinsic connectivity networks for salience processing and executive control. *Journal of Neuroscience.* 2007; **27**(9): 2349–56.

58. Jacobs R, Barba A, Gowins J, et al. Decoupling of the amygdala to other salience network regions in adolescent-onset recurrent major depressive disorder. *Psychological Medicine.* 2016; **46**(5): 1055–1067.

59. Packard MG, Cahill L. Affective modulation of multiple memory systems. *Current Opinion in Neurobiology.* 2001; **11**(6): 752–756.

60. Burianova H, McIntosh AR, Grady CL. A common functional brain network for autobiographical, episodic, and semantic memory retrieval. *Neuroimage.* 2010; **49**(1): 865–874.

61. Noulhiane M, Piolino P, Hasboun D, et al. Autobiographical memory after temporal lobe resection: neuropsychological and MRI volumetric findings. *Brain.* 2007; **130**(12): 3184–3199.

62. Aggleton JP, Brown MW. Episodic memory, amnesia, and the hippocampal–anterior thalamic axis. *Behavioral and Brain Sciences.* 1999; **22**(3): 425–444.

63. Young KD. Effects of amygdala neurofeedback on depressive symptoms. Identification No. NCT02709161. Retrieved from https://clinical trials.gov/ct2/show/NCT02709161. 2016.

64. Young KD. Neurofeedback for treatment resistant depression. Identification No. NCT03428828.

Retrieved from https://clinicaltrials.gov/ct2/show/ NCT03428828. 2018.

65. Engen HG, Bernhardt BC, Skottnik L, Ricard M, Singer T. Structural changes in socio-affective networks: Multi-modal MRI findings in long-term meditation practitioners. *Neuropsychologia.* 2018; **116**: 26–33.

66. Young KD, Misaki M, Harmer CJ, et al. Real-time functional magnetic resonance imaging amygdala neurofeedback changes positive information processing in major depressive disorder. *Biological Psychiatry.* 2017; **82**(8): 578–586.

67. Mathiak K. Symptom based treatment affects brain plasticity – cognitive training in patients with affective symptoms (APIC-II). Identification No. NCT03183947. Retrieved from https://clinicaltrials .gov/ct2/show/NCT03183947. 2017.

68. Hamilton JP, Etkin A, Furman DJ, et al. Functional neuroimaging of major depressive disorder: A meta-analysis and new integration of baseline activation and neural response data. *American Journal of Psychiatry.* 2012; **169**(7): 693–703.

69. Caria A, Sitaram R, Veit R, Begliomini C, Birbaumer N. Volitional control of anterior insula activity modulates the response to aversive stimuli. A real-time functional magnetic resonance imaging study. *Biological Psychiatry.* 2010; **68**(5): 425–432.

70. Herwig U, Lutz J, Scherpiet S, et al. Training emotion regulation through real-time fMRI neurofeedback of amygdala activity. *NeuroImage.* 2019; **184**: 687–696.

71. Perlman G, Simmons AN, Wu J, et al. Amygdala response and functional connectivity during emotion regulation: a study of 14 depressed adolescents. *Journal of Affective Disorders.* 2012; **139**(1): 75–84.

72. Carballedo A, Scheuerecker J, Meisenzahl E, et al. Functional connectivity of emotional processing in depression. *Journal of Affective Disorders.* 2011; **134**(1–3): 272–279.

73. de Almeida JRC, Versace A, Mechelli A, et al. Abnormal amygdala-prefrontal effective connectivity to happy faces differentiates bipolar from major depression. *Biological Psychiatry.* 2009; **66**(5): 451–459.

74. Zahn R, Weingartner J, Basilio R, et al. 30 *Blame Rebalance fMRI Feedback Proof-of-Concept Trial in Major Depressive Disorder.* BMJ Publishing Group Ltd; 2017.

75. Greicius MD, Flores BH, Menon V, et al. Resting-state functional connectivity in major depression: Abnormally increased contributions from subgenual cingulate cortex and thalamus. *Biological Psychiatry.* 2007; **62**(5): 429–437.

76. Sheline YI, Price JL, Yan Z, Mintun MA. Resting-state functional MRI in depression unmasks increased connectivity between networks via the dorsal nexus. *Proceedings of the National Academy of Sciences*. 2010; **107**(24): 11020–11025.

77. Veer IM, Beckmann C, Van Tol M-J, et al. Whole brain resting-state analysis reveals decreased functional connectivity in major depression. *Frontiers in Systems Neuroscience*. 2010; **4**: 41.

78. Drysdale AT, Grosenick L, Downar J, et al. Resting-state connectivity biomarkers define neurophysiological subtypes of depression. *Nature Medicine*. 2017; **23**(1): 28.

79. Dinga R, Schmaal L, Penninx B, et al. Evaluating the evidence for biotypes of depression: Methodological replication and extension of. *NeuroImage: Clinical*. 2019; **22**: 101796.

80. Yamada T, Hashimoto R-i, Yahata N, et al. Resting-state functional connectivity-based biomarkers and functional MRI-based neurofeedback for psychiatric disorders: a challenge for developing theranostic biomarkers. *International Journal of Neuropsychopharmacology*. 2017; **20**(10): 769–781.

81. Moll J, Weingartner JH, Bado P, et al. Voluntary enhancement of neural signatures of affiliative emotion using fMRI neurofeedback. *PloS One*. 2014; **9**(5): e97343.

82. Sokhadze EM, El-Baz AS, Tasman A, et al. Neuromodulation integrating rTMS and neurofeedback for the treatment of autism spectrum disorder: an exploratory study. *Applied Psychophysiology and Biofeedback*. 2014; **39**(3–4): 237–257.

83. Koganemaru S, Mikami Y, Maezawa H, et al. Neurofeedback control of the human GABAergic system using non-invasive brain stimulation. *Neuroscience*. 2018; **380**: 38–48.

84. Siepmann M, Aykac V, Unterdörfer J, Petrowski K, Mueck-Weymann M. A pilot study on the effects of heart rate variability biofeedback in patients with depression and in healthy subjects. *Applied Psychophysiology and Biofeedback*. 2008; **33**(4): 195–201.

85. Karavidas MK, Lehrer PM, Vaschillo E, et al. Preliminary results of an open label study of heart rate variability biofeedback for the treatment of major depression. *Applied Psychophysiology and Biofeedback*. 2007; **32**(1): 19–30.

86. Gevirtz R. The promise of heart rate variability biofeedback: Evidence-based applications. *Biofeedback*. 2013; **41**(3): 110–120.

87. Tang Y, Posner MI, Rothbart MK. Meditation improves self-regulation over the life span. *Annals of the New York Academy of Sciences*. 2014; **1307**(1): 104–111.

88. Tang Y, Ma Y, Wang J, et al. Short-term meditation training improves attention and self-regulation. *Proceedings of the National Academy of Sciences*. 2007; **104**(43): 17152–17156.

89. Baird B, Mrazek MD, Phillips DT, Schooler JW. Domain-specific enhancement of metacognitive ability following meditation training. *Journal of Experimental Psychology: General*. 2014; **143**(5): 1972.

90. Hofmann SG, Sawyer AT, Witt AA, Oh D. The effect of mindfulness-based therapy on anxiety and depression: A meta-analytic review. *Journal of Consulting and Clinical Psychology*. 2010; **78**(2): 169.

91. Peciña M. Study of neural responses induced by antidepressant effects (SONRISA). Identification No. NCT02674529. Retrieved from https://clinicaltrials.gov/ct2/show/NCT02674529. 2016.

92. Scharnowski F. Neural correlates of neurofeedback training. Identification No. NCT03165578. Retrieved from https://clinicaltrials.gov/ct2/show/NCT03165578. 2017.

93. Sorger B, Scharnowski F, Linden DE, Hampson M, Young KD. Control freaks: Towards optimal selection of control conditions for fMRI neurofeedback studies. *NeuroImage*. 2019; **186**: 256–265.

94. Randell E, McNamara R, Subramanian L, Hood K, Linden D. *Current Practices in Clinical Neurofeedback with Functional MRI-Analysis of a Survey Using the TIDieR Checklist*. Eur Psychiatry; 2018.

95. Grossberg, S, On the dynamics of operant conditioning. *Journal of Theoretical Biology*. 1971 November; **33**(2): 225–255.

96. Staddon JER, Cerutti DT. Operant Conditioning. *Annu Rev Psychol*. 2003; **54**: 115–144.

Chapter 13

Functional Near-Infrared Spectroscopy Studies in Mood Disorders

Koji Matsuo and Toshio Matsubara

13.1 Introduction

In 1977, Frans F Jöbsis pioneered a noninvasive method for measuring the hemodynamic oxygenation of biological tissue using near-infrared light (1). This method fostered a new era of near-infrared spectroscopy (NRIS) studies in the field of neuroscience. Over the last two decades, functional NIRS (fNIRS) has been applied to evaluate brain activation in humans in vivo and functional abnormalities in patients with psychiatric illnesses. Along with other functional neuroimaging modalities, such as functional MRI (fMRI), single-photon emission computed tomography (SPECT), and positron emission tomography (PET), studies using fNIRS to investigate mood disorders have been accumulating given the increasingly widespread use of NIRS in the study of psychiatric disorders. Novel and distinct imaging methods, such as fNIRS, will likely contribute to an increased understanding of brain pathophysiology in mood disorders. In this chapter, we discuss the principals of NIRS and its application in the study of mood disorders.

13.2 Principle of Near-Infrared Spectroscopy

Here, we summarize the principles of NIRS. Details of physiological, technical, and theoretical principles ((1–7)), and the main characteristics of NIRS ((8–10)) are described elsewhere.

Briefly, NIRS can measure the absorbance of light in certain tissues at several wavelengths in the 650–1,000 nm spectral range. It can also noninvasively and continuously quantify alterations in oxygenated (oxy-Hb) and deoxygenated (deoxy-Hb) hemoglobin. In the NIR spectral window (650–1,000 nm), which is called an "optical window," human tissues are mainly transparent to light. Near-infrared light travels and scatters across tissues and is absorbed into them. The

tissue oxymetry in NIRS was based on the modified Beer–Lambert law (1):

$$\text{Attenuation(OD)} = -\log(I/I_0) = \varepsilon c L B + G,$$

where OD represents optical densities, I_0 represents the incident light intensity, I represents the detected light intensity, ε represents the absorption coefficient of the chromophore ($\text{mM}^{-1}\ \text{cm}^{-1}$), c represents the concentration of chromophore (mM), L represents the physical distance between the points where light enters and leaves the tissue (cm), B represents a "path-length factor," which takes into account the scattering of light into the tissue, and G represents a factor related to the measurement geometry and type of tissue. The absorption coefficients of oxy-Hb and deoxy-Hb have been measured in pure hemoglobin solutions.

For the measurement of brain tissue, NIR light diffusely penetrates the tissue layers of the head (skin, skull, and cerebrospinal fluid) beneath an optical probe. NIR light, attenuated in tissue, indicates the quantity of chromophore hemoglobin (the oxygen transport red blood cell protein) located in microcirculation vessels (<1 mm in diameter), such as capillary, arteriolar, and venular beds. The blood vessels >1 mm absorb the majority of NIR light. Then, a small amount of NIR light returns to the surface through the tissues of the head. Such an NIR light tract appears to form a "banana-shape" ((3)). Adequate depth of NIR light penetration (approximately one-half of the source-detector distance) can be achieved using a source-detector distance of around 30 mm. The detector optode detects NIR signals of hemodynamic changes in the cerebral cortex, as well as the skin ((11)). This signal depends on the distance between the source of NIR light and the detectors. If the distance of the source-detector is 20, 30, and 40 mm, the oxygenated change, resulting from cerebral activation, would be estimated to contribute 33.0, 54.8, and 68.5% of NIR signals detected, respectively ((12)). The units for oxy-Hb and deoxy-Hb signal changes should be expressed as μmolar*cm or mmolar*mm when the optical path-length of tissue is longer than the distance between the source and the detector, since the scattering effects of different tissue layers in the brain are unknown ((4)).

NIRS gauges changes in oxy-Hb and deoxy-Hb relevant to brain activity while excluding most of the effects of skin blood flow ((2)). An increase in oxy-Hb and corresponding decrease in deoxy-Hb, when linked with neural activity, is thought to indicate an increase in local arteriolar vasodilatation, local cerebral blood flow, and cerebral blood volume. This mechanism has been termed "neurovascular coupling." Oxy-Hb is transported excessively to brain tissues where neuronal cells utilize the oxygen for their activity, resulting in an overabundance of cerebral blood oxygenation in the activated brain tissues ((13)). Oxy-Hb change, measured by NIRS, has been shown to be highly correlated with changes in regional cerebral blood flow, as determined by PET ((14)), and blood-oxygen-level-dependent (BOLD) signals, as determined by fMRI ((15–18)).

There are noteworthy strengths and weaknesses in the use of NIRS to evaluate brain function. The strengths include (1) near-infrared light is noninvasive to the brain and body, which means it is able to be used safely and repeatedly; (2) NIRS has high time-resolution of Hb data on the order of 100 ms; (3) participants are able to undergo NIRS examinations without stabled or restricted body positioning (e.g., measurements can be taken in a comfortable position in a chair or at the bedside); (4) NIRS devices are relatively compact and portable compared to MRI and CT devices; and (5) NIRS does not require a sealed and purpose-built room. The weaknesses include (1) NIRS only measures relative changes in Hb concentration; (2) NIRS only assesses the function of the inner surface of brain (e.g., dorsolateral prefrontal area), but not of deep brain structures (e.g., cingulate, subcortical area, and hippocampus/amygdala); (3) NIRS uses a target task combined with control tasks to eliminate confounding factors that may impact absorption of hemoglobin (e.g., skin, muscle, skull absorption); and (4) NIRS has a low spatial resolution on the order of 10–30 mm. It is of note that the low spatial resolution indicates that NIRS evaluates brain function in a specific area (e.g., inferior prefrontal "area"), but not anatomically accurate brain cortical structures or regions (e.g., inferior prefrontal "cortex"). However, a probable brain map for use with NIRS has been created ((19)). Thus, within this chapter, we describe anatomical locations using the term "area," although some studies cited here within use the term "cortex."

13.3 Application to Mood Disorders

To our knowledge, the first fNIRS study for patients with mood disorders was reported by Okada et al. ((20)). They examined brain activation in the left and right frontal areas during a mirror-drawing task, to assess visuospatial function, and found that patients with major depressive disorder (MDD) showed lower brain activation during the task than healthy subjects. To date, there are around fifty NIRS studies investigating mood disorders. Twenty-four studies (around 50%) used a single verbal fluency task (VFT), with letter version, eight used a single other cognitive task, and eleven used a combination of tasks including VFT and other cognitive and physiological tasks. Twenty-seven studies (57%) were conducted in patients with MDD versus healthy subjects, eight (17%) were conducted in patients with bipolar disorder (BD) versus healthy subjects, and twelve (26%) compared patients with MDD and BD and patients with other mood disorders and psychiatric illnesses.

Many fNIRS studies using the VFT, with letter version, were conducted in Japan. VFT, with letter version requires subjects to produce words beginning with a certain letter of the alphabet, usually "F," "A," and "S." This task has been preinstalled in certain NIRS devices since 2009 because the physiological examination of fNIRS in the frontal area, using this task, was approved by the Japanese health ministry as an "advanced medical technology" to assist psychiatric diagnoses in 2009. As such, fNIRS was covered by public health insurance in Japan, since 2014, as a supplementary laboratory test for the differential diagnosis of BD and schizophrenia from that of MDD. The *Nature News* reports such diagnostic assisting methods in fascination ((21)).

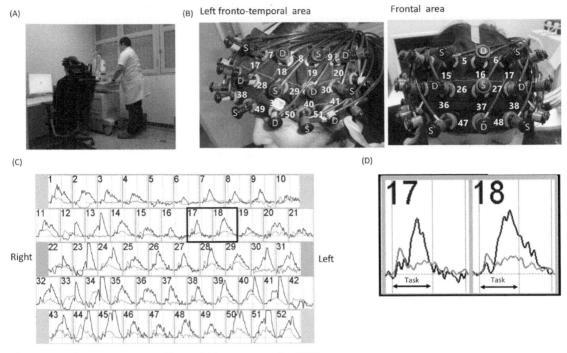

Figure 13.1 Change in oxygenated hemoglobin as measured by fNIRS

(a) A scene from an experiment using an NIRS device (ETG-4000, Hitachi Medical Co., Japan) in our laboratory. (b) Position of the probes for the source and detector and fifty-two channels in the frontotemporal area. The letter "S" represents a source probe, "D" represents a detector probe, and the number between S and D represents one of the channels measured. (c) A typical time course of oxygenated hemoglobin (oxy-Hb) change during a verbal fluency task, with letter version. The number represents one of the channels measured. (d) Expanding of the oxy-Hb change in the channel numbers 17 and 18, where it is estimated to be anatomically set in the left middle frontal area. A large increase of oxy-Hb change in a forty-eight-year-old healthy subject (black line) and small increase in oxy-Hb change in a thirty-five-year-old patient with major depressive disorder during a depressed state (gray line)

Very recently, a meta-analytic study of fNIRS in MDD provided some evidence that patients at remitted and depressed states showed increased oxy-Hb during cognitive activation of the prefrontal areas compared to healthy participants (22). However, this analysis did not reveal a significant difference in change of oxy-Hb during cognitive activation between remitted and depressed patients.

13.3.1 Major Depressive Disorder versus Healthy Subjects

13.3.1.1 VFT, Letter Version

To the best of our knowledge, the first study of NIRS using the VFT was done by Matsuo et al. ((23)), and a modified and simplified version was used by Fukuda and his colleagues ((24)). This modified version is easier to use and has been broadly distributed (Figure 13.1). Thus, the procedure of VFT, with letter version, is very similar across recent studies in Japan ((25–39)). The VFT, with letter version, activates the frontal, and in particular, dorsolateral prefrontal cortex ((40, 41)) and is thought to assess cognitive response generation, working memory, and cognitive speed in the neuropsychological field ((42)). Cross-sectional fNIRS studies using the VFT often compare clinical features in depressed or euthymic patients with MDD such as melancholic versus non-melancholic ((30, 33)), suicidal versus non-suicidal ((39)), suicidal ideation versus non-suicidal ideation ((34)), vascular depression versus nonvascular depression ((29)), menopausal depression versus MDD ((43)), selective serotonin reuptake inhibitor responders versus nonresponders ((36)), positive and negative autonomic thought ((26)), and discrepancy between self-measured and observer-measured depression severity ((32)). The VFT studies also demonstrated associations between brain activation during the task with clinical variables such as depression severity ((27)), sleep quality ((37)), obsessive symptoms ((44)), dose of psychotropic medication [38], and stress-coping style ((45)). Furthermore, there are five longitudinal fNIRS that have investigated response to biological treatments including antidepressants ((31, 35, 36)) and electroconvulsive therapy ((25)). For instance, Tomioka et al. examined oxy-Hb changes during the VFT in medication-naive patients with MDD in the pre- and post-phase of antidepressant administration ((35)). They found that patients with MDD demonstrated blunted brain activation in frontotemporal areas, during the task, in both phases compared to healthy subjects. Although depressive symptoms were improved by the treatment, MDD patients in the pre-phase did not demonstrate differential brain activation compared to the same patients in the post-phase, which suggested that low frontotemporal activation during the task may be a trait characteristic of MDD. However, the results of fNIRS studies that use the VFT should be interpreted cautiously because these studies investigated similar comparison of a subset of patients and similar correlations with clinical variables, used the same task paradigm, and measured very similar areas (frontotemporal or frontal areas) due to them often being conducted for Japanese public health insurance-related reasons. Significant changes in oxy-Hb in the frontal and/or temporal brain areas were a common finding across studies regardless of the clinical characteristic found to be associated with this activation, which could indicate that a clinical characteristic implicated in a subgroup in one study may confound the results of a different study. For instance, wide frontotemporal area activation was significantly different between MDD patients with suicide ideas and healthy subjects ((34)); this same area, to some extent, also showed activation differences between MDD patients with melancholic features and healthy subjects ((33)). Further, NIRS studies using the VFT are required to replicate previous findings and to validate and further evaluate the effect of, or interaction between, these potentially confounding factors.

13.3.1.2 Other Tasks

Five cross-sectional and two longitudinal studies were conducted in patients with MDD using other tasks such as mirror drawing ((20, 46)), n-back ((45, 47)) to assess working memory and executive function, rock–paper–scissors ((48)) to evaluate cognitive inhibition ((49)), and arithmetic task ((46)). The other tasks included were physiological tasks used to evaluate microvascular sclerosis; these task included hyperventilation and paper-bag breathing ((50)), and carbon dioxide inhalation ((51)).

Matsuo et al. used an in-house VFT, with letter version, and carbon dioxide inhalation in older MDD patients during the full remission ((51)). The results demonstrated poor activation during the VFT and blunted hemodynamic response to carbon dioxide inhalation in frontal areas in patients when compared to healthy subjects. The authors suggested that prefrontal microvascular dysregulation, as shown in fNIRS, is involved in the trait pathophysiology of frontal hypofunction in later-life depression because the patients were at remitted state. This study demonstrates the effectiveness of fNIRS when combined with different tasks at the bedside. The use of different tasks to stimulate brain function may not be as easily done in other imaging modalities such as fMRI.

13.3.2 Bipolar Disorder versus Healthy Subjects

To date, four fNIRS studies have been conducted in BD patients using the VFT, with letter version ((52–55)), and four other studies have investigated BD using other tasks such as the Iowa Gambling task ((56)), various physiological tasks ((57, 58)), and multiple cognitive tasks ((59)). Three studies were conducted during the depressed phase ((52, 54, 56)), two were conducted during the remitted phase ((57, 58)), and three were conducted during a variety of mood phases ((53, 55, 59)). For instance, one study examined frontal activation during multiple cognitive tasks in patients with BD during various mood states ((59)); tasks included VFT, with category and letter version, Raven's Colored Progressive Matrices (set at A and B) to assess nonverbal visual function, and letter cancellation test to evaluate attention. This study found that patients with BD demonstrated an abnormal pattern of prefrontal activation across all tasks and a larger oxy-Hb change during the Raven's Colored Progressive Matrices (set at B) and letter cancellation test compared to healthy subjects, although patients were in euthymic, depressed, and hypomanic states. This study demonstrated one of the strengths of fNIRS, which is that multiple tasks can be continuously administered while measuring brain activation. Moreover, another study by Nishimura et al. showed, cross-sectionally, that hypomanic patients demonstrated more activation in ventrolateral prefrontal areas during the VFT, with letter version, than depressed patients. They also demonstrated, longitudinally, that when the hypomanic patients were in a non-hypomanic state after treatment, they showed diminished activation in the dorsolateral prefrontal area ((55)).

13.3.3 Comparisons with Mood Disorders and Other Psychiatric Illnesses

Twelve fNIRS studies compared brain activation across psychiatric diagnoses, such as MDD, BD, schizophrenia, and anxiety disorders. Seven studies used the VFT, with letter version, from Japan ((24, 60–65)), and the others studies used the n-back ((66)), respiration ((50)), emotional Stroop ((67)), muscular pressure pain ((68)), and conversation ((69)) task.

In a multicenter fNIRS study by Takizawa et al., using the VFT, with letter version, the brain activation of 185 depressed patients (74 with MDD, 45 with BD, and 66 with schizophrenia) and 529 healthy subjects was studied. Brain activation was assessed using two indicators of oxy-Hb change: the integral value to describe the size of the hemodynamic response during the activation task period and the centroid value to serve as a parameter of time-course changes throughout the task ((63)). The receiver-operating curve of the centroid value of the frontal area was correctly classified in MDD and in the other diagnoses, with 74.6% accuracy for MDD and 85.5% accuracy for the others. These results suggest that assessing brain activation using fNIRS may assist the differential diagnosis of major psychiatric disorders, and could provide a promising biomarker for personalized care in clinical settings. Furthermore, these findings validate the use of fNIRS for this purpose, permitting it to be covered by Japanese public health insurance, as discussed in the former section.

A few fNIRS studies have used emotional tasks. Matsubara and his colleagues examined fronto-temporal brain activation during the Stroop task, using emotional words, in MDD and BD patients during a remitted state ((67)). During presentation of emotional words with a negative valence, patients with both diagnoses showed similar increases in activation of the left frontal areas compared to healthy subjects. In contrast, during presentation of the emotional words with a positive valence, BD patients showed reduced activation in the left and right frontal areas compared to MDD patients and healthy subjects, and MDD patients and healthy subjects did not significantly differ in task-induced brain activation. These results suggest that hyperactivation of the left frontal area in response to negative emotional stimuli is shared between mood disorders. On the other hand, hypoactivation of the frontal region, bilaterally, in response to positive emotional stimuli is distinct to specific mood disorders, indicating that it may represent a trait characteristic of certain mood disorders and can help elucidate the neural mechanisms within the bipolar/major depressive disorder continuum.

Of interest, one study tested frontotemporal brain activation during face-to-face conversation in MDD patients, BD patients, and healthy subjects ((69)). The participants talked, face-to-face, to a research interviewer sitting in a chair. Two parameters were measured during NIRS: one parameter assessed global function required to interact with another person and have a conversation and the other parameter assessed speech-related function. The patients with BD and those with MDD showed lower activation in the left dorsolateral prefrontal area and fronto-polar area during the task compared to healthy subjects. This study is well designed to emphasize the strength of fNIRS, that is, to measure brain activation in a relaxed upright posture in a quotidian condition.

13.4 Conclusions and Future Directions

fNIRS is a novel and distinct neuroimaging method. Its strengths include user-friendliness, participant-friendliness, noninvasiveness, and compact device size. Its weaknesses include low spatial resolution and inability to measure relative brain function beneath the surface of the brain. Future fNIRS studies should aim to technically improve these shortcomings and to continue investigating brain abnormalities in mood disorders. Considering both the strengths and weaknesses of fNIRS, this method may be suitable to screen for functional abnormalities in patients in clinical settings such as at the bedside, rather than investigating brain mechanisms in a research setting, like is currently done in fMRI studies. Hopefully, fNIRS may provide a physiological test to assess whether brain activity during illness may act as a diagnostic biomarker and whether brain activity during recovery may act as a treatment biomarker. In our conjectural opinion, fNIRS could potentially link subjective complaints relevant to symptoms with objective brain activation patterns, and, ultimately, aid psychiatrists and primary physicians in disease diagnosis and treatment.

References

1. Jobsis FF. Noninvasive, infrared monitoring of cerebral and myocardial oxygen sufficiency and circulatory parameters. *Science*. 1977; **198**(4323): 1264–1267.

2. Villringer A, Planck J, Hock C, Schleinkofer L, Dirnagl U. Near infrared spectroscopy (NIRS): A new tool to study hemodynamic changes during activation of brain function in human adults. *Neurosci Lett*. 1993; **154**(1–2): 101–104.

3. Gratton G, Maier JS, Fabiani M, Mantulin WW, Gratton E. Feasibility of intracranial near-infrared optical scanning. *Psychophysiology*. 1994; **31**(2): 211–215.

4. Maki A, Yamashita Y, Ito Y, et al. Spatial and temporal analysis of human motor activity using noninvasive NIR topography. *Med Phys*. 1995; **22**(12): 1997–2005.

5. Villringer A, Chance B. Non-invasive optical spectroscopy and imaging of human brain function. *Trends Neurosci*. 1997; **20**(10): 435–442.

6. Obrig H. et al. Near-infrared spectroscopy: Does it function in functional activation studies of the adult brain? *Int J Psychophysiol*. 2000; **35**(2–3): 125–142.

7. Yamashita Y, Maki A, Koizumi H. Wavelength dependence of the precision of noninvasive optical measurement of oxy-, deoxy-, and total-hemoglobin concentration. *Med Phys*. 2001; **28**(6): 1108–1114.

8. Ferrari M, Quaresima V. A brief review on the history of human functional near-infrared spectroscopy (fNIRS) development and fields of application. *Neuroimage*. 2012; **63**(2): 921–935.

9. Strangman G, Boas DA, Sutton JP. Non-invasive neuroimaging using near-infrared light. *Biol Psychiatry*. 2002; **52**(7): 679–693.

10. Elwell CE. et al. Measurement of adult cerebral haemodynamics using near infrared spectroscopy. *Acta Neurochir Suppl (Wien)*. 1993; **59**: 74–80.

11. Takahashi T, Takikawa Y, Kawagoe R, et al. Influence of skin blood flow on near-infrared spectroscopy signals measured on the forehead during a verbal fluency task. *Neuroimage*. 2011; **57**(3): 991–1002.

12. Kohri S, Hoshi Y, Tamura M, et al. Quantitative evaluation of the relative contribution ratio of cerebral tissue to near-infrared signals in the adult human head: A preliminary study. *Physiol Meas*. 2002; **23**(2): 301–312.

13. Fox PT, Raichle ME. Focal physiological uncoupling of cerebral blood flow and oxidative metabolism during somatosensory stimulation in human subjects. *Proc Natl Acad Sci U S A*. 1986; **83**(4): 1140–1144.

14. Hock C. et al. Decrease in parietal cerebral hemoglobin oxygenation during performance of a verbal fluency task in patients with Alzheimer's disease monitored by means of near-infrared spectroscopy (NIRS)–correlation with simultaneous rCBF-PET measurements. *Brain Res*. 1997; **755**(2): 293–303.

15. Sato H. et al. A NIRS-fMRI investigation of prefrontal cortex activity during a working memory task. *Neuroimage*. 2013; **83**: 158–173.

16. Cui X, Bray S, Bryant DM, Glover GH, Reiss AL. A quantitative comparison of NIRS and fMRI across multiple cognitive tasks. *Neuroimage*. 2011; **54**(4): 2808–2821.

17. Strangman G, Culver JP, Thompson JH, Boas DA. A quantitative comparison of simultaneous BOLD fMRI and NIRS recordings during functional brain activation. *Neuroimage*. 2002; **17**(2): 719–731.

18. Moriguchi Y. et al. Validation of brain-derived signals in near-infrared spectroscopy through multivoxel analysis of concurrent functional magnetic resonance imaging. *Hum Brain Mapp*. 2017; **38**(10): 5274–5291.

19. Tsuzuki D, Jurcak V, Singh AK, et al. Virtual spatial registration of stand-alone fNIRS data to MNI space. *Neuroimage*. 2007; **34**(4): 1506–1518.

20. Okada F, Takahashi N, Tokumitsu Y. Dominance of the 'nondominant' hemisphere in depression. *J Affect Disord.* 1996; **37**(1): 13–21.

21. Cyranoski D. Neuroscience: Thought experiment. *Nature.* 2011; **469**(7329): 148–149.

22. Zhang H. et al. Near-infrared spectroscopy for examination of prefrontal activation during cognitive tasks in patients with major depressive disorder: A meta-analysis of observational studies. *Psychiatry Clin Neurosci.* 2015; **69**(1): 22–33.

23. Matsuo K, Kato T, Fukuda M, Kato N. Alteration of hemoglobin oxygenation in the frontal region in elderly depressed patients as measured by near-infrared spectroscopy. *J Neuropsychiatry Clin Neurosci.* 2000; **12**(4): 465–471.

24. Suto T, Fukuda M, Ito M, Uehara T, Mikuni M. Multichannel near-infrared spectroscopy in depression and schizophrenia: cognitive brain activation study. *Biol Psychiatry.* 2004; **55**(5): 501–511.

25. Hirano J. et al. Frontal and temporal cortical functional recovery after electroconvulsive therapy for depression: A longitudinal functional near-infrared spectroscopy study. *J Psychiatr Res.* 2017; **91**: 26–35.

26. Koseki S. et al. The relationship between positive and negative automatic thought and activity in the prefrontal and temporal cortices: A multi-channel near-infrared spectroscopy (NIRS) study. *J Affect Disord.* 2013; **151**(1): 352–359.

27. Noda T. et al. Frontal and right temporal activations correlate negatively with depression severity during verbal fluency task: A multi-channel near-infrared spectroscopy study. *J Psychiatr Res.* 2012; **46**(7): 905–912.

28. Pu S. et al. The relationship between the prefrontal activation during a verbal fluency task and stress-coping style in major depressive disorder: A near-infrared spectroscopy study. *J Psychiatr Res.* 2012; **46**(11): 1427–1434.

29. Pu S. et al. Reduced frontopolar activation during verbal fluency task associated with poor social functioning in late-onset major depression: Multi-channel near-infrared spectroscopy study. *Psychiatry Clin Neurosci.* 2008; **62**(6): 728–737.

30. Tsujii N. et al. Relationship between prefrontal hemodynamic responses and quality of life differs between melancholia and non-melancholic depression. *Psychiatry Res.* 2016; **253**(30): 26–35.

31. Usami M, Iwadare Y, Kodaira M, Watanabe K, Saito K. Near infrared spectroscopy study of the frontopolar hemodynamic response and depressive mood in children with major depressive disorder: A pilot study. *PLoS One.* 2014; **9**(1): e86290.

32. Akashi H, Tsujii N, Mikawa W, et al. Prefrontal cortex activation is associated with a discrepancy between self- and observer-rated depression severities of major depressive disorder: A multichannel near-infrared spectroscopy study. *J Affect Disord.* 2015; **174**(15): 165–172.

33. Tsujii N. et al. Right temporal activation differs between melancholia and nonmelancholic depression: A multichannel near-infrared spectroscopy study. *J Psychiatr Res.* 2014; **55**: 1–7.

34. Pu S. et al. Suicidal ideation is associated with reduced prefrontal activation during a verbal fluency task in patients with major depressive disorder. *J Affect Disord.* 2015; **18**: 9–17.

35. Tomioka H. et al. A longitudinal functional neuroimaging study in medication-naive depression after antidepressant treatment. *PLoS One.* 2015; **10**(3): e0120828.

36. Masuda K. et al. Different functioning of prefrontal cortex predicts treatment response after a selective serotonin reuptake inhibitor treatment in patients with major depression. *J Affect Disord.* 2017; **214**: 44–52.

37. Nishida M, Kikuchi S, Matsumoto K, et al. Sleep complaints are associated with reduced left prefrontal activation during a verbal fluency task in patients with major depression: A multi-channel near-infrared spectroscopy study. *J Affect Disord.* 2017; **207**: 102–109.

38. Takamiya A. et al. High-dose antidepressants affect near-infrared spectroscopy signals: A retrospective study. *Neuroimage Clin.* 2017; **14**: 648–655.

39. Tsujii N. et al. Reduced left precentral regional responses in patients with major depressive disorder and history of suicide attempts. *PLoS One.* 2017; **12**(4): e0175249.

40. Schlosser R. et al. Functional magnetic resonance imaging of human brain activity in a verbal fluency task. *J Neurol Neurosurg Psychiatry.* 1998; **64**(4): 492–498.

41. Cuenod CA, Bookheimer SY, Hertz-Pannier L, et al. Functional MRI during word generation, using conventional equipment: A potential tool for language localization in the clinical environment,. *Neurology.* 1995; **45**(10): 1821–1827.

42. Strauss E, Sherman EMS, Spreen O, Spreen O. *A Compendium of Neuropsychological Tests : Administration, Norms, and Commentary.* Oxford; New York: Oxford University Press, 2006.

43. Ma XY. et al. Near-infrared spectroscopy reveals abnormal hemodynamics in the left dorsolateral prefrontal cortex of menopausal depression patients. *Dis Markers*. 2017; (2017): 1695930. DOI: 10.1155/2017/1695930

44. Liu X. et al. Relationship between the prefrontal function and the severity of the emotional symptoms during a verbal fluency task in patients with major depressive disorder: A multi-channel NIRS study. *Prog Neuropsychopharmacol Biol Psychiatry*. 2014; **54**: 114–121.

45. Pu S. et al. Reduced prefrontal cortex activation during the working memory task associated with poor social functioning in late-onset depression: Multi-channel near-infrared spectroscopy study. *Psychiatry Res*. 2012; **203** (2–3): 222–228.

46. Eschweiler GW. et al. Left prefrontal activation predicts therapeutic effects of repetitive transcranial magnetic stimulation (rTMS) in major depression. *Psychiatry Res*. 2000; **99**(3): 161–172.

47. Pu S. et al. A multi-channel near-infrared spectroscopy study of prefrontal cortex activation during working memory task in major depressive disorder. *Neurosci Res*. 2011; **70**(1): 91–97.

48. Onishi Y, Kikuchi S, Watanabe E, Kato S. Alterations in prefrontal cortical activity in the course of treatment for late-life depression as assessed on near-infrared spectroscopy. *Psychiatry Clin Neurosci*. 2008; **62**(2): 177–184.

49. Kikuchi S. et al. Prefrontal cerebral activity during a simple "rock, paper, scissors" task measured by the noninvasive near-infrared spectroscopy method. *Psychiatry Res*. 2007; **156** (3): 199–208.

50. Matsuo K, Kato N, Kato T. Decreased cerebral haemodynamic response to cognitive and physiological tasks in mood disorders as shown by near-infrared spectroscopy. *Psychol Med*. 2002; **32**(6): 1029–1037.

51. Matsuo K, Onodera Y, Hamamoto T, et al. Hypofrontality and microvascular dysregulation in remitted late-onset depression assessed by functional near-infrared spectroscopy. *Neuroimage*. 2005; **26**(1): 234–242.

52. Ono Y. et al. Prefrontal oxygenation during verbal fluency and cognitive function in adolescents with bipolar disorder type II. *Asian J Psychiatr*. 2017; **25**: 147–153.

53. Mikawa W, Tsujii N, Akashi H, et al. Left temporal activation associated with depression severity during a verbal fluency task in patients with bipolar disorder: A multichannel near-infrared spectroscopy study. *J Affect Disord*. 2015; **173**: 193–200.

54. Nishimura Y. et al. Social function and frontopolar activation during a cognitive task in patients with bipolar disorder. *Neuropsychobiology*. 2015; **72**(2): 81–90.

55. Nishimura Y, Takahashi K, Ohtani T, et al. Dorsolateral prefrontal hemodynamic responses during a verbal fluency task in hypomanic bipolar disorder. *Bipolar Disord*. 2015; **17**(2): 172–183.

56. Ono Y. et al. Reduced prefrontal activation during performance of the Iowa gambling task in patients with bipolar disorder. *Psychiatry Res*. 2015; **233**(1): 1–8.

57. Matsuo K. et al. A near-infrared spectroscopy study of prefrontal cortex activation during a verbal fluency task and carbon dioxide inhalation in individuals with bipolar disorder. *Bipolar Disord*. 2007; **9**(8): 876–883.

58. Matsuo K, Watanabe A, Onodera Y, Kato N, Kato T. Prefrontal hemodynamic response to verbal-fluency task and hyperventilation in bipolar disorder measured by multi-channel near-infrared spectroscopy. *J Affect Disord*. 2004; **82**(1): 85–92.

59. Kubota Y. et al. Altered prefrontal lobe oxygenation in bipolar disorder: A study by near-infrared spectroscopy. *Psychol Med*. 2009; **39**(8): 1265–1275.

60. Ohi K. et al. Impact of familial loading on prefrontal activation in major psychiatric disorders: A near-infrared spectroscopy (NIRS) study. *Sci Rep*. 2017; **7**: 44268.

61. Ohta H. et al. Hypofrontality in panic disorder and major depressive disorder assessed by multi-channel near-infrared spectroscopy. *Depress Anxiety*. 2008; **25**(12): 1053–1059.

62. Kameyama M. et al. Frontal lobe function in bipolar disorder: A multichannel near-infrared spectroscopy study. *Neuroimage*. 2006; **29**(1): 172–184.

63. Takizawa R. et al. Neuroimaging-aided differential diagnosis of the depressive state. *Neuroimage*. 2014; **85**(Pt 1): 498–507.

64. Kinou M. et al. Differential spatiotemporal characteristics of the prefrontal hemodynamic response and their association with functional impairment in schizophrenia and major depression. *Schizophr Res*. 2013; **150**(2–3): 459–467.

65. Ohtani T, Nishimura Y, Takahashi K, et al. Association between longitudinal changes in prefrontal hemodynamic responses and social adaptation in patients with bipolar disorder and major depressive disorder. *J Affect Disord*. 2015; **176**: 78–86.

66. Zhu Y. et al. Prefrontal activation during a working memory task differs between patients with unipolar and bipolar depression: A preliminary exploratory study. *J Affect Disord.* 2018 January 1; **225**: 64–70.

67. Matsubara T. et al. Prefrontal activation in response to emotional words in patients with bipolar disorder and major depressive disorder. *Neuroimage.* 2014; **85**(Pt 1): 489–497.

68. Uceyler N, Zeller J, Kewenig S, et al. Increased cortical activation upon painful stimulation in fibromyalgia syndrome. *BMC Neurol.* 2015; **15**: 210.

69. Takei Y. et al. Near-infrared spectroscopic study of frontopolar activation during face-to-face conversation in major depressive disorder and bipolar disorder. *J Psychiatr Res.* 2014; **57**: 74–83.

Electrophysiological Biomarkers for Mood Disorders

Nithya Ramakrishnan, Nicholas Murphy, Sudhakar Selvaraj, and Raymond Y. Cho

14.1 Introduction

To more effectively investigate, diagnose, and treat mood disorders, there is a need to move beyond standard clinical characterizations. While symptom-based nosology has provided a reliable and pragmatic framework for clinical practice, advances in neuroimaging research have permitted the possibility of identifying neurophysiologic biomarkers that index underlying pathophysiologic processes and provide an effective complement to clinical symptoms. Functional magnetic resonance imaging (fMRI) is one of the common state-of-the-art neuroimaging approaches for investigating brain disorders and has been very useful in providing a functional neuroanatomic account of neural disturbances in mood disorders. However, while it excels in providing a fine, spatial resolution (1–3 mm), fMRI lacks in temporal resolution to characterize neurophysiologic disturbances at the timescale of neural activations.

While having a poorer spatial resolution (2 cm) than fMRI, electroencephalography (EEG) can track cortical activity at the millisecond timescale of neural networks. In addition to tracking measurement of spontaneous resting activity, through concurrent recording during cognitive task performance, it is possible to study EEG activity time-locked to the onset of stimulus or behavioral events. The EEG consists of time-varying electrical signals generated by cortical postsynaptic potentials. The signals mostly derived from the electrical potential gradients along the apical dendrites of cortical pyramidal neurons whose parallel alignments oriented perpendicular to the cortical surface, permit spatial summation when synchronously active. Due to the folding of cortical tissue, and the transmission across other tissues including the white matter and skull, the electrical activity becomes distorted and broadly

projected across the scalp electrodes. This traversing of electrical signals through different tissues with complex geometry is known as volume conduction and impedes our ability to pinpoint the anatomical locus of a signal of interest. Magnetoencephalography (MEG), which detects magnetic fields that are orthogonal to the direction of the current and optimally sensitive to sulcal sources, is less prone to such smearing effects and as such allows for better localization of sources.

In the realm of clinical research, the focus of biomarker exploration has primarily been centered on event-related potentials (ERPs) and quantitative EEG (qEEG) analysis. ERPs are a measure of average time-locked EEG activity relative to the onset of a stimulus or behavioral response event Fig 14.1. Measurement of the amplitudes and latencies of these components offers insights into the nature and order of the physiological processes that occur during the engagement of the given perceptual or cognitive processes. The timing of ERP components indicates the stage of information processing, with early responses, such as the N1 or P100, typically signifying early sensory processing (1). Components at greater latencies generally reflect higher-order sensory and cognitive processing (1). Measurement of the amplitudes provides a summary index of excitatory and inhibitory activations across local neuronal networks. Whereas ERPs provide a summary index of spatiotemporal changes in the electrical field in the time domain, qEEG measures are derived from the spectral decomposition of the EEG into its frequency content using a mathematical operation called Fourier transformation. This approach breaks down the M/EEG signal into its contributing oscillatory components, providing information about the activity at different frequency bands (delta [1–3 Hz], theta [4–7 Hz], alpha [8–12 Hz], beta [13–25 Hz], and gamma [>26 Hz]). These oscillations reflect the rate at which a given population of neurons becomes depolarized and can be useful for identifying specific patterns of communication.

Whereas structural, functional, and molecular imaging have helped to draw a detailed atlas of the effects of mood disorder pathology on larger spatial scale, the implementation of neurophysiological techniques has aided us in the discovery of more detailed functional biomarkers. These biomarkers are more cost-effective to research, and can be broken down to observe highly specific subcomponents of a cognitive function, or observe changes in response to medication at a fine timescale. Neurophysiological biomarkers hold great potential for use as frontline tools to aid in diagnosis. In this chapter, we describe the current progress in identifying robust electrophysiological correlates and biomarkers of major depressive disorder (MDD) and bipolar disorder (BD).

14.1.1 Event-Related Potentials

14.1.2 P300

The P300 component is a positive deflection in the EEG signal associated with the process of item discrimination in attention and working memory. P300 is commonly measured by the auditory "oddball paradigm" during which participants are presented with a common tone that is infrequently replaced with a deviant tone stimulus. P300 research has revealed it is, in fact, multidimensional with separate subcomponents reflecting the detection of novel stimuli (P3a) and discrimination of task-relevant versus irrelevant information (P3b). This critical distinction between components of the P300 complex has been brought to bear on elucidating the electrophysiological correlates of the cognitive profile seen in depressive disorders.

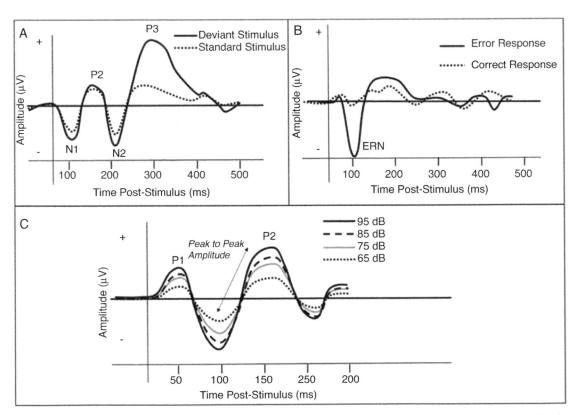

Figure 14.1 Schematic examples of event-related potentials (ERPs) commonly described in studies of major depressive disorder (MDD). (a) Example of the grand average ERPs during an auditory oddball experiment. (b) An example of the response difference between correct and incorrect task performance. (c) The N1 and P2 components of the auditory evoked potential are increased in response to increased stimulus amplitude (in decibels). The slope of the peak to peak amplitudes over the stimulus conditions is used as a metric for the excitability of central serotonergic pathways

14.1.3 Diagnosis

In patients with MDD, there is a tendency for a reduction in the amplitude and increase in the latency of the P3a in response to auditory and visual oddball stimuli (2–6). In contrast, the P3b in MDD does not typically demonstrate any difference from healthy controls (7, 8). These findings point toward the disturbance of a perceptual orienting response but emphasize the retention of higher-level cognition (9, 10). However, when studied in patients with BD, the P300 measurements tend to vary depending on the phase of the illness. During the depressive episodes, the P300 profile behaves similarly to MDD patients. As individuals recover toward a euthymic state, there is a gradual improvement in the measurement of the P300 (11, 12), highlighting the state dependency of the P300 profile of BD patients. In a review by Bruder and colleagues (13), the authors describe the consistency of P300 findings across thirty years of research, however, emphasizing that there are a number of negative findings, and that positive findings typically had weak effect sizes. The response to this has been to break down patient groupings into subgroups that separate the individuals along important cognitive and neurophysiological distinctions (7). Cognitive deterioration has been shown to increase P300 latency in auditory oddball paradigms (2), and to decrease the N2b–P3a complex amplitude during choice-reaction time tasks (7). In MDD patients with psychotic features, the P300 amplitude in response to auditory oddball stimuli was lower than controls and MDD patients without psychotic features (14), whereas the opposite is true in patients with comorbid anxiety (7, 15, 16).

14.1.4 Treatment Prediction

Treatment with selective serotonin reuptake inhibitor (SSRI) antidepressants is typically associated with a normalizing of the P300 response toward that of controls (14, 17, 18). In tandem, the response to treatment with serotonergic agents has been shown to be greatest in patients with more impaired P3a and P3b characteristics (both amplitude and latency)(2, 19). This finding has also been mirrored in the study of predictors of treatment response to repetitive transcranial magnetic current stimulation (rTMS) for MDD. The multisite study found that P300 amplitude at baseline had significantly predicted the likelihood of response (20). In each of these studies, the patients who typically experienced the greatest response to treatment had the most deteriorated P300 profile, which suggests a greater severity of depression (21). From these findings it would appear that P300 might represent a candidate for identifying patients with poor frontal regulation of the serotonergic system. However, future research would benefit from more rigorous study design including a focus on the interaction between P300 and other neural correlates of depression to understand their unique contributions and causal relationships to pathophysiologic mechanisms and therapeutic responses.

14.2 Error-Related Negativity

The error-related negativity (ERN) is a negative deflection in the EEG following the commission of an error during a cognitive task, typically requiring a motor response. The response peaks between 50 and 150 ms and is maximal at fronto-central electrodes (22). The component is believed to represent the dopaminergic disinhibition of the anterior cingulate cortex (ACC)(23) following an error and is viewed as part of a response monitoring process for regulating cognitive control of behavior.

14.2.1 Diagnosis

Based on the cognitive and physiological profiles of patients with MDD, their ERN should theoretically be distinct from healthy controls. However, the literature presents mixed findings, which likely reflect differences in the experimental design between studies. Varying task conditions will alter the network engaged during task performance and contribute to the efficiency of error monitoring. For example, in depressive disorders, where the processing of affective information is altered relative to controls, the ERN amplitude in response to errors committed during affective go/no-go trials was reduced in MDD patients relative to controls but remained equivalent during cognitive trials (24). Likewise, there is evidence of a blunted ERN in response to flanker tasks with a monetary reward component (25). Both tasks engage dopaminergic pathways that are known to be dysfunctional in patients with MDD and typically scale with the severity of the disease (26–29).

Conversely during neutral and punish trials of a flanker task, the ERN amplitude has been shown to increase relative to controls (30), possibly emphasizing a biasing toward a heightened focus on negative information (31).

14.2.2 Treatment Prediction

In a study of geriatric depression patients, one of the few investigations of ERN found that those who achieved remission from depression following citalopram treatment demonstrated a reduction in ERN amplitude, a finding not present in those who failed to achieve remission (32). In contrast, Schrijvers and colleagues (28) found similarities between controls and MDD patients in ERN amplitude at the start and after seven weeks of antidepressant intervention. However, they observed a correlation between the ERN amplitude and absolute change in symptom severity score. A valuable insight to this was provided by Weinberg and colleagues (29) through their investigation of the ERN in patients with melancholic features of depression. They found that even compared with patients with an otherwise similar profile of disease severity those with melancholia exhibited a blunted ERN that also carried over into remission. Although not being improved through pharmacological intervention, patients showed increased ERN amplitude after a course of mindfulness therapy, albeit in the absence of symptom changes (33). The lack of consistent ERN findings in depression may question the use of the ERN in monitoring depression and treatment response. Future investigations could investigate whether this may reflect differential impact due to severity or subtype of depression.

14.3 Loudness Dependence of the Auditory Evoked Potential

The loudness dependence of the auditory evoked potential (LDAEP) is a metric derived from the changing of the auditory evoked potential amplitude in response to the increasing intensity of an auditory stimulus. The LDAEP is typically taken by measuring the peak to peak amplitude of the N1/P2 complex and then measuring the slope of the line that results from plotting the amplitude as a function of intensity, though sometimes broken down to individual N1 and P2 components. The

functional basis of the LDAEP has been linked to serotonergic innervation of the primary auditory cortex (34–36) and is believed to represent a mechanism for cortical homeostasis via the control of neuronal gain response (37, 38). In several animal studies, there is substantial evidence supporting a relationship between the LDAEP and serotonergic activity levels in response to 5HT1a and 5HT2 influencing drugs (35, 36, 39), which suggest that it is feasible to consider the LDAEP as a diagnostic marker of central serotonergic activity. This claim is further supported by a study in rodents in response to citalopram treatment (40), which found a negative relationship between epidural LDAEP recordings and posttreatment primary auditory cortex serotonin levels. Based on empirical support from basic neuroscience studies, the LDAEP is a reliable marker for neurochemical activity in mood disorders that are characterized by alterations of serotonergic pathways.

14.3.1 Diagnosis

In patients with depression, the N1/P2 LDAEP has consistently been found to be increased relative to control subjects reflecting the findings of serotonergic suppression on LDAEP in animals (41, 42). However, this concept is contested by some studies that either have found no differences between patients and controls (43, 44) or have observed a dimensional effect of disease subtype on LDAEP properties. For example, Gopal and colleagues (42) noted that the amplitude of the N1/P2 complex was higher with increasing disease severity, and similarly, patients who had reported a history of suicidality had steeper LDAEP slopes than MDD patients without any suicidality (45). Conversely, MDD patients with melancholic symptoms have been shown to demonstrate a shallower LDAEP slope than non-melancholic patients (46). A similar counterintuitive finding was made by Jaworska and colleagues (47), who identified a negative correlation between the N1/P2 LDAEP slope and Montgomery-Asberg Depression Rating Scale (MADRS) score. Both studies highlight the importance of considering treatment history and the potential effects of interventions on the monoaminergic systems being targeted. For example, the use of high doses of drugs that affect levels of serotonergic neurotransmitters will alter what is considered the baseline state of that individual.

14.3.2 Treatment Prediction

Despite some conflicting findings regarding the LDAEP as a diagnostic marker of MDD, there has been a strikingly consistent pattern of reports suggesting that the LDAEP is highly predictive of treatment response. Patients with a greater baseline LDAEP tend to show a more significant improvement in depression symptom scores following both short- and long-term treatment with a variety of serotonergic agents (48–50). The pretreatment LDAEP slope has also been shown to predict treatment response, with high baseline LDAEP being complicit with a positive response to pharmacological intervention (51).

There have also been a series of recent LDAEP investigations with rTMS as a treatment for MDD. The mechanism of action for rTMS at the left dorsolateral prefrontal cortex (DLPFC) for MDD appears to include downstream desensitization of 5HT1a receptors in the raphe nucleus and the hypothalamus of rats (52, 53). rTMS has also been shown to improve the metabolism of 5-HT in the human limbic system (54). The LDAEP has demonstrated a similar predictive relationship with rTMS, with higher baseline LDAEP slope correlated with greater improvements in HAMD scores post-intervention (55). Unlike pharmacological interventions, patients did not exhibit a posttreatment effect on the LDAEP slope implying that the resulting changes to 5-HT1a activity are more acute following rTMS. This potentially implies that symptom improvement is due in part to regulation of serotonergic activity in tandem with improved emotional regulation arising from the alteration of the DLPFC neuron firing. Through functional connectivity studies, we understand that there is a pattern of communication between the DLPFC and the subgenual ACC (SGACC), which is related to the control of affective cognition (56). Therefore, symptom improvement is likely stemming from a more complicated pattern of system-level changes.

Overall, the LDAEP may be a robust marker for treatment response due to it reflecting gross central serotonergic activity, while inadvertently highlighting the dimensionality of the neurophysiological profile associated with depression through its variations across subtypes of dementia.

14.3.2.1 Quantitative EEG

Early studies of qEEG in MDD predominantly examined spectral power from scalp electrode recordings, demonstrating differences in the delta, theta, alpha, and beta bands between depressed subjects and healthy controls (57). However, most of the studies were not consistent in their findings and did not demonstrate regional differences (58). More recently, larger-scale, more methodologically sound EEG studies have shed some light on the utility of qEEG measures as biomarkers for both diagnosis and prognosis of MDD.

14.4 Alpha Activity

The EEG alpha rhythm is believed to be generated by corticothalamic feedback loops (59, 60), and is typically associated with the regulation and modulation of synaptic gain (61). Alpha oscillations increase over the cortical areas representing unattended or task-irrelevant information (61). This means that there exists an inverse relationship between alpha power and cortical activity, where lower alpha power represents a higher state of cortical excitability (62–65). Resting EEG alpha-band power is largely stable within individuals over time (66, 67), suggesting that alpha-power might reflect a trait-like variable. Disrupted alpha rhythms are a product of dysfunctional thalamic activity, which is partly associated with dopaminergic imbalance (68, 69).

14.4.1 Diagnosis

One of the most well-replicated EEG findings in the diagnosis of depressed patients is elevated alpha activity during rest where maximum amplitudes are observed at parieto-occipital locations in the eyes-closed condition (70). Several studies have reported elevated alpha power in depressed patients compared to healthy controls (71–73). A number of studies have localized elevated alpha activity to parietal, occipital, and frontal regions (73–75). Another well-replicated finding derived from alpha power as a biomarker for MDD is alpha asymmetry with decreased alpha power in the frontal right hemisphere regions compared to the left frontal regions, also known as frontal alpha asymmetry (FAA)(73, 76–86). FAA is thought to relate to the finding that MDD is characterized by a hyperactive right prefrontal cortex and hypoactive left prefrontal cortex (82, 87). The essential features of emotional affect can be described using the diathesis model developed by Davidson and Tomarken (82), where two fundamental motivational systems in response to external stimuli exist, namely appetitive (approach) and aversive (withdrawal)(88). The differential hemispheric activity in EEG can be attributed to the balance in the activations of these two systems (88). Left frontal activation is thought to index appetitive behavior (approach), and right frontal activation is thought to index aversive behavior (withdrawal) (89, 90). Elevated frontal left versus right alpha activity (73, 78, 84–86, 91–93) (Inferred as reduced frontal left versus right activation) thus indexes reduced approach motivation and sensitivity to reward. Stewart and colleagues (94) found that depressed individuals exhibited a similar pattern of reduced relative left frontal activity during all facial expressions, regardless of valence or approach/withdrawal related. This suggests a trait-like mechanism of emotional responding that is similar to most of the resting EEG asymmetry literature on depression (94, 95). However, many studies, including large sample studies failed to replicate the findings of the FAA in MDD (96–108). The uniformity and generalizability of most studies measuring frontal alpha asymmetry are lacking, owing to differences in technical aspects of EEG data collection and analysis as well as subject profiles. This necessitates meta-analysis and larger-scale studies (88).

14.4.2 Treatment Prediction

FAA and alpha power have shown some promise in differentiating responders and nonresponders to tricyclic antidepressants (TCA) such as clomipramine and imipramine, and with SSRIs(96, 109–113). In the International Study to Predict Optimized Treatment in Depression (iSPOT-D), a multicenter, randomized, prospective open-label trial, 1,008 MDD participants were randomized to eight-week treatment with escitalopram, sertraline, or venlafaxine-extended release (96). The patients were compared to 336 healthy controls (96). From the baseline EEG measures, a gender and drug-class interaction effect was found for FAA (96), with FAA associated with response to the SSRI escitalopram and sertraline, but in females only (96). In a study by Bruder and colleagues (109), MDD

patients were treated with fluoxetine for twelve weeks. They found that nonresponders showed greater activation (less alpha) over the right hemisphere, but responders did not. Again, the difference was significant in females but not males. This study was replicated by the same group (75) where they found that occipital alpha asymmetry could be used to differentiate responders from nonresponders to SSRIs where responders showed greater alpha (less activity) over right than left hemisphere and nonresponders showed the opposite. They also found greater alpha power in treatment of responders compared with nonresponders and healthy controls at occipital sites (75), and hypothesized that increased pretreatment alpha activity might be indicative of the relationship between low serotonergic activity and low arousal. This is because serotonergic activity mediates behavioral arousal; thus, low serotonergic activity could reflect the reduced activity of the mesencephalic raphe nuclei and cortical afferents. Also, it is known that depression may be related to dysfunction of temporoparietal mechanisms, which may play a role in mediating emotional arousal (114, 115). Increased alpha power and alpha asymmetry found in SSRI responders could be due to this biological mechanism (114). In rTMS studies, a slow alpha peak frequency has been consistently found to be a predictor for nonresponse (20, 116).

14.5 Theta Activity

In depressive disorders, particularly MDD, there is a profile of frontal and limbic system dysfunction, particularly attributed to the DLPFC, medial prefrontal cortex (mPFC), orbitofrontal cortex (OFC), and the ACC (57, 117–120). The hippocampus is a predominant source of theta waves in the frontal areas (121), with many studies reporting frontal midline theta frequency and their correlation with anxiety (122). Also, MDD psychopathology involves hippocampal symptoms (123 124). With MDD, changes in the theta band activity are implicated primarily in altered emotional regulation (125). This has been observed in studies combining MEG–EEG measures (126, 127) with correlations of scalp EEG theta rhythms recorded from prefrontal channels with MEG activity from the ACC. Cortical theta activity is considered to serve as a gating function on information processing in the limbic regions (128).

14.5.1 Diagnosis

A number of earlier studies reported increased theta band activity in MDD (71, 129–131), with more recently, localized to frontal regions including ACC (57, 73, 132). Recently, Grin-Yatsenko and colleagues (133) found increased alpha (and theta power) in a large cohort of patients in the early stages of depression. A recent review of BD literature has found increased theta as one of the most robust findings for resting EEG (134). However, there are many mixed findings where some studies have either reported no differences between MDD and controls or decreased ACC activity in MDD (128, 135, 136). Thus, there are no promising findings to conclude elevated theta activity as a diagnostic biomarker and future studies need to follow stringent methodological considerations such as different mood states and medication status of patients.

14.5.2 Treatment Prediction

Changes in theta activity have shown to correspond with treatment with various antidepressants (110, 113) and with electroconvulsive therapy (137). However, there are mixed findings in these studies investigating pretreatment and early changes in the theta band. Reduced pretreatment theta band activity has been observed for TCA, imipramine, and open-label SSRIs at eight weeks with 63% accuracy (113, 114, 138), and high frontal theta activity is associated with nonresponse to antidepressant treatments (139). With a 60% accuracy, Iosifescu and colleagues (138) showed that reduced frontal theta relative power at one-week posttreatment was predictive of treatment response at eight weeks. However, the same finding, but in the opposite direction was found by Spronk and colleagues (140), who reported higher pretreatment theta power as predictive of a higher decrease in depressive symptoms after antidepressant treatment. It may be useful to note that the widespread report on frontal (not midline) theta activity could be due to "drowsiness" theta power. These findings are in line with PET and fMRI studies, where low metabolic activity in the ACC is demonstrated to be associated with worse treatment outcome. Another study reported increased rostral ACC and frontal theta activity to be associated with nonresponse (132), but not with non-remission. Noteworthy is that these results are mostly driven by antidepressant treatment resistance. This suggests that future studies should also investigate the role of treatment resistance for the association of rostral ACC and treatment outcome (132). Increased pretreatment theta current density localized to the rostral ACC has been associated with responses to nortriptyline, citalopram, reboxetine, fluoxetine, or venlafaxine, in depressed patients (141–143).

14.6 Gamma Activity

Gamma rhythms correlate with increased neuronal action potential generation, including when individuals receive and process sensory stimuli (144–148) and have been associated with attention, memory, and perceptual organization (149), and found to facilitate hippocampal-cortical coordination (150–152).

14.6.1 Diagnosis

Gamma rhythms could be a novel biomarker for major depression with more recent results that provide some objective information on major depressive disease status (148). In a review of gamma disturbances in MDD, Fitzgerald and Watson (148) concluded that depending on the task, gamma rhythms could be either elevated or reduced in depressed patients compared to healthy controls and can also be used to distinguish unipolar depression from bipolar depression. One study found that gamma activity increased in frontal and temporal regions during spatial and arithmetic tasks (153) while other studies found decreased gamma in the frontal region during emotional tasks (154, 155). Another study found reduced gamma in the ACC in MDD patients compared to healthy controls at baseline (156). However, these results need to be replicated with larger-scale controlled studies to identify the underlying pathophysiology that is probed by each task and how the changes in gamma activity can inform the dysfunction. Future studies should also combine profiles of gamma band power across the brain to assess ratios of activity across regions (148). Differentiating MDD and bipolar disorder (BD) can still be a clinical challenge (157). Numerous studies have identified neuroimaging biomarkers that can differentiate between MDD and BD (157), but neurophysiological studies benefit from the ability to measure direct consequences of the electrical activity of neurons at a high temporal resolution (157) and thus can be used to probe gamma activity. One of the most widely investigated tasks with respect to gamma oscillations is the auditory steady-state response (ASSR) task. A recent MEG study found that subjects with unipolar depression had greater gamma power than those with bipolar disorder (157) globally across the whole brain. Another study found that BD patients showed decreased auditory-evoked gamma in a variety of brain regions compared to healthy controls (158). A few studies found that emotional tasks can be used to differentiate unipolar and bipolar depression. Compared to bipolar disorder, patients with unipolar depression showed increased gamma power in temporal regions and decreased frontal gamma power (148, 154, 155, 159).

14.6.2 Treatment Prediction

Serotonergic and noradrenergic drugs have opposing effects on gamma power in different brain regions (148), with serotonergic antidepressants suppressing gamma and noradrenergic antidepressants increasing gamma in animal models. This finding serves as a potentially important guide to pinpoint how the pathophysiology of depression involves altered signaling in different circuits, which could be used to better understand the individual's biotype of depression. Ketamine is another therapeutic agent that has recently gained much interest concerning understanding its role in depressive circuitry and electrophysiological effect due to its reported rapid and potentially durable effects (148, 160). A significant increase of gamma power as soon as ketamine is administered, preceding most mood effects implies that gamma power could play an important role in the mechanism of action of ketamine (161–163). A recent MEG study found that ketamine had an antidepressant effect in depressed patients and induced a mild depression in healthy controls (164). This study also noted that in patients who had lower baseline gamma, higher drug-induced gamma power across various brain regions was associated with the improved response. This was the opposite for patients with a higher baseline gamma. This study posited an "inverted U" relationship with optimal gamma power being associated with euthymia (148). However, it is still uncertain if gamma activity is causally related to the therapeutic actions of ketamine and monoaminergic antidepressants (148). Noninvasive, non-

pharmaceutical treatments like TMS show increased gamma signaling after recovery from depression, and this is especially the case with baseline gamma (165–167). Specifically, a study (165) found that treatment response can be associated with increases in prefrontal gamma power as well as measures of theta gamma coupling.

14.7 Limitations and Recommendations to the Field

MDD is a heterogeneous disorder with unclear pathophysiological mechanisms, a highly variable course, and an inconsistent treatment response (168). Thus, there is a necessity for objective biological indices that can be used for diagnosis and treatment monitoring and response prediction. EEG has many advantages in identifying potential biomarkers, and the numerous studies have identified various EEG characteristics as biomarkers and investigated its use. However, there are some limitations, including low spatial resolution. Advanced source localization techniques are often used to infer the brain regions that are generating EEG recorded at the scalp, but only provide an approximate location for the source. More studies could either use MEG or multimodal approaches such as a combination of EEG and fMRI to provide additional information on anatomical specificity. Also, EEG generally differs from intracranial or intra-brain recordings (148), due to low-pass filtering and volume averaging effects by tissue before reaching the scalp (148), thus, better reflective of cortical signals rather than deeper, subcortical structures. This is especially an issue when using EEG measures to study deeper regions and structures implicated in depression such as the ACC or the amygdala. One of the other limitations in the field is that the experimental approaches used to measure the EEG biomarker vary, with some measuring during a cognitive or sensory task and others measuring at rest or baseline (148). Thus, EEG measures should be considered in the context of the brain state of the patients. One major limitation in the field is the lack of specificity of EEG biomarkers in the diagnosis of MDD or BD, for instance, gamma activity anomalies implicated in MDD are also affected in schizophrenia, perhaps due to overlapping genetics, pathophysiology, and symptomatology (169). Though limiting their diagnostic value, a lack of specificity does not preclude utility in treatment response and prediction. In this regard, there should be distinctions of stable trait markers of mood disorders versus electrophysiological markers of state that track clinical symptom severity. Finally, there have been promising studies of treatment response through biotyping, for instance, fMRI connectivity patterns used to biotype MDD were successful in predicting response to rTMS treatment (170). A similar approach employing EEG biomarkers could strengthen both diagnostic specificity and treatment prediction within a precision medicine framework.

References

1. Woodman GF. A brief introduction to the use of event-related potentials in studies of perception and attention. *Atten Percept Psychophys* [Internet]. 2010 November; **72**(8): 2031–2046. Available from: www .ncbi.nlm.nih.gov/pubmed/21097848

2. Vandoolaeghe E, van Hunsel F, Nuyten D, Maes M. Auditory event related potentials in major depression: prolonged P300 latency and increased P200 amplitude. *J Affect Disord*. 1998 March; **48** (2–3): 105–113.

3. Pfefferbaum A, Wenegrat BG, Ford JM, Roth WT, Kopell BS. Clinical application of the P3 component of event-related potentials. II. Dementia, depression and schizophrenia. *Electroencephalogr Clin Neurophysiol*. 1984 April; **59**(2): 104–124.

4. Diner BC, Holcomb PJ, Dykman RA. P300 in major depressive disorder. *Psychiatry Res*. 1985 July; **15**(3): 175–184.

5. Bange F, Bathien N. Visual cognitive dysfunction in depression: An event-related potential study. *Electroencephalogr Clin Neurophysiol*. 1998 September; **108**(5): 472–481.

6. Schlegel S, Nieber D, Herrmann C, Bakauski E. Latencies of the P300 component of the auditory event-related potential in depression are related to the Bech-Rafaelsen melancholia scale but not to the Hamilton Rating Scale for Depression. *Acta Psychiatr Scand*. 1991 June; **83**(6): 438–440.

7. Pierson A, Ragot R, Van Hooff J, et al. Heterogeneity of information-processing alterations according to dimensions of depression: an event-related potentials study. *Biol Psychiatry*. 1996; **40**(2): 98–115.

8. Bruder GE, Kroppmann CJ, Kayser J, et al. Reduced brain responses to novel sounds in depression: P3

9. Friedman D, Simpson G, Hamberger M. Age-related changes in scalp topography to novel and target stimuli. *Psychophysiology*. 1993; **30**(4): 383–396.

10. Tenke CE, Kayser J, Stewart JW, Bruder GE. Novelty P3 reductions in depression: characterization using principal components analysis (PCA) of current source density (CSD) waveforms. *Psychophysiology*. 2010; **47**(1): 133–146.

11. Fu L, Xiang D, Subodh D, et al. Auditory P300 study in patients with convalescent bipolar depression and bipolar depression. *Neuroreport*. 2018 August; **29**(11): 968–973.

12. Bersani FS, Minichino A, Fattapposta F, et al. P300 component in euthymic patients with bipolar disorder type I, bipolar disorder type II and healthy controls: A preliminary event-related potential study. *Neuroreport*. 2015 March; **26**(4): 206–210.

13. Bruder GE, Kayser J, Tenke CCE. Event-related brain potentials in depression: clinical, cognitive and neurophysiologic implications. *Oxford Handb event-related potential components* [Internet]. 2012; **2012**: 563–592. Available from: http://psy chophysiology.cpmc.columbia.edu/pdf/bru der2009a.pdf

14. Karaaslan F, Gonul AS, Oguz A, Erdinc E, Esel E. P300 changes in major depressive disorders with and without psychotic features. *J Affect Disord*. 2003; **73**(3): 283–287.

15. Li Y, Hu Y, Liu T, Wu D. Dipole source analysis of auditory P300 response in depressive and anxiety disorders. *Cogn Neurodyn*. 2011; **5**(2): 221–229.

16. Li Y, Wang W, Liu T, et al. Source analysis of P3a and P3b components to investigate interaction of depression and anxiety in attentional systems. *Sci Rep*. 2015; **5**: 17138.

17. Hetzel G, Moeller O, Evers S, et al. The astroglial protein S100B and visually evoked event-related potentials before and after antidepressant treatment. *Psychopharmacology (Berl)*. 2005; **178**(2–3): 161–166.

18. Hansenne M, Ansseau M. P300 event-related potential and serotonin-1A activity in depression. *Eur psychiatry*. 1999; **14**(3): 143–147.

19. Jaworska N, Protzner A. Electrocortical features of depression and their clinical utility in assessing antidepressant treatment outcome. *Can J Psychiatry*. 2013; **58**(9): 509–514.

20. Arns M, Drinkenburg WH, Fitzgerald PB, Kenemans JL. Neurophysiological predictors of

non-response to rTMS in depression. *Brain Stimul* [Internet]. 2012; **5**(4): 569–576. Available from: h ttp://dx.doi.org/10.1016/j.brs.2011.12.003

21. Tripathi SM, Mishra N, Tripathi RK, Gurnani KC. P300 latency as an indicator of severity in major depressive disorder. *Ind Psychiatry J.* 2015; **24**(2): 163–167.

22. Scheffers MK, Coles MGH. Performance monitoring in a confusing world: Error-related brain activity, judgments of response accuracy, and types of errors. Vol. **26**, *Journal of Experimental Psychology: Human Perception and Performance*. US: American Psychological Association; 2000. 141–151.

23. Olvet DM, Hajcak G. The error-related negativity (ERN) and psychopathology: Toward an Endophenotype. *Clin Psychol Rev* [Internet]. 2008 December 9; **28**(8): 1343–1354. Available from: www.ncbi.nlm.nih.gov/pmc/articles/PMC2615243/

24. Schoenberg PLA. The error processing system in major depressive disorder: Cortical phenotypal marker hypothesis. *Biol Psychol.* 2014 May; **99**: 100–114.

25. Ruchsow M, Herrnberger B, Wiesend C, et al. The effect of erroneous responses on response monitoring in patients with major depressive disorder: A study with event-related potentials. *Psychophysiology.* 2004 November; **41**(6): 833–840.

26. Schrijvers D, Hulstijn W, Sabbe BGC. Psychomotor symptoms in depression: A diagnostic, pathophysiological and therapeutic tool. *J Affect Disord.* 2008 July; **109**(1–2): 1–20.

27. Schrijvers D, de Bruijn ERA, Maas Y, et al. Action monitoring in major depressive disorder with psychomotor retardation. *Cortex.* 2008 May; **44**(5): 569–579.

28. Schrijvers D, De Bruijn ERA, Maas YJ, et al. Action monitoring and depressive symptom reduction in major depressive disorder. *Int J Psychophysiol.* 2009 March; **71**(3): 218–224.

29. Weinberg A, Liu H, Shankman SA. Blunted neural response to errors as a trait marker of melancholic depression. *Biol Psychol.* 2016 January; **113**: 100–107.

30. Chiu PH, Deldin PJ. Neural evidence for enhanced error detection in major depressive disorder. *Am J Psychiatry.* 2007; **164**(4): 608–616.

31. Gorka SM, Lieberman L, Shankman SA, Phan KL. Startle potentiation to uncertain threat as a psychophysiological indicator of fear-based psychopathology: An examination across multiple internalizing disorders. *J Abnorm Psychol.* 2017; **126**(1): 8.

32. Alexopoulos GS. The vascular depression hypothesis: 10 years later. Vol. **60**, *Biological Psychiatry*. United States; 2006. pp. 1304–1305.

33. Fissler M, Winnebeck E, Schroeter TA, et al. Brief training in mindfulness may normalize a blunted error-related negativity in chronically depressed patients. *Cogn Affect Behav Neurosci.* 2017 December; **17**(6): 1164–1175.

34. Hegerl U, Juckel G. Intensity dependence of auditory evoked potentials as an indicator of central serotonergic neurotransmission: A new hypothesis* 1. *Biological Psychiatry.* 1993; **33**: 173–187.

35. Juckel G, Molnar M, Hegerl U, Csepe V, Karmos G. Auditory-evoked potentials as indicator of brain serotonergic activity–first evidence in behaving cats. *Biol Psychiatry.* 1997 June; **41**(12): 1181–1195.

36. Juckel G, Hegerl U, Molnar M, Csepe V, Karmos G. Auditory evoked potentials reflect serotonergic neuronal activity–a study in behaving cats administered drugs acting on 5-HT1A autoreceptors in the dorsal raphe nucleus. *Neuropsychopharmacology.* 1999 December; **21**(6): 710–716.

37. Jacobs BL, Wilkinson LO, Fornal CA. The role of brain serotonin: A neurophysiologic perspective. *Neuropsychopharmacology.* 1990; **3**(5–6): 473–479.

38. Aghajanian GK, Vandermaelen CP. Specific Systems of the Reticular Core: Serotonin [Internet]. Comprehensive Physiology. 2011. (Major Reference Works). Available from: https://doi.org/10.1002/cphy.cp010404

39. Lewis DA, Campbell MJ, Foote SL, Morrison JH. The monoaminergic innervation of primate neocortex. *Hum Neurobiol* [Internet]. 1986; **5**(3): 181–188. Available from: http://europepmc.org/a bstract/MED/3533864

40. Wutzler A, Winter C, Kitzrow W, et al. Loudness dependence of auditory evoked potentials as indicator of central serotonergic neurotransmission: Simultaneous electrophysiological recordings and in vivo microdialysis in the rat primary auditory cortex. *Neuropsychopharmacology* [Internet]. 2008 May 7; **33**: 3176. Available from: http://dx.doi.org/10.1038/npp.2008.42

41. Ruohonen EM, Astikainen P. Brain responses to sound intensity changes dissociate depressed participants and healthy controls. *Biol Psychol* [Internet]. 2017; **127**: 74–81. Available from: www.sciencedirect.com/science/article/pii/S0301051117301060

42. Gopal K V, Bishop CE, Carney L. Auditory measures in clinically depressed individuals. II.

Auditory evoked potentials and behavioral speech tests. *Int J Audiol.* 2004 October; **43**(9): 499–505.

43. Linka T, Sartory G, Bender S, Gastpar M, Müller BW. The intensity dependence of auditory ERP components in unmedicated patients with major depression and healthy controls. An analysis of group differences. *J Affect Disord* [Internet]. 2007; **103**(1): 139–145. Available from: www.sciencedirect.com/science/article/pii/S0165032707000201

44. Park Y-M, Lee S-H, Kim S, Bae S-M. The loudness dependence of the auditory evoked potential (LDAEP) in schizophrenia, bipolar disorder, major depressive disorder, anxiety disorder, and healthy controls. *Prog Neuro-Psychopharmacology Biol Psychiatry.* 2010; **34**(2): 313–316.

45. Chen T-J, Yu YW-Y, Chen M-C, et al. Serotonin dysfunction and suicide attempts in major depressives: An auditory event-related potential study. *Neuropsychobiology.* 2005; **52**(1): 28–36.

46. Fitzgerald PB, Mellow TB, Hoy KE, et al. A study of intensity dependence of the auditory evoked potential (IDAEP) in medicated melancholic and non-melancholic depression. *J Affect Disord.* 2009; **117**(3): 212–216.

47. Jaworska N, Blier P, Fusee W, Knott V. Scalp- and sLORETA-derived loudness dependence of auditory evoked potentials (LDAEPs) in unmedicated depressed males and females and healthy controls. *Clin Neurophysiol* [Internet]. 2012 September; **123**(9): 1769–1778. Available from: http://dx.doi.org/10.1016/j.clinph.2012.02.076

48. Lee B-H, Park Y-M, Lee S-H, Shim M. Prediction of long-term treatment response to selective serotonin reuptake inhibitors (SSRIs) using scalp and source loudness dependence of auditory evoked potentials (LDAEP) Analysis in patients with major depressive disorder. *Int J Mol Sci* [Internet]. 2015; **16**(3): 6251–6265. Available from: www.mdpi.com/1422-0067/16/3/6251

49. Mulert C, Juckel G, Augustin H, Hegerl U. Comparison between the analysis of the loudness dependency of the auditory N1/P2 component with LORETA and dipole source analysis in the prediction of treatment response to the selective serotonin reuptake inhibitor citalopram in major depression. *Clin Neurophysiol* [Internet]. 2002; **113**(10): 1566–1572. Available from: www.sciencedirect.com/science/article/pii/S1388245702002523

50. Jaworska N, Blondeau C, Tessier P, et al. Response prediction to antidepressants using scalp and source-localized loudness dependence of auditory evoked potential (LDAEP) slopes. *Prog Neuro-Psychopharmacology Biol Psychiatry* [Internet].

2013; **44**: 100–107. Available from: www.sciencedirect.com/science/article/pii/S0278584613000146

51. Gallinat J, Bottlender R, Juckel G, et al. The loudness dependency of the auditory evoked N1/P2-component as a predictor of the acute SSRI response in depression. *Psychopharmacology (Berl)* [Internet]. 2000 March; **148**(4): 404–411. Available from: https://doi.org/10.1007/s002130050070

52. Gur E, Lerer B, Dremencov E, Newman ME. Chronic repetitive transcranial magnetic stimulation induces subsensitivity of presynaptic serotonergic autoreceptor activity in rat brain. *Neuroreport* [Internet]. 2000; **11**(13). Available from: https://journals.lww.com/neuroreport/Fulltext/2000/09110/Chronic_repetitive_transcranial_magnetic.19.aspx

53. Gur E, Lerer B, Van de Kar LD, Newman ME. Chronic rTMS induces subsensitivity of post-synaptic 5-HT1A receptors in rat hypothalamus. *Int J Neuropsychopharmacol* [Internet]. 2004 September 1; **7**(3): 335–340. Available from: http://dx.doi.org/10.1017/S1461145703003985

54. Sibon I, Strafella AP, Gravel P, et al. Acute prefrontal cortex TMS in healthy volunteers: Effects on brain 11 C-αMtrp trapping. *Neuroimage* [Internet]. 2007; **34**(4): 1658–1664. Available from: www.sciencedirect.com/science/article/pii/S1053811906008846

55. Lee S, Jang K-I, Chae J-H. Association of the loudness dependence of auditory evoked potentials with clinical changes to repetitive transcranial magnetic stimulation in patients with depression. *J Affect Disord.* 2018 October; **238**: 451–457.

56. Fox MD, Buckner RL, White MP, Greicius MD, Pascual-Leone A. Efficacy of transcranial magnetic stimulation targets for depression is related to intrinsic functional connectivity with the subgenual cingulate. *Biol Psychiatry.* 2012 October; **72**(7): 595–603.

57. Korb AS, Cook IA, Hunter AM, Leuchter AF. Brain electrical source differences between depressed subjects and healthy controls. *Brain Topogr.* 2008; **21**(2): 138–146.

58. Pollock VE, Schneider LS. Topographic quantitative EEG in elderly subjects with major depression. *Psychophysiology* [Internet]. 1990 July 1; **27**(4): 438–444. Available from: https://doi.org/10.1111/j.1469-8986.1990.tb02340.x

59. Lopes da Silva F., Vos J., Mooibroek J, Rotterdam A van. Relative contributions of intracortical and thalamo-cortical processes in the generation of alpha rhythms, revealed by partial

coherence analysis. *Electroencephalogr Clin Neurophysiol.* 1980; **50**(5–6): 449–456.

60. Suffczynski P. Computational model of thalamo-cortical networks: dynamical control of alpha rhythms in relation to focal attention. *Int J Psychophysiol.* 2001; **43**(1): 25–40.

61. Chaumon M, Busch NA. Prestimulus neural oscillations inhibit visual perception via modulation of response gain. *J Cogn Neurosci* [Internet]. 2014 April 17; **26**(11): 2514–2529. Available from: https://doi.org/10.1162 /jocn_a_00653

62. Laufs H, Krakow K, Sterzer P, et al. Electroencephalographic signatures of attentional and cognitive default modes in spontaneous brain activity fluctuations at rest. 2003;(October) PNAS September 16, 2003 100 (19) 11053–11058.

63. Gonçalves SI. Correlating the alpha rhythm to BOLD using simultaneous EEG/fMRI: inter-subject variability. *NeuroImage (Orlando, Fla).* 2006; **30**(1): 203–213.

64. Laufs H, Holt J, Elfont R, et al. Where the BOLD signal goes when alpha EEG leaves. *NeuroImage (Orlando, Fla).* 2006; **31**(4): 1408–1418.

65. de Munck JC. The hemodynamic response of the alpha rhythm: An EEG/fMRI study. *NeuroImage (Orlando, Fla).* 2007; **35**(3): 1142–1151.

66. Klimesch W, Sauseng P, Hanslmayr S. EEG alpha oscillations : The inhibition – timing hypothesis. 2006; 3. Brain Research Reviews. Volume 53, Issue 1, January 2007, Pages 63–88.

67. Näpflin M, Wildi M, Sarnthein J. Test-retest reliability of resting EEG spectra validates a statistical signature of persons. Vol. **118**, *Clinical Neurophysiology.* Sarnthein, Johannes: Universitatsspital Zurich, Zurich, Switzerland, CH-8091, johannes.sarnthein@usz.ch: Elsevier Science; 2007. pp. 2519–2524.

68. Begić DD, Mahnik-Miloš M, Grubišin J. EEG characteristics in depression, "negative" and "positive" schizophrena. *Psychiatr Danub.* 2009; **21**(4): 579–584.

69. Carlsson A. The dopamine theory revisited. *Schizophrenia.* 1995; 379–400.

70. Olbrich S, Van Dinteren R, Arns M. Personalized medicine: Review and perspectives of promising baseline EEG biomarkers in major depressive disorder and attention deficit hyperactivity disorder. *Neuropsychobiology.* 2016; **72**(3–4): 229–240.

71. Roemer RA, Shagass C, Dubin W, Jaffe R, Siegal L. Quantitative EEG in elderly depressives. *Brain Topogr.* 1992; **4**(4): 285–290.

72. Begic D, Popovic-Knapic V, Grubisin J, et al. Quantitative electroencephalography in schizophrenia and depression. *Psychiatr Danub.* 2011 December; **23**(4): 355–362.

73. Jaworska N, Blier P, Fusee W, Knott V. α Power, α asymmetry and anterior cingulate cortex activity in depressed males and females. *J Psychiatr Res* [Internet]. 2012; **46**(11): 1483–1491. Available from: www.pubmedcentral.nih.gov/articlerender.fcgi?arti d=3463760&tool=pmcentrez&rendertype=abstract

74. Grin-Yatsenko V a, Baas I, Ponomarev V a, Kropotov JD. EEG power spectra at early stages of depressive disorders. *J Clin Neurophysiol.* 2009; **26** (6): 401–406.

75. Bruder GE, Sedoruk JP, Stewart JW, et al. Electroencephalographic alpha measures predict therapeutic response to a selective serotonin reuptake inhibitor antidepressant: Pre- and post-treatment findings. *Biol Psychiatry.* 2008; **63** (12): 1171–1177.

76. Davidson RJ. Cerebral asymmetry, emotion, and affective style. In: *Brain asymmetry.* Cambridge, MA, US: The MIT Press; 1995. pp. 361–387.

77. Davidson RJ, Henriques J. Regional brain function in sadness and depression. In: *The Neuropsychology of Emotion.* New York, NY, US: Oxford University Press; 2000. pp. 269–297. (Series in affective science.).

78. Davidson RJ, Lewis DA, Alloy LB, et al. Neural and behavioral substrates of mood and mood regulation. *Biol Psychiatry* [Internet]. 2002; **52**(6): 478–502. Available from: www.sciencedirect.com /science/article/pii/S0006322302014580

79. Tomarkenand AJ, Keener AD. Frontal brain asymmetry and depression: A self-regulatory perspective. *Cogn Emot* [Internet]. 1998 May 1; **12**(3): 387–420. Available from: https://doi.org/10 .1080/026999398379655

80. Micoulaud-Franchi J-A, Richieri R, Cermolacce M, et al. Parieto-temporal alpha EEG band power at baseline as a predictor of antidepressant treatment response with repetitive transcranial magnetic stimulation: A preliminary study. *J Affect Disord* [Internet]. 2012; **137**(1): 156–160. Available from: www.sciencedirect.com /science/article/pii/S0165032711007932

81. Chang JS, Yoo CS, Yi SH, et al. An integrative assessment of the psychophysiologic alterations in young women with recurrent major depressive disorder. *Psychosom Med.* 2012 June; **74**(5): 495–500.

82. Henriques JB, Davidson RJ. Left frontal hypoactivation in depression. *J Abnorm Psychol.* 1991 November; **100**(4): 535–545.

83. Schaffer CE, Davidson RJ, Saron C. Frontal and parietal electroencephalogram asymmetry in depressed and nondepressed subjects. *Biol Psychiatry*. 1983 July; **18**(7): 753–762.

84. Kemp AH, Griffiths K, Felmingham KL, et al. Disorder specificity despite comorbidity: Resting EEG alpha asymmetry in major depressive disorder and post-traumatic stress disorder. *Biol Psychol* [Internet]. 2010; **85**(2): 350–354. Available from: http://dx.doi.org/10.1016/j.biopsycho.2010.08.001

85. Beeney JE, Levy KN, Gatzke-Kopp LM, Hallquist MN. EEG asymmetry in borderline personality disorder and depression following rejection. *Personal Disord Theory, Res Treat*. 2014; **5**(2): 178–185.

86. Gollan JK, Hoxha D, Chihade D, et al. Frontal alpha EEG asymmetry before and after behavioral activation treatment for depression. *Biol Psychol* [Internet]. 2014; **99**: 198–208. Available from: www.sciencedirect.com/science/article/pii/S0301051114000623

87. Olbrich S, Arns M. EEG biomarkers in major depressive disorder: Discriminative power and prediction of treatment response. *Int Rev Psychiatry*. 2013; **25**(5): 604–618.

88. van der Vinne N, Vollebregt MA, van Putten MJAM, Arns M. Frontal alpha asymmetry as a diagnostic marker in depression: Fact or fiction? A meta-analysis. *NeuroImage Clin*. 2017; **16**(July): 79–87.

89. Davidson RJ. Affect, cognition, and hemispheric specialization. In: *Emotions, Cognition, and Behavior*. New York, NY, US: Cambridge University Press; 1985. pp. 320–365.

90. Kelley NJ, Hortensius R, Schutter DJLG, Harmon-Jones E. The relationship of approach/avoidance motivation and asymmetric frontal cortical activity: A review of studies manipulating frontal asymmetry. *Int J Psychophysiol* [Internet]. 2017; **119**: 19–30. Available from: www.sciencedirect.com/science/article/pii/S0167876017301770

91. Debener S, Beauducel A, Nessler D, et al. Is resting anterior EEG alpha asymmetry a trait marker for depression? Findings for healthy adults and clinically depressed patients. *Neuropsychobiology*. 2000; **41**(1): 31–37.

92. Pizzagalli DA, Nitschke JB, Oakes TR, et al. Brain electrical tomography in depression: the importance of symptom severity, anxiety, and melancholic features. *Biol Psychiatry* [Internet]. 2002; **52**(2): 73–85. Available from: www.sciencedirect.com/science/article/pii/S0006322302013136

93. Allen JJB, Coan JA, Nazarian M. Issues and assumptions on the road from raw signals to metrics of frontal EEG asymmetry in emotion. *Biol Psychol* [Internet]. 2004; **67**(1): 183–218. Available from: www.sciencedirect.com/science/article/pii/S0301051104000377

94. Stewart JL, Coan JA, Towers DN, Allen JJB. Frontal EEG asymmetry during emotional challenge differentiates individuals with and without lifetime major depressive disorder. *J Affect Disord* [Internet]. 2011; **129**(1–3): 167–174. Available from: http://dx.doi.org/10.1016/j.jad.2010.08.029

95. Thibodeau R, Jorgensen RS, Kim S. Depression, anxiety, and resting frontal EEG asymmetry: A meta-analytic review. *J Abnorm Psychol*. 2006; **115**(4): 715–729.

96. Arns M, Bruder G, Hegerl U, et al. EEG alpha asymmetry as a gender-specific predictor of outcome to acute treatment with different antidepressant medications in the randomized iSPOT-D study. *Clin Neurophysiol* [Internet]. 2016; **127**(1): 509–519. Available from: http://dx.doi.org/10.1016/j.clinph.2015.05.032

97. Carvalho A, Moraes H, Silveira H, et al. EEG frontal asymmetry in the depressed and remitted elderly: Is it related to the trait or to the state of depression? *J Affect Disord* [Internet]. 2011; **129**(1): 143–148. Available from: www.sciencedirect.com/science/article/pii/S0165032710005598

98. Gold C, Fachner J, Erkkilä J. Validity and reliability of electroencephalographic frontal alpha asymmetry and frontal midline theta as biomarkers for depression. *Scand J Psychol* [Internet]. 2013 April 1; **54**(2): 118–126. Available from: https://doi.org/10.1111/sjop.12022

99. Reid SA, Duke LM, Allen JJB. Resting frontal electroencephalographic asymmetry in depression: Inconsistencies suggest the need to identify mediating factors. *Psychophysiology* [Internet]. 1998 July 1; **35**(4): 389–404. Available from: https://doi.org/10.1111/1469-8986.3540389

100. Segrave RA, Cooper NR, Thomson RH, et al. Individualized Alpha Activity and Frontal Asymmetry in Major Depression. *Clin EEG Neurosci* [Internet]. 2011 January 1; **42**(1): 45–52. Available from: https://doi.org/10.1177/155005941104200110

101. M. Kentgen L, Tenke C, Pine D, et al. Electroencephalographic asymmetries in adolescents with major depression: Influence of comorbidity with anxiety disorders. *Journal of Abnormal Psychology*. 2000; **109**: 797–802.

102. Knott V, Mahoney C, Kennedy S, Evans K. EEG power, frequency, asymmetry and coherence in male depression. *Psychiatry Res Neuroimaging* [Internet]. 2001; **106**(2): 123–140. Available from: www.sciencedirect.com/science/article/pii/S0925492700000809

103. Deldin PJ, Chiu P. Cognitive restructuring and EEG in major depression. *Biol Psychol* [Internet]. 2005; **70**(3): 141–151. Available from: www.sciencedirect.com/science/article/pii/S030105110500027X

104. Mathersul D, Williams LM, Hopkinson PJ, Kemp AH. Investigating models of affect: Relationships among EEG alpha asymmetry, depression, and anxiety. Vol. 8, *Emotion*. Kemp, Andrew H.: The Brain Dynamics Centre, Westmead Hospital, Acacia House, Hawkesbury Road, Westmead, NSW, Australia, 2145, akemp@usyd.edu.au: American Psychological Association; 2008. 560–572.

105. Quraan MA, Protzner AB, Daskalakis ZJ, et al. EEG power asymmetry and functional connectivity as a marker of treatment effectiveness in DBS surgery for depression. *Neuropsychopharmacology* [Internet]. 2013 November 28; **39**: 1270. Available from: https://doi.org/10.1038/npp.2013.330

106. Price GW, Lee JW, Garvey C, Gibson N. Appraisal of sessional EEG features as a correlate of clinical changes in an rTMS treatment of depression. *Clin EEG Neurosci* [Internet]. 2008 July 1; **39**(3): 131–138. Available from: https://doi.org/10.1177/155005940803900307

107. Allen JJB, Kline JP. Frontal EEG asymmetry, emotion, and psychopathology: The first, and the next 25 years. *Biol Psychol* [Internet]. 2004; **67**(1): 1–5. Available from: www.sciencedirect.com/science/article/pii/S0301051104000304

108. Kaiser AK, Doppelmayr M, Iglseder B. Electroencephalogram alpha asymmetry in geriatric depression. *Z Gerontol Geriatr* [Internet]. 2018; **51**(2): 200–205. Available from: https://doi.org/10.1007/s00391-016-1108-z

109. Bruder GE, Stewart JW, Tenke CE, et al. Electroencephalographic and perceptual asymmetry differences between responders and nonresponders to an SSRI antidepressant. *Biol Psychiatry*. 2001; **49**(5): 416–425.

110. Knott V, Mahoney C, Kennedy S, Evans K. Pretreatment EEG and it's relationship to depression severity and paroxetine treatment outcome. *Pharmacopsychiatry*. 2000; 33: 201–205.

111. Ulrich G, Haug H-J, Stieglietz R-D, Fahndrich E. EEG characteristics of clinically defined on-drug-responders and non-responders – A comparison clomipramine vs. maprotiline. *Pharmacopsychiatry* [Internet]. 1988; **21**(6): 367–368. Available from: www.scopus.com/inward/record.uri?eid=2-s2.0-0024213743&partnerID=40&md5=73803912ace9ccfcd8af4ee36646e933

112. Baskaran A, Farzan F, Milev R, et al. The comparative effectiveness of electroencephalographic indices in predicting response to escitalopram therapy in depression: A pilot study. *J Affect Disord* [Internet]. 2017; **227** (October 2017): 542–549. Available from: https://doi.org/10.1016/j.jad.2017.10.028

113. Knott VJ, I. Telner J, D. Lapierre Y, et al. Quantitative EEG in the prediction of antidepressant response to imipramine. *J Affect Disord*. 1996 August 1; **39**(3): 175–184.

114. Baskaran A, Milev R, McIntyre RS. The neurobiology of the EEG biomarker as a predictor of treatment response in depression. *Neuropharmacology*. 2012; **63**(4): 507–513.

115. Heller W, A. Etienne M, A. Miller G. Patterns of perceptual asymmetry in depression and anxiety: Implications for neuropsychological models of emotion and psychopathology. Journal of Abnormal Psychology. 1995; **104**: 327–333.

116. Arns M, Spronk D, Fitzgerald PB. Potential differential effects of 9 Hz rTMS and 10 Hz rTMS in the treatment of depression. *Brain Stimul*. 2010; **3**(2): 124–126.

117. Bench CJ, Friston KJ, Brown RG, et al. The anatomy of melancholia–focal abnormalities of cerebral blood flow in major depression. *Psychol Med* [Internet]. 1992; **22**(3): 607–615. Available from: www.ncbi.nlm.nih.gov/pubmed/1410086

118. Drevets WC, Videen TO, Price JL, et al. A functional anatomical study of unipolar depression. *J Neurosci*. 1992 September; **12**(9): 3628–3641.

119. Mayberg HS, Lewis PJ, Regenold W, Wagner HNJ. Paralimbic hypoperfusion in unipolar depression. *J Nucl Med*. 1994 June; **35** (6): 929–934.

120. Seminowicz DA, Mayberg HS, McIntosh AR, et al. Limbic-frontal circuitry in major depression: a path modeling metanalysis. *Neuroimage*. 2004 May; **22**(1): 409–418.

121. Klimesch W. EEG alpha and theta oscillations reflect cognitive and memory performance: a review and analysis. *Brain Res Rev [Internet]*. 1999 April [cited 2014 August 15]; **29**(2–3): 169–195. Available from: www.sciencedirect.com/science/article/pii/S0165017398000563

122. Dharmadhikari AS, Tandle AL, Jaiswal S V, et al. Frontal theta asymmetry as a biomarker of

depression. *East Asian Arch Psychiatry* [Internet]. 2018; **28**(1): 17–22. Available from: www .easap.asia/index.php/find-issues/current-issue/i tem/795-1803-v28n1-p17

123. Kempermann G, Kronenberg G. Depressed new neurons – Adult hippocampal neurogenesis and a cellular plasticity hypothesis of major depression. *Biol Psychiatry*. 2003; **54**(5): 499–503.

124. Fingelkurts AA, Fingelkurts AA, Rytsälä H, et al. Composition of brain oscillations in ongoing EEG during major depression disorder. *Neurosci Res*. 2006; **56**(2): 133–144.

125. Iosifescu DV. Electroencephalography-derived biomarkers of antidepressant response. *Harv Rev Psychiatry*. 2011; **19**(3): 144–154.

126. Ishii R, Shinosaki K, Ukai S, et al. Medial prefrontal cortex generates frontal midline theta rhythm. *Neuroreport*. 1999; **10**(4): 675–679.

127. Asada H, Fukuda Y, Tsunoda S, Yamaguchi M, Tonoike M. Frontal midline theta rhythms reflect alternative activation of prefrontal cortex and anterior cingulate cortex in humans. *Neurosci Lett*. 1999; **274**(1): 29–32.

128. Pizzagalli DA, Oakes TR, Davidson RJ. Coupling of theta activity and glucose metabolism in the human rostral anterior cingulate cortex: An EEG/ PET study of normal and depressed subjects. *Psychophysiology*. 2003; **40**(6): 939–949.

129. Kwon JS, Youn T, Jung HY. Right hemisphere abnormalities in major depression: Quantitative electroencephalographic findings before and after treatment. *J Affect Disord*. 1996; **40**(3): 169–173.

130. Nystrom C, Matousek M, Hallstrom T. Relationships between EEG and clinical characteristics in major depressive disorder. *Acta Psychiatr Scand*. 1986; **73**(4): 390–394.

131. Lieber AL. Diagnosis and subtyping of depressive disorders by quantitative electroencephalography: II. Interhemispheric measures are abnormal in major depressives and frequency analysis may discriminate certain subtypes. *The Hillside Journal of Clinical Psychiatry*. 1988; **10**: 84–97.

132. Arns M, Etkin A, Hegerl U, et al. Frontal and rostral anterior cingulate (rACC) theta EEG in depression: Implications for treatment outcome? *Eur Neuropsychopharmacol* [Internet]. 2015; **25** (8): 1190–1200. Available from: http://dx.doi.org /10.1016/j.euroneuro.2015.03.007

133. Grin-Yatsenko VA, Baas I, Ponomarev VA, Kropotov JD. Independent component approach to the analysis of EEG recordings at early stages of depressive disorders. *Clin Neurophysiol* [Internet]. 2010; **121**(3): 281–289. Available from: http://dx.doi.org/10.1016/j .clinph.2009.11.015

134. Degabriele R, Lagopoulos J. A review of EEG and ERP studies in bipolar disorder. *Acta Neuropsychiatr* [Internet]. 2014/06/24. 2009; **21** (2): 58–66. Available from: www.cambridge.org/ core/article/review-of-eeg-and-erp-studies-in-bipolar-disorder /C7825AAA07D3119CF55C54A4563ABCA2

135. Mientus S, Gallinat J, Wuebben Y, et al. Cortical hypoactivation during resting EEG in schizophrenics but not in depressives and schizotypal subjects as revealed by low resolution electromagnetic tomography (LORETA). *Psychiatry Res – Neuroimaging*. 2002; **116**(1–2): 95–111.

136. Lubar JF, Congedo M, Askew JH. Low-resolution electromagnetic tomography (LORETA) of cerebral activity in chronic depressive disorder. *Int J Psychophysiol*. 2003 September; **49**(3): 175–185.

137. Heikman P, Salmelin R, Mäkelä JP, et al. Relation between frontal 3–7 Hz MEG activity and the efficacy of ECT in major depression. *J ECT*. 2001; **17**(2): 136–140.

138. Iosifescu D V., Greenwald S, Devlin P, et al. Frontal EEG predictors of treatment outcome in major depressive disorder. *Eur Neuropsychopharmacol* [Internet]. 2009; **19**(11): 772–777. Available from: http://dx.doi.org/10 .1016/j.euroneuro.2009.06.001

139. Pizzagalli DA. Frontocingulate dysfunction in depression: Toward biomarkers of treatment response. *Neuropsychopharmacology* [Internet]. 2011; **36**(1): 183–206. Available from: http://dx .doi.org/10.1038/npp.2010.166

140. Spronk D, Arns M, Barnett KJ, Cooper NJ, Gordon E. An investigation of EEG, genetic and cognitive markers of treatment response to antidepressant medication in patients with major depressive disorder: A pilot study. *J Affect Disord* [Internet]. 2011; **128**(1–2): 41–48. Available from: http://dx.doi.org/10.1016/j .jad.2010.06.021

141. Korb AS, Hunter AM, Cook IA, Leuchter AF. Rostral anterior cingulate cortex theta current density and response to antidepressants and placebo in major depression. *Clin Neurophysiol* [Internet]. 2009; **120**(7): 1313–1319. Available from: http://dx.doi.org/10.1016/j .clinph.2009.05.008

142. Mulert C, Juckel G, Brunnmeier M, et al. Prediction of treatment response in major depression: Integration of concepts. *J Affect Disord*. 2007; **98**(3): 215–225.

143. Pizzagalli DA, Pascual-Marqui RD, Nitschke JB, et al. Anterior cingulate activity as a predictor of degree of treatment response in major depression: Evidence from brain electrical tomography analysis. *Am J Psychiatry* [Internet]. 2001; **158**(3): 405–415. Available from: http://ajp .psychiatryonline.org.myaccess.library.utoronto .ca/doi/abs/10.1176/appi.ajp.158.3.405%5Cnfiles/ 523/Pizzagalli et al. – 2001 – Anterior Cingulate Activity as a Predictor of Degr.pdf

144. Watson BO, Ding M, Buzsáki G. Temporal coupling of field potentials and action potentials in the neocortex. *Eur J Neurosci* [Internet]. 2018 October 1; **48**(7): 2482–2497. Available from: ht tps://doi.org/10.1111/ejn.13807

145. Nir Y, Fisch L, Mukamel R, et al. Coupling between neuronal firing rate, gamma LFP, and BOLD fMRI is related to interneuronal correlations. *Curr Biol.* 2007; **17**(15): 1275–1285.

146. Fries P, Reynolds JH, Rorie AE, Desimone R. Modulation of oscillatory neuronal synchronization by selective visual attention. *Science.* 2001 February; **291**(5508): 1560–1563.

147. Kim H, Ährlund-Richter S, Wang X, Deisseroth K, Carlén M. Prefrontal parvalbumin neurons in control of attention. *Cell.* 2016; **164** (1–2): 208–218.

148. Fitzgerald PJ, Watson BO. Gamma oscillations as a biomarker for major depression: an emerging topic. *Transl Psychiatry* [Internet]. 2018; **8**(1): 177. Available from: https://doi.org/10.1038/s41 398-018-0239-y

149. Uhlhaas PJ, Haenschel C, Nikolić D, Singer W. The role of oscillations and synchrony in cortical networks and their putative relevance for the pathophysiology of schizophrenia. *Schizophr Bull* [Internet]. 2008 September [cited 2014 October 1]; **34**(5): 927–943. Available from: www .pubmedcentral.nih.gov/articlerender.fcgi?artid =2632472&tool=pmcentrez&rendertype= abstract

150. Colgin LL, Denninger T, Fyhn M, et al. Frequency of gamma oscillations routes flow of information in the hippocampus. *Nature* [Internet]. 2009 November 19; **462**: 353. Available from: https://doi.org/10.1038/nature08573

151. Fernández-Ruiz A, Oliva A, Nagy GA, et al. Entorhinal-CA3 dual-input control of spike timing in the hippocampus by theta-gamma coupling. *Neuron* [Internet]. 2017; **93**(5): 1213–1226.e5. Available from: www .sciencedirect.com/science/article/pii/ S0896627317301010

152. Spellman T, Rigotti M, Ahmari SE, et al. Hippocampal–prefrontal input supports spatial encoding in working memory. *Nature [Internet].* 2015 June 8; **522**: 309. Available from: https://doi .org/10.1038/nature14445

153. Strelets VB, Garakh Z V, Novototskiĭ-Vlasov VI. Comparative study of the gamma-rhythm in the norm, pre-examination stress and patients with the first depressive episode. *Zh Vyssh Nerv Deiat Im I P Pavlova [Internet].* 2006; **56**(2): 219–227. Available from: www.ncbi.nlm.nih.gov/pubmed/ 16756129

154. Lee PS, Chen YS, Hsieh JC, Su TP, Chen LF. Distinct neuronal oscillatory responses between patients with bipolar and unipolar disorders: A magnetoencephalographic study. *J Affect Disord [Internet].* 2010; **123**(1–3): 270–275. Available from: http://dx.doi.org/10.1016/j .jad.2009.08.020

155. Liu TY, Chen YS, Su TP, Hsieh JC, Chen LF. Abnormal early gamma responses to emotional faces differentiate unipolar from bipolar disorder patients. *Biomed Res Int.* 2014; **2014**.

156. Pizzagalli DA, Peccoralo LA, Davidson RJ, Cohen JD. Resting anterior cingulate activity and abnormal responses to errors in subjects with elevated depressive symptoms: A 128-channel EEG study. *Hum Brain Mapp [Internet].* 2006 March 1; **27**(3): 185–201. Available from: https:// doi.org/10.1002/hbm.20172

157. Isomura S, Onitsuka T, Tsuchimoto R, et al. Differentiation between major depressive disorder and bipolar disorder by auditory steady-state responses. *J Affect Disord.* 2016; **190**(2016): 800–806.

158. Oda Y, Onitsuka T, Tsuchimoto R, Hirano S, Oribe N, Ueno T, et al. Gamma band neural synchronization deficits for auditory steady state responses in bipolar disorder patients. *PLoS One [Internet].* 2012 July; **7**(7): e39955. Available from: http://dx.doi.org/10.1371/journal .pone.0039955

159. Liu T-Y, Hsieh J-C, Chen Y-S, et al. Different patterns of abnormal gamma oscillatory activity in unipolar and bipolar disorder patients during an implicit emotion task. *Neuropsychologia [Internet].* 2012 June [cited 2014 October 3]; **50**(7): 1514–1520. Available from: www .ncbi.nlm.nih.gov/pubmed/22406691

160. Berman RM, Cappiello A, Anand A, et al. Antidepressant effects of ketamine in depressed patients. *Biol Psychiatry.* 2000 February; **47**(4): 351–354.

161. Hong LE, Summerfelt A, Buchanan RW, et al. Gamma and delta neural oscillations and association with clinical symptoms under subanesthetic ketamine.

Neuropsychopharmacology [Internet]. 2009 November 4; **35**: 632. Available from: https://doi .org/10.1038/npp.2009.168

162. Muthukumaraswamy SD, Shaw AD, Jackson LE, et al. Evidence that subanesthetic doses of Ketamine cause sustained disruptions of NMDA and AMPA-mediated frontoparietal connectivity in humans. *J Neurosci [Internet].* 2015 August 19; **35**(33): 11694LP–11706. Available from: www .jneurosci.org/content/35/33/11694.abstract

163. Shaw AD, Saxena N, Jackson LE, et al. Ketamine amplifies induced gamma frequency oscillations in the human cerebral cortex. *Eur Neuropsychopharmacol [Internet].* 2015; **25**(8): 1136–1146. Available from: http://dx.doi.org/10 .1016/j.euroneuro.2015.04.012

164. Nugent AC, Ballard ED, Gould TD, et al. Ketamine has distinct electrophysiological and behavioral effects in depressed and healthy subjects. *Mol Psychiatry [Internet].* 2018; Available from: https:// doi.org/10.1038/s41380-018-0028-2

165. Noda Y, Zomorrodi R, Saeki T, et al. Resting-state EEG gamma power and theta–gamma coupling enhancement following high-frequency left dorsolateral prefrontal rTMS in patients with depression. *Clin Neurophysiol [Internet].* 2017; **128**(3): 424–432. Available from: http://dx .doi.org/10.1016/j.clinph.2016.12.023

166. Bailey NW, Hoy KE, Rogasch NC, et al. Responders to rTMS for depression show increased fronto-midline theta and theta connectivity compared to non-responders. *Brain Stimul [Internet].* 2018; **11**(1): 190–203. Available from: https://doi.org/10.1016/j .brs.2017.10.015

167. Pathak Y, Salami O, Baillet S, Li Z, Butson CR. *Longitudinal Changes in Depressive Circuitry in Response to Neuromodulation Therapy [Internet].* Vol. **10**, Frontiers in Neural Circuits; 2016. p. 50. Available from: www.frontiersin.org/article/10 .3389/fncir.2016.00050

168. Belmaker RH, Agam G. Major depressive disorder. *N Engl J Med [Internet].* 2008 January 3; **358**(1): 55–68. Available from: https://doi.org/10 .1056/NEJMra073096

169. Gandal MJ, Haney JR, Parikshak NN, et al. Shared molecular neuropathology across major psychiatric disorders parallels polygenic overlap. *Science (80-) [Internet].* 2018 February 9; **359**(6376): 693LP–697. Available from: http://science.sciencemag.org/content/359/ 6376/693.abstract

170. Drysdale AT, Grosenick L, Downar J, et al. *HHS Public Access.* 2017; **23**(1): 28–38.

Chapter 15

Magnetoencephalography Studies in Mood Disorders

Allison C. Nugent

15.1 Introduction to Magnetoencephalography

Magnetoencephalography (MEG) has emerged as an important tool in the study of mood disorders. Although electroencephalography (EEG) is much more widely utilized, largely due to its low cost and ease of use, MEG has the distinct advantage of enabling accurate localization of brain structures. Although a full discussion of the methodology of MEG is beyond the scope of this brief chapter, we will present a brief overview of the technique and refer the reader to several excellent volumes (1–3) for more information.

While EEG measures the electric potentials on the surface of the scalp, MEG measures the magnetic fields produced by brain activity. Electric potentials are conducted by the scalp, smearing the signals, while magnetic fields are not attenuated in this way. It is believed that the fields measured by both EEG and MEG reflect the summed local field potentials of large populations of parallel pyramidal cells in the cortex. It is often repeated that MEG is not sensitive to sources oriented radially to the surface of the skull (i.e., on gyri) and can only detect fields from sources parallel to the surface (i.e., sulci). This would only be true were the head a perfect sphere, and for sources that are perfectly radial.

The magnetic fields produced by the human brain are extraordinarily small, on the order of femtotesla. To detect fields of this magnitude, extremely sensitive detectors must be used. Commercial MEG devices make use of superconducting quantum interference devices, or SQUIDs. Briefly, each SQUID is a superconducting loop broken by two insulators, known as Josephson junctions. Small magnetic fields can be detected by SQUIDs because the current flowing in a SQUID will reverse each

time a half quantum of magnetic flux passes through the loop. In order to measure the fields, the SQUIDs must be coupled to a flux transformer or a coil sensitive to magnetic fields. There are multiple potential orientations of flux transformers, including magnetometers, and axial and planar gradiometers, each with a different sensitivity pattern. It is a common misconception that MEG systems are insensitive to deep sources. Axial gradiometers have greater sensitivity to deep sources than do planar gradiometers. Numerous studies of axial gradiometer MEG systems have demonstrated the ability to localize activity to subcortical regions, given sufficient signal to noise.

A consequence of the superconducting nature of SQUIDs is that they must be immersed in liquid helium, at 4 kelvin. This makes MEG systems large, cumbersome, and expensive to operate. MEG systems also must be housed in a magnetically shielded room (MSR), made of multiple layers of mu-metal designed to eliminate ambient fields as much as possible. An alternative to SQUIDs are optically pumped magnetometers (OPMs). These devices excite rubidium atoms in a vapor, then measure the opacity of that vapor, which is affected by local magnetic fields. While OPM-based systems have been prominently featured in scientific publications (4), a commercially viable system requires solving issues with sensitivity, the breadth of frequencies that can be measured, and interference of neighboring channels.

Modern MEG platforms utilize hundreds of channels, arrayed more or less evenly around the head. Sophisticated electronics systems are required to translate the reversing currents of the SQUIDs into magnetic field values. Changes in the field are captured by the system at a high frequency in order to obtain measures of brain activity into the gamma range (30 Hz and above). MEG recordings can be captured at rest, or during performance of tasks similar to those administered during functional magnetic resonance imaging (fMRI) exams. Some tasks will evoke responses that are time-locked to the delivery of the stimulus. These evoked response fields (ERFs, in contrast to evoked response potentials, or ERPs, measured by EEG) can be compared between diagnostic groups or task condition in terms of their amplitude or latency to peak. Other tasks may induce changes in oscillatory power, which can be compared between groups or task conditions. These induced power changes may occur in the canonical frequency bands, including delta, theta, alpha, beta, and gamma. Different frequencies of oscillation have different mechanisms and functional significance, and some are better understood than others; an in-depth treatment on this subject can be found in Buzsaki's *Rhythms of the Brain* (5).

While MEG signals can be analyzed without source localization (referred to as "sensor space"), the power of MEG comes from transforming the signals to the space of the subject's brain, usually with the addition of a high-resolution MRI. There are multiple ways to project MEG data into source space, and all are approximations. Some methods localize a small number of sources with high accuracy, which may work well when dealing with simple sensory inputs (i.e. localizing the response to an auditory stimulus to auditory cortex). Other methods will produce maps of the fields measured at all points on the surface of the cortex or within the full brain volume. Broadly speaking, these algorithms generally require minimization of a measure of overall power. An excellent discussion of methods for projection into source space can be found in *MEG: An Introduction to the Methods* (1).

15.2 MEG in Mood Disorders

Although the application of MEG to the study of mood disorders has been steadily increasing, there are still less than 100 peer-reviewed studies. Unfortunately, most of these studies have small sample sizes, and the majority utilizes medicated patients, complicating generalization and interpretation. We will review most published works here, in order to inform the reader of the full extent of the literature. Most studies involve patients with major depressive disorder (MDD), although there is a growing literature on bipolar disorder (BD). We will cover the studies by topic, beginning with studies involving sensory evoked fields. We'll move on to more complex task-based studies, including those investigating emotional processing, as well as resting-state studies. Finally, we will cover the field of neuromodulation treatments and MEG.

15.3 Sensory Evoked Fields

Synchronized, time-locked responses are evoked in primary sensory cortices in response to a multitude of stimuli – robust visual, auditory, motor, and somatosensory fields can be measured and localized with MEG. These fields are of particular interest in mood disorders because they are measures of neuronal excitability, and thus may reflect synaptic plasticity. As mood disorders are increasingly characterized as disorders of homeostatic plasticity, interest is growing in interventions which result in synaptic potentiation, which can be measured by pre- versus posttreatment measures of sensory evoked responses. Furthermore, underlying abnormalities in basic cortical sensory responses may reflect global alterations in brain function, rather than system/circuit level dysfunction.

15.3.1 Motor and Somatosensory Evoked Fields

Somatosensory evoked fields (SEFs) are generated in somatosensory cortex in response to median nerve stimulation at 20 and 30 ms poststimulation. Although one study found reduced M20 amplitudes in MDD compared to healthy controls (6), another small study in a partially euthymic group reported no differences (7). The idea that neuronal excitability may be attenuated in MDD is consistent with a series of studies examining the SEFs to tactile stimulation and treatment with ketamine. First, Cornwell et al. (8) found that patients with MDD who responded to ketamine showed an increase in the evoked gamma band response to a somatosensory stimulus; nonresponders to ketamine showed no increases. A follow-up study in both MDD and healthy subjects using a placebo control found no differences in groups at baseline, but an increase in the evoked gamma response in responders, and a linear relationship between response and the difference in evoked gamma power between ketamine and placebo conditions

(Figure 15.1a and b)(9). Basic sensory tasks are also ideal for analysis using dynamic causal modeling (DCM). DCM uses Bayesian priors to estimate structural models given endogenous interregional connections, modulatory connections influenced by task state, and a driving stimulus. Indeed, a DCM analysis of these data revealed that post-ketamine, NMDA-mediated backward connections were elevated in MDD compared to healthy subjects (Figure 15.1 c–e)(10). The enhancement of

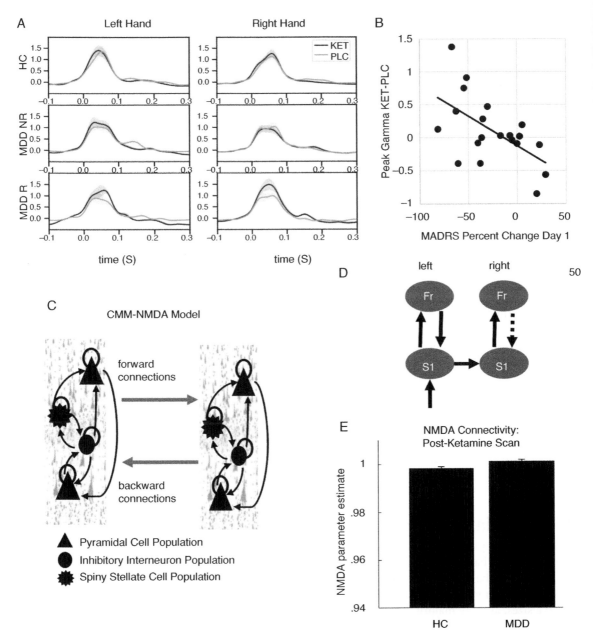

Figure 15.1 Panel (a) shows averaged evoked response fields from contralateral somatosensory cortex for left- and right-handed stimulation. The increase-evoked response post-ketamine is evident in patients who respond to ketamine (MDD-R) but not nonresponders (MDD-NR) or healthy subjects (HC). Panel (b) illustrates that a large increase in peak gamma power between ketamine and placebo sessions is associated with a favorable antidepressant response to ketamine. Panel (c) illustrates the DCM model including multiple cell layers, and (d) illustrates the specific model used incorporating bilateral prefrontal cortex (Fr) and primary somatosensory cortex (S1), along with a driving input. Panel (e) shows the between-subjects difference in NMDA-mediated connectivity post-ketamine infusion in the backward connection from right Fr to S1 (dashed line in panel d). Figure modified from previously published work (10)

backward connections post-ketamine in MDD is consistent with the idea that successful antidepressant treatment enhances prefrontal modulation of basic sensory and limbic processes. In total, these studies not only provide more evidence for reduced neuronal excitability in MDD, but also demonstrate that synaptic plasticity may be a crucial mechanism of action of ketamine, and possibly other antidepressants.

15.3.2 Auditory Evoked Fields

Auditory stimuli evoke a field at approximately 100 ms poststimulus (M100), generated in Heschl's gyrus. Smaller auditory evoked fields (AEFs) are also generated at approximately 50 ms (M50) and 200 ms (M200) poststimulus (11); other fields may be generated by more complex task designs. While many studies have found alterations in early auditory processing in mood disorders, the available results do not converge on a single, reliable marker for MDD or BD. In MDD, decreased latency (12) or no differences (13) in M100 have been reported; in BD, one study found reduced M100 and M200 fields bilaterally compared to healthy subjects (11), although another study found no differences in the M100 (14, 15). Notably, it has been hypothesized that the sensitivity of the M100 and M200 to stimulus intensity may be related to serotonergic function (16), making studies in medicated patients particularly problematic.

One widely used class of auditory paradigms are "oddball" tasks. Classically, these tasks present a series of tones, most of a single frequency, with intermittent tones presented at a different frequency. The mismatch negativity (MMN) is derived by subtracting the evoked field of the frequent event from that of the rare event, typically producing a negative deflection. MMN is thought to represent processing that occurs before conscious attention to the stimulus (14). Lower MMN amplitudes have been reported in MDD (13, 17) and BD, with amplitudes of MMN in BD correlated with a measure of mania (18). Shorter latencies to MMN have also been reported in MDD (17), with longer latencies observed in BD (14), potentially indicating a possible diagnostic marker. At least one study found no changes in MMN in MDD (12).

Periodic stimuli, either oscillating tones or click-trains, elicit an auditory steady-state response (ASSR) synchronized to the stimulus in phase and frequency. Patients with BD have demonstrated significantly reduced ASSR amplitudes and phase locking values to gamma frequency stimuli (19, 20). Interestingly, MDD patients demonstrated significantly greater ASSR amplitudes than BD patients, with controls falling between MDD and BD patients (although MDD patients did not significantly differ from healthy volunteers). It is thought that ASSR reflects the efficiency of GABAergic interneuron activity in response to rhythmic stimuli (20). Previous reports have related decreased ASSR to increased spontaneous gamma power (21), although none of the studies reviewed here examined spontaneous gamma power in auditory cortex. Nevertheless, if the greater ASSR amplitudes in MDD are reflective of lower basal gamma power, this would be consistent with findings from MEG and EEG that increasing gamma power in patients with MDD using either ketamine (22) or TMS (23) will relieve symptoms of depression. Likewise, there is some evidence from EEG that gamma power is elevated in BD (24).

Although other auditory paradigms have been employed, the evidence is insufficient to support firm conclusions. Studies investigating the typical left-right asymmetry in the location of either M100 evoked responses (15) or ASSR (25) find evidence for reduced asymmetry in BD subjects, potentially indicating alterations in brain development. Paired stimulus paradigms where two stimuli (S1 and S2) are presented can be used to study inhibitory gating mechanisms, whereby an initial stimulus invokes inhibitory mechanisms, attenuating the response evoked by the second stimulus. Increased M50 responses to S2 in BD compared to controls been found, along with greater S2/S1 ratios for both the M50 and M100(26). This may indicate a failure in sensory gating by inhibitory neuronal pathways, potentially resulting from neuronal hyperexcitability (26). Auditory stimuli can also induce coherent oscillations, and there is evidence that patients with BD demonstrate increased evoked power in the beta and gamma ranges, at least in response to speech sounds (27).

Taken together, the literature examining basic sensory processing in mood disorders points toward systemic dysfunction. There is evidence from auditory, motor, and somatosensory studies supporting the notion that neuronal excitability is attenuated in MDD as compared to healthy subjects. In contrast, multiple studies in BD suggest an increase in neuronal excitability, although results are inconsistent, potentially due to medication effects or effects of current mood state (i.e., manic vs. depressed). These abnormalities in basic sensory processing are significant, because they implicate fundamental neurophysiological processes, rather than deficits in specific monoaminergic neurotransmitter systems or isolated functional networks and/or brain regions.

15.4 Emotional Paradigms

Given that mood disorders are clinically disorders of emotion regulation, numerous studies have compared patient groups in both behavioral and neurophysiological responses to emotional tasks. As in fMRI, many paradigms have been used, and responses to similar paradigms may be quite different. Evoked response paradigms typically measure modulation of either visual evoked fields (VEFs) or evoked response fields to faces (M170) by the affective valance of the stimulus. Induced oscillations in response to more complex emotional tasks can also be examined. The primary limitations of these studies are the lack of replication, especially given that studies with slightly different paradigms may produce discrepant results.

15.4.1 Evoked Responses to Affective Stimuli

Several studies have utilized the VEF to emotionally arousing visual stimuli to examine a potential bias toward negative stimuli and modulation of affective arousal systems. In a study of twenty-five healthy volunteers and twenty-five unmedicated patients with MDD, subjects showed significantly attenuated VEFs in response to emotional stimuli across the parietal cortex, and stronger VEFs to negative rather than positively valanced images (healthy subjects showed a trend toward greater response to positive stimuli). Both the VEF amplitude in the right temporoparietal junction and the difference in VEF amplitude to negative vs. positive stimuli in the dorsolateral prefrontal cortex (DLPFC) were correlated with depression severity. A subset of fifteen patients underwent repeat scanning after treatment with mirtazapine and showed partial normalization of the parietal VEF, although the neural bias toward aversive

stimuli was unchanged (28). A similar negative bias was observed in the occipital M300 response to faces in an affective oddball-type paradigm in dysphoric patients, some with a diagnosis of MDD (29). Affective stimuli can also be subjected to intensity modulation to evoke rhythmic steady-state visual evoked fields (ssVEFs). Similar to prior findings (28), MDD patients exhibited attenuated ssVEF amplitudes compared to healthy subjects in right temporoparietal cortex, although with reduced modulation by valance rather than a negative bias (30). A replication study demonstrated that this effect may have been driven by patients who had a family history of mood disorders (31). These results are consistent with the findings of reductions in evoked fields in other sensory modalities, as well as substantial behavioral and fMRI evidence supporting a bias toward negative stimuli in MDD (32).

Another type of task utilized in fMRI involves repeated presentation of emotional stimuli to examine habituation, the normal decrease of neuronal activity in response to a repeated stimulus. Unmedicated MDD patients demonstrated increasing amplitudes of the evoked responses to repeated negative faces in the pregenual area of ACC (pgACC), while healthy subjects showed decreasing amplitudes; this was true only for the first of two face sets presented. The change in both pgACC and amygdala activity correlated with subsequent antidepressant response to ketamine (33).

Several studies carried out by the same research group examined a task utilizing short videos of emotional facial expressions, where subjects were asked to respond if the expression shown was sad. Data were analyzed using several different methods for connectivity, including DCM (discussed earlier), Granger causality, and coherence. Granger causality calculates directed connectivity by modeling the signal in a given region as predicted by the signal in other regions at earlier time points. Coherence can intuitively be interpreted as a version of correlation including the dimension of frequency. Overall, these studies pointed to the importance of the amygdala in network models, and generally found enhanced connectivity from amygdala to prefrontal cortical areas, and decreased connectivity from prefrontal cortex to amygdala in MDD patients compared to controls (34–36). One additional study using the same paradigm and both MEG and DTI found that coupling between the salience network and ventral attention network was elevated in depressed patients compared to controls (37). In total, these results echo the simpler affective VEF results, suggesting a bias toward negative stimuli, as well as the importance of the ACC and amygdala in emotional face processing. These results also support the notion that depression involves impaired top-down control of the limbic system by prefrontal areas.

15.4.2 Induced Oscillatory Responses to Affective Stimuli

Few studies have been performed examining induced changes in power in response to emotional paradigms in MEG, despite the obvious parallels to fMRI paradigms. One study used the above-described emotional identification task (34–36), and applied a multichannel matching pursuit (MMP) algorithm to extract the principle signal elements, from which oscillatory power amplitudes were calculated. These values were used to determine if a support vector machine could discriminate MDD patients from healthy subjects. Elevated alpha and beta power, primarily in frontal and central sensors, was found to provide the greatest discriminatory power, though reduced theta power was also noted (38). An implicit version of this task has also been employed, where subjects respond with the gender of the face rather than the valence. While both MDD and BD patients exhibited focal areas of increased alpha power in response to angry faces, with some regions discriminating between groups, these regions did not map onto specific known functional networks (39). A study using the same paradigm, but collapsing over all stimulus emotions, found reduced gamma power in both MDD and BD compared to controls in widespread brain areas, with activity in parieto-occipital sensors differentiating MDD from BD subjects (40). Unfortunately, the lack of convergent evidence from these studies limits their broader interpretation.

15.4.3 Other Cognitive Tasks

Numerous cognitive domains are impaired in mood disorders, and several studies have used cognitive tasks and MEG to elucidate the neural mechanisms behind these deficits.

Reduced hippocampal volume is one of the most robust structural findings in MDD (41), motivating studies of spatial navigation, a domain in which the hippocampus plays a vital role. A virtual Morris water maze navigation task was administered to nineteen unmedicated patients with MDD. Behaviorally, the MDD patients showed longer latencies to find a hidden platform than healthy subjects. Hippocampal theta activity during hidden platform searching was significantly lower in the depressed subjects, and parahippocampal cortex theta power was correlated with longer latency to navigate to the platform (42).

Working memory processes are also disrupted in mood disorders, and a study of patients with MDD found that beta desynchronization in response to increasing task load in the sgACC and pgACC was associated with subsequent antidepressant response to ketamine. Patients who showed the greatest desynchronization, which may be associated with greater neuronal engagement, were most likely to respond to ketamine (43). Notably, the region identified overlapped with previous findings using an emotional processing task (33, 43). Furthermore, connectivity between the pgACC and the amygdala was negatively correlated with antidepressant response (43). A follow-up study showed that differences in beta power between healthy and MDDs were driven by the subset of patients who had significant anxiety. These anxious depressed patients showed greater beta power in the cuneus/precuneus, insula, and inferior and middle frontal cortex during the highest cognitive load condition (2-back) compared to the easier condition (1-back)(44).

As with the emotional processing results, MEG results from cognitive processing studies are difficult to interpret due to the relative lack of replication data. However, the MEG findings are consistent with the well documented behavioral effects, and these preliminary data suggest that MEG may provide information beyond that offered by fMRI, in that the added dimension of frequency may better pinpoint what neuronal processes are responsible for behavioral dysfunction.

15.5 Resting-State MEG

Due to the inherent richness in electrophysiological signals, a broad array of metrics can be used to describe the resting state in MEG. In addition to measures of spectral power, there are a variety of linear and nonlinear metrics, as well as connectivity metrics. While some measures have been used to derive resting-state networks similar to those seen in fMRI, other measures derive features unique to electrophysiological networks. While the demonstration that the canonical fMRI resting-state networks can be observed in MEG data has elevated the profile of MEG in the greater neuroimaging community, it is our contention that MEG data provide crucial validation for the fMRI findings, rather than the other way around. While the fMRI signal represents a neuronal signal convolved with a hemodynamic response function, MEG data are a direct measure of neuronal function. Thus, MEG may be interpreted as closer to the ground truth than other methods, despite the relatively lower spatial resolution.

15.5.1 Spectral Power

Although few studies exist that examine only spectral density, many resting-state studies include an examination of power in the canonical bands, most frequently in sensor space. The reader may know that alpha asymmetry is one of the most widely reported EEG findings in MDD; this value is unreliable in MEG, since apparent asymmetry may result if the cortex is not perfectly centered in the imaging device. We will discuss each canonical frequency band later, though the frequency ranges for each band are not standardized and differ slightly across studies.

Although studies of infra-slow wavelengths exist, most studies consider delta (2–4 Hz) to be the lower end of physiological oscillatory processes. Delta waves dominate during deep sleep; prominent delta waves during waking generally indicate serious neurological dysfunction. Frontal delta may be corrupted by artifacts from eye blinks or movements, which is particularly problematic when studying connectivity. Although source reconstruction methods should localize the artifact to the eyes, there is inevitably some signal leakage and results in orbital cortex should be interpreted with caution. Elevated delta activity, correlated with severity, has been reported in MDD as compared to healthy subjects over the right occipital cortex (45), while another study showed elevated 2–6 Hz activity over the left hemisphere (46). Elevated delta power has also been observed in BD posteriorly (47). Theta oscillations

(4–8 Hz) are also considered slow waves and their measurement can also be corrupted by eye blinks or movements. Reductions in theta power in MDD compared to controls has been noted in frontal areas (48) as well as in occipital parietal and right temporo-central regions (49); elevated theta has been noted in posterior sensors in BD compared to healthy subjects (47).

Alpha oscillations (8–12 Hz) are the most prominent in the human brain, particularly when the eyes are closed, and are hypothesized to be related to the default mode network. Reduced parietal alpha has been noted in MDD as compared to healthy subjects, with decreased alpha associated with greater depressive symptoms (48). Desynchronization of beta frequency oscillations (12–30 Hz), resulting in reduced beta power, has been associated with attention and cognitive demands. At rest, stronger frontal and parietal beta power has been observed in MDD compared to healthy subjects (48).

Gamma oscillations, at frequencies above 30 Hz, are generated through recurrent inhibition in networks of GABAergic interneurons, or through feedback networks of GABAergic interneurons and parvalbumin-expressing glutamatergic pyramidal cells (50). Gamma oscillations are reflective of inhibition/excitation balance and may be a proxy measure for synaptic homeostasis (51). Despite the importance of these oscillations, few studies have directly measured basal gamma power in patients with mood disorders, surprising given the mounting evidence that alterations in homeostasis underlie depression (52). Several EEG studies have reported increased gamma power in MDD (53, 54) and BD (24), although MEG studies in both BD (47) and MDD patients (22, 48) have failed to find significant differences relative to controls. Gamma power oscillations are readily contaminated by muscular artifacts, which may be particularly problematic in EEG recordings where spatial localization is usually not performed. Once MEG data have been projected into source space, artifactual increases in gamma power due to muscular activity will be readily apparent along the edges of temporal cortex (due to muscular activity in the jaw) and cerebellum (due to muscular activity in the neck).

The rapid acting antidepressant ketamine has been shown to produce robust increases in gamma power in both animal models and in MEG studies in healthy subjects (55, 56). A study in both patients with MDD and healthy controls showed that gamma power is increased in widespread areas across the cortex up to 6–9 hours post ketamine infusion (Figure 15.2a–c)(22). Elevated gamma power hours after the acute infusion may reflect glutamatergic modulatory activity of an active metabolite of ketamine (2 R,6 R; 2S,6S Hydroxynorketamine, or HNK). The relationship of the increase in gamma power to the antidepressant response is not linear, however, and there is evidence that basal inhibition/excitation balance is a key factor. Indeed, post-ketamine infusion gamma power demonstrated a significant interaction of baseline gamma and the antidepressant response to ketamine. Patients with low baseline gamma power demonstrating large increases in gamma power post-ketamine tended to show favorable antidepressant responses; patients with high baseline gamma power demonstrating large increases in gamma power post-ketamine tended

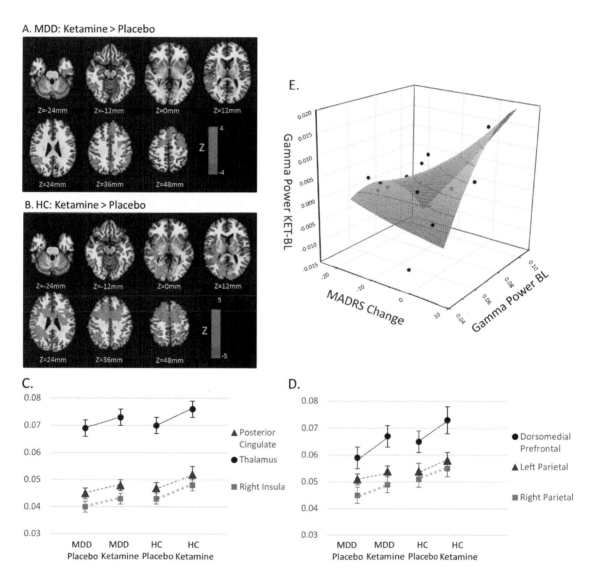

Figure 15.2 Panels a and b illustrate increases in gamma power observed in the ketamine session relative to the placebo session, in patients with MDD and healthy controls, respectively. Panels c and d show data from cluster peaks, in order to qualitatively illustrate the relative magnitude of increases in patients and controls in regions known to be implicated in the pathophysiology of MDD. Panel e shows a three-dimensional surface fitted to data from a mixed model examining how baseline gamma power mediates the relationship between the increase in gamma power post-ketamine and the antidepressant response. Patients with low baseline gamma who show large increases in gamma power tend to respond favorably to ketamine. Patients with high baseline gamma who show large increases in gamma power tend to respond poorly to ketamine. Figure modified from previously published work (22)

to show poor responses (Figure 15.2e)(22). These results provide further support for alterations in homeostatic regulation in MDD, and potentially point to gamma oscillations as a fundamental metric of homeostasis.

15.5.2 Nonlinear Measures

Numerous nonlinear measures exist to quantify features such as information carriage (entropy and mutual information), long-range temporal autocorrelations (detrended fluctuation analysis, or DFA), and signal complexity (Lempel-Ziv complexity, or LZC). While the brain is undoubtedly a nonlinear system (57), interpretation of nonlinear metrics is not straightforward. Additionally, although we have some understanding of how cortical oscillations or local field potentials are generated mechanistically, we have only rudimentary understanding of how nonlinear properties are generated. Thus, even though abnormalities in nonlinear metrics may be identified, it is doubtful given our current knowledge that these findings could be translated into targets for intervention.

DFA involves calculating exponents that reflect the "memory" of the system, determining the temporal range of past events to influence future events. Reduced DFA exponents, correlated with depressive symptoms, have been observed in MDD subjects in theta oscillations, indicating a lack of long-range temporal autocorrelations as compared to healthy subjects. The authors suggest these findings are consistent with other findings of altered hippocampal structure and function in MDD, as the hippocampus is a known generator of theta oscillations (49). Another metric, LZC, is essentially a measure of the repetitiveness of a signal. A study of twenty unmedicated patients with MDD showed elevated LZC compared to controls across all MEG sensors, which was reduced after six months of antidepressant treatment to an extent concomitant with the antidepressant effect (58), although another study found no significant differences (although values in MDD subjects were nominally larger compared to healthy controls). LZC increases with age in healthy subjects, but not in MDD subjects (58, 59), and may decrease with age in BD patients (59).

15.5.3 Connectivity

Resting-state connectivity is a growing field in MEG. A fundamental problem is signal leakage,

the phenomenon by which spurious connectivity can be observed due to "leakage" of the signal into neighboring areas (60). Numerous methods have been derived to deal with the problem of signal leakage, but most work by removing zero phase-lag correlations. Some connectivity metrics, such as phase locking value (PLV) are naturally insensitive to zero-lag connectivity. A particularly common method to investigate connectivity in MEG is amplitude envelope connectivity. First, the time series is filtered for a specific band, and then the Hilbert envelope is calculated to obtain a measure of the fluctuations in band limited power. The resultant time series is typically downsampled to 0.5–1 Hz and has spectral properties similar to the BOLD time series. In order to remove zero-lag correlation when building connectivity matrices for amplitude envelope time series, a simple regression-based orthogonalization can be performed between regions in a pair-wise fashion before the Hilbert envelope is calculated (61). Alternatively, all the time series data can be orthogonalized simultaneously (62); other methods of leakage reduction also exist.

We know of only one study investigating resting-state connectivity in BD subjects using MEG. In this study, a quantity related to nonlinear synchronization or similarity was calculated between pairs of frontal sensors. Delta band similarity was elevated in patients with BD compared to healthy controls, but reduced in alpha and beta bands (63). The functional significance of a shift in connectivity to lower frequency bands is unknown.

As noted before, the Hilbert envelope time series has similar properties to the resting-state fMRI time series. Indeed, Brookes and colleagues in 2009 found that a temporal independent components analysis (ICA) on beta-band data could be used to extract resting-state networks remarkably similar to those seen in spatial ICA analyses of fMRI data. Building upon this result, a study with similar methods found significantly reduced connectivity in MDD patients compared to controls between a bilateral precentral network and both the sgACC and hippocampus/parahippocampal gyrus. In addition, increased connectivity in MDD between left and right insula/temporal cortex and the ipsilateral amygdala was found. Notably, these findings were replicated in independent data collected in the same session from a subset of patients and controls (64). A subset of these patients went on to receive ketamine infusions; the abnormally increased connectivity between insular-temporal cortex and amygdala observed at baseline was reduced following ketamine. In addition, the reduced connectivity noted between bilateral precentral cortices and sgACC observed at baseline was further reduced following ketamine; notably, the decrease correlated with the change in the metabolic rate of glucose consumption as measured by positron emission tomography (PET). These results may suggest that ketamine reduces connectivity globally, which is consistent with widespread alterations in spectral power (22, 65).

One more recent study looked only at connectivity within nodes of the default mode network (DMN) using alpha-band Hilbert envelope data. The study found overall reduced connectivity within the DMN in MDD compared to healthy subjects, as well as changes in dynamical microstates, such that MDD patients spent less time in the dominant connected microstate and more time in the supplemental disconnected state (66). Given that MDD patients spent closer to equal amounts of time in the two states while healthy subjects spent a greater proportion of time in the dominant state, this may be consistent with findings from fMRI that DMN connectivity is more variable in MDD patients compared to controls (67), but it is difficult to compare studies with such disparate methods.

Given that symptoms of mood disorders are present regardless of task performance, the resting state may be the ideal condition to study. Indeed, it has been suggested that aberrant connectivity in the DMN may underlie symptoms such as ruminations and maladaptive interoceptive processes (68, 69). Alterations in the neurophysiology of network nodes may provide potential targets for neuromodulatory therapies, as reviewed in the next section.

15.6 MEG and Neuromodulation

Electroconvulsive therapy (ECT) is one of the most highly effective treatments for depression. Unfortunately, this frequently comes at the price of adverse effects on memory and cognition. Modern stimulation methods have reduced these adverse effects, but the development of more targeted treatments will require additional knowledge into the mechanism by which ECT relieves the symptoms of depression. Repetitive transcranial magnetic stimulation (rTMS) has been proven to be a safe and effective treatment for MDD (70), although likely not as broadly effective as ECT. The choice of stimulation location, as well as the amplitude, frequency, and duration of the applied pulses is largely empiric, and there remains a vast parameter space to be explored. The electrophysiological imaging techniques are uniquely suited to determine the optimal parameters for neuromodulation.

There is a growing body of literature seeking to use MEG to understand the neurobiological correlates of rTMS, as well as markers that may predict response. In the most commonly used protocol, twenty trains of 5 s duration, 10 Hz pulses are delivered to the left DLPFC. Two studies have investigated changes in spectral power pre- and post-TMS. One study showing increased 2–6 Hz activity in the left frontal cortex in MDD compared to healthy subjects at baseline demonstrated normalization after ten TMS sessions (46). Another study administering five sessions over four weeks found that beta and gamma power increased in the left DLPFC following treatment, with power correlating with MADRS scores over the course of the trial (71). The same study also investigated connectivity as a mechanism of action of TMS, and showed that delta band coherence between DLPFC and amygdala increased posttreatment, while gamma band coherence between DLPFC and sgACC decreased (71). These results may suggest enhanced prefrontal control of limbic areas following treatment, although coherence does not provide information regarding the directionality of connections.

Another study administering ten TMS sessions over two weeks collected both MEG and FDG-PET, to measure glucose metabolism. At baseline, healthy subjects showed strong correlations between frontal alpha power and glucose metabolism in the thalamus, precuneus, and middle cingulate. Prior to TMS, patients showed correlations between frontal alpha power and both medial prefrontal and dorsal cingulate cortex; after successful TMS treatment patients showed a similar pattern to controls, with correlations between frontal alpha and glucose metabolism in the thalamus, precuneus, and middle cingulate (72). Unfortunately, this study did not utilize source localization of the MEG signals, making the results more difficult to interpret.

We know of only one study to investigate the effects of ECT using MEG. Twenty healthy subjects and twenty patients with MDD underwent baseline MEG recording. Following four weeks of three-times-weekly ECT treatment, patients underwent repeat MEG recordings. During each MEG session, participants passively viewed affective pictures from the IAPS picture set. Before treatment, patients showed significantly decreased amplitude of evoked activity to the affective images compared to controls, to an extent that correlated with depression severity. These pretreatment findings are consistent with above-reviewed work, showing reduced visual evoked fields to similar emotional tasks (28, 30). Post treatment, patients exhibited increased evoked responses to the emotional images, suggestive of normalization.

As noted earlier, the use of MEG to both predict response to and evaluate the mechanism of action of neuromodulation would seem to be a natural fit. Additionally, MEG could potentially hold the key to optimizing treatment. Theoretically, MEG could be used to identify aberrant brain rhythms, and then neuromodulation methods such as TMS could be used to target those rhythms directly and potentially provide personalized treatment.

15.7 Conclusions

In this chapter, we have attempted to summarize the use of MEG in mood disorders. MEG is still a developing technology, but holds significant advantages over EEG for mechanistic studies, given that activity can be localized to brain regions. Further developments in OPM technology may one day make MEG deployable in the clinic, although such developments are many years away.

There is a small but growing body of work exploring the electrophysiological abnormalities in mood disorders. Studies of evoked fields in primary sensory cortices have generally shown reductions in neuronal excitability in MDD, indicating that synaptic plasticity is a potential target for treatment. Studies of patients with BD have been less consistent, and controlling for both mood state and medication is challenging. There is some evidence that alterations in amplitudes or

latencies of evoked fields may serve as markers to distinguish between MDD and BD patients.

A large body of work has used MEG to investigate both evoked responses and induced oscillatory activity during the performance of affective and other cognitive tasks. In general, these studies have added additional evidence of an increased bias toward negative stimuli in mood disorders, as well as the idea that patients with mood disorders exhibit inadequate prefrontal cortical control over limbic processes. MEG adds to these studies by providing information about the basic neuronal processes that underlie these abnormalities. Resting-state studies have also provided vital information to understanding mood disorders, by demonstrating alterations in power or connectivity in specific frequency bands. Treatment with the antidepressant ketamine is known to produce robust increases in gamma power, and other pharmacologic or neuromodulatory treatments could potentially be designed to address abnormalities in other frequency bands.

Overall, MEG has made a significant contribution to our understanding of mood disorders and their treatment and will likely continue to make such contributions in the future. As new hardware and analysis methods are developed, MEG will be able to map the brain with greater accuracy and reliability. MEG is uniquely suited to evaluating therapies that produce alterations in neuronal processes, and its use may someday enable more personalized psychiatric treatments.

Acknowledgments

Thanks to Dr. Carlos Zarate for leading the team that carried out the research performed at the NIMH, and Dr. Jessica Gilbert for her crucial role in MEG studies and her editorial assistance. I am also grateful for the patients who participated in the described research and their families.

References

1. Hansen PC, Kringelbach ML, Salmelin R, editors. *MEG: An Introduction to Methods*. Oxford: Oxford University Press; 2010.

2. Hari R, Puce A, editors. *MEG-EEG Primer*. Oxford: Oxford University Press; 2017.

3. Supek S, Aine CJ, editors. *Magnetoencephalography: From Signals to Dynamic Cortical Networks*. Berlin: Springer-Verlag; 2014.

4. Boto E, Holmes N, Leggett J, et al. Moving magnetoencephalography towards real-world applications with a wearable system. *Nature*. 2018; **555**(7698): 657–661.

5. Buzsáki G. *Rhythms of the Brain*. Oxford: Oxford University Press; 2006.

6. Salustri C, Tecchio F, Zappasodi F, et al. Cortical excitability and rest activity properties in patients with depression. *Journal of Psychiatry and Neuroscience*. 2007; **32**(4): 259–266.

7. Kurita S, Takei Y, Maki Y, et al. Magnetoencephalography study of the effect of attention modulation on somatosensory processing in patients with major depressive disorder. *Psychiatry and Clinical Neurosciences*. 2016; **70**(2): 116–125.

8. Cornwell BR, Salvadore G, Furey M, et al. Synaptic potentiation is critical for rapid antidepressant response to ketamine in treatment-resistant major depression. *Biological Psychiatry*. 2012; **72**(7): 555–561.

9. Nugent AC, Wills KE, Gilbert JR, Zarate Jr CA. Synaptic Potentiation and Rapid Antidepressant Response to Ketamine in Treatment-Resistant Major Depression: A Replication Study. In Revision.

10. Gilbert JR, Yarrington JS, Wills KE, Nugent AC, Zarate CA, Jr. Glutamatergic signaling drives ketamine-mediated response in depression: Evidence from dynamic causal modeling. *Int J Neuropsychopharmacol*. 2018; **21**(8): 740–747.

11. Wang Y, Jia Y, Feng Y, et al. Overlapping auditory M100 and M200 abnormalities in schizophrenia and bipolar disorder: A MEG study. *Schizophrenia Research*. 2014; **160**(1–3): 201–207.

12. Kähkönen S, Yamashita H, Rytsälä H, et al. Dysfunction in early auditory processing in major depressive disorder revealed by combined MEG and EEG. *Journal of Psychiatry and Neuroscience*. 2007; **32**(5): 316–222.

13. Takei Y, Kumano S, Hattori S, et al. Preattentive dysfunction in major depression: A magnetoencephalography study using auditory mismatch negativity. *Psychophysiology*. 2009; **46**(1): 52–61.

14. Takei Y, Kumano S, Maki Y, et al. Preattentive dysfunction in bipolar disorder: A MEG study using auditory mismatch negativity. *Progress in Neuro-Psychopharmacology and Biological Psychiatry*. 2010; **34**(6): 903–912.

15. Wang Y, Feng Y, Jia Y, et al. Absence of auditory M100 source asymmetry in schizophrenia and bipolar disorder: A MEG study. *PLoS ONE*. 2013; **8**(12).

16. Hegerl U, Juckel G. Intensity dependence of auditory evoked potentials as an indicator of central serotonergic neurotransmission: A new hypothesis. *Biol Psychiatry*. 1993; **33**(3): 173–187.

17. Hirakawa N, Hirano Y, Nakamura I, et al. Right hemisphere pitch-mismatch negativity reduction in patients with major depression: An MEG study. *Journal of Affective Disorders*. 2017; **215**: 225–229.

18. Shimano S, Onitsuka T, Oribe N, et al. Preattentive dysfunction in patients with bipolar disorder as revealed by the pitch-mismatch negativity: A magnetoencephalography (MEG) study. *Bipolar Disorders*. 2014; **16**(6): 592–599.

19. Isomura S, Onitsuka T, Tsuchimoto R, et al. Differentiation between major depressive disorder and bipolar disorder by auditory steady-state responses. *Journal of Affective Disorders*. 2016; **190**: 800–806.

20. Oda Y, Onitsuka T, Tsuchimoto R, et al. Gamma band neural synchronization deficits for auditory steady state responses in bipolar disorder patients. *PLoS ONE*. 2012; 7(7).

21. Hirano Y, Oribe N, Kanba S, et al. Spontaneous gamma activity in schizophrenia. *JAMA Psychiatry*. 2015; **72**(8): 813–821.

22. Nugent AC, Ballard ED, Gould TD, et al. Ketamine has distinct electrophysiological and behavioral effects in depressed and healthy subjects. *Mol Psychiatry*. 2018; **24**(7): 1040–1052.

23. Noda Y, Zomorrodi R, Saeki T, et al. Resting-state EEG gamma power and theta-gamma coupling enhancement following high-frequency left dorsolateral prefrontal rTMS in patients with depression. *Clin Neurophysiol*. 2017; **128**(3): 424–432.

24. Kam JW, Bolbecker AR, O'Donnell BF, Hetrick WP, Brenner CA. Resting state EEG power and coherence abnormalities in bipolar disorder and schizophrenia. *J Psychiatr Res*. 2013; **47**(12): 1893–1901.

25. Reite M, Teale P, Rojas DC, et al. MEG auditory evoked fields suggest altered structural/functional asymmetry in primary but not secondary auditory cortex in bipolar disorder. *Bipolar Disorders*. 2009; **11**(4): 371–381.

26. Wang Y, Feng Y, Jia Y, et al. Auditory M50 and M100 sensory gating deficits in bipolar disorder: A MEG study. *Journal of Affective Disorders*. 2014; **152–154**(1): 131–138.

27. Oribe N, Onitsuka T, Hirano S, et al. Differentiation between bipolar disorder and schizophrenia revealed by neural oscillation to speech sounds: An MEG study. Bipolar Disorders. 2010; **12**(8): 804–812.

28. Domschke K, Zwanzger P, Rehbein MA, et al. Magnetoencephalographic correlates of emotional processing in major depression before and after pharmacological treatment. *International Journal of Neuropsychopharmacology.* 2016; **19**(2): 1–9.

29. Xu Q, Ruohonen EM, Ye C, et al. Automatic processing of changes in facial emotions in dysphoria: A magnetoencephalography study. *Frontiers in Human Neuroscience.* 2018; **12**.

30. Moratti S, Rubio G, Campo P, Keil A, Ortiz T. Hypofunction of right temporoparietal cortex during emotional arousal in depression. *Archives of General Psychiatry.* 2008; **65**(5): 532–541.

31. Moratti S, Strange B, Rubio G. Emotional arousal modulation of right temporoparietal cortex in depression depends on parental depression status in women: First evidence. *Journal of Affective Disorders.* 2015; **178**: 79–87.

32. Disner SG, Beevers CG, Haigh EA, Beck AT. Neural mechanisms of the cognitive model of depression. *Nat Rev Neurosci.* 2011; **12**(8): 467–477.

33. Salvadore G, Cornwell BR, Colon-Rosario V, et al. Increased anterior cingulate cortical activity in response to fearful faces: A neurophysiological biomarker that predicts rapid antidepressant response to ketamine. *Biological Psychiatry.* 2009; **65**(4): 289–295.

34. Lu Q, Bi K, Liu C, et al. Predicting depression based on dynamic regional connectivity: A windowed Granger causality analysis of MEG recordings. *Brain Research.* 2013; **1535**: 52–60.

35. Lu Q, Li H, Luo G, et al. Impaired prefrontal-amygdala effective connectivity is responsible for the dysfunction of emotion process in major depressive disorder: A dynamic causal modeling study on MEG. *Neuroscience Letters.* 2012; **523**(2): 125–130.

36. Lu Q, Wang Y, Luo G, Li H, Yao Z. Dynamic connectivity laterality of the amygdala under negative stimulus in depression: A MEG study. *Neuroscience Letters.* 2013; **547**: 42–47.

37. Bi K, Hua L, Wei M, et al. Dynamic functional-structural coupling within acute functional state change phases: Evidence from a depression recognition study. *Journal of Affective Disorders.* 2016; **191**: 145–155.

38. Lu Q, Jiang H, Luo G, Han Y, Yao Z. Multichannel matching pursuit of MEG signals for discriminative oscillation pattern detection in depression. *International Journal of Psychophysiology.* 2013; **88**(2): 206–212.

39. Lee PS, Chen YS, Hsieh JC, Su TP, Chen LF. Distinct neuronal oscillatory responses between patients with bipolar and unipolar disorders: A magnetoencephalographic study. *Journal of Affective Disorders.* 2010; **123**(1–3): 270–275.

40. Liu TY, Hsieh JC, Chen YS, et al. Different patterns of abnormal gamma oscillatory activity in unipolar and bipolar disorder patients during an implicit emotion task. *Neuropsychologia.* 2012; **50**(7): 1514–1520.

41. McKinnon MC, Yucel K, Nazarov A, MacQueen GM. A meta-analysis examining clinical predictors of hippocampal volume in patients with major depressive disorder. *J Psychiatry Neurosci.* 2009; **34**(1): 41–54.

42. Cornwell BR, Salvadore G, Colon-Rosario V, et al. Abnormal hippocampal functioning and impaired spatial navigation in depressed individuals: Evidence from whole-head magnetoencephalography. *American Journal of Psychiatry.* 2010; **167**(7): 836–844.

43. Salvadore G, Cornwell BR, Sambataro F, et al. Anterior cingulate desynchronization and functional connectivity with the amygdala during a working memory task predict rapid antidepressant response to ketamine. *Neuropsychopharmacology.* 2010; **35**(7): 1415–1422.

44. Ionescu DF, Nugent AC, Luckenbaugh DA, et al. Baseline working memory activation deficits in dimensional anxious depression as detected by magnetoencephalography. *Acta Neuropsychiatrica.* 2015; **27**(3): 143–152.

45. Fernández A, Rodriguez-Palancas A, López-Ibor M, et al. Increased occipital delta dipole density in major depressive disorder determined by magnetoencephalography. *Journal of Psychiatry and Neuroscience.* 2005; **30**(1): 17–23.

46. Maihöfner C, Ropohl A, Reulbach U, et al. Effects of repetitive transcranial magnetic stimulation in depression: A magnetoencephalographic study. *NeuroReport.* 2005; **16**(16): 1839–1842.

47. Al-Timemy AH, Fernandez A, Escudero J, editors. *Spectral Analysis of Resting State Magnetoencephalogram Activity in Patients with Bipolar Disorder.* 2014.

48. Jiang H, Popov T, Jylänki P, et al. Predictability of depression severity based on posterior alpha oscillations. *Clinical Neurophysiology.* 2016; **127**(4): 2108–2114.

49. Linkenkaer-Hansen K, Monto S, Rytsälä H, et al. Breakdown of long-range temporal correlations in theta oscillations in patients with major depressive disorder. *Journal of Neuroscience.* 2005; **25**(44): 10131–10137.

50. Buzsaki G, Wang XJ. Mechanisms of gamma oscillations. *Annu Rev Neurosci.* 2012; **35**: 203–225.

51. Gandal MJ, Sisti J, Klook K, et al. GABAB-mediated rescue of altered excitatory-inhibitory balance, gamma synchrony and behavioral deficits following constitutive NMDAR-hypofunction. *Transl Psychiatry*. 2012; **2**: e142.

52. Duman RS, Aghajanian GK. Synaptic dysfunction in depression: Potential therapeutic targets. *Science*. 2012; **338**(6103): 68–72.

53. Bachmann M, Paeske L, Kalev K, et al. Methods for classifying depression in single channel EEG using linear and nonlinear signal analysis. *Comput Methods Programs Biomed*. 2018; **155**: 11–17.

54. Strelets VB, Garakh Zh V, Novototskii-Vlasov VY. Comparative study of the gamma rhythm in normal conditions, during examination stress, and in patients with first depressive episode. *Neurosci Behav Physiol*. 2007; **37**(4): 387–394.

55. Shaw AD, Saxena N, Jackson LE, et al. Ketamine amplifies induced gamma frequency oscillations in the human cerebral cortex. *European Neuropsychopharmacology*. 2015; **25**(8): 1136–1146.

56. Zanos P, Moaddel R, Morris PJ, et al. NMDAR inhibition-independent antidepressant actions of ketamine metabolites. *Nature*. 2016; **533**(7604): 481–486.

57. Stam CJ. Nonlinear dynamical analysis of EEG and MEG: review of an emerging field. *Clin Neurophysiol*. 2005; **116**(10): 2266–2301.

58. Méndez MA, Zuluaga P, Hornero R, et al. Complexity analysis of spontaneous brain activity: Effects of depression and antidepressant treatment. *Journal of Psychopharmacology*. 2012; **26**(5): 636–643.

59. Fernández A, Al-Timemy AH, Ferre F, Rubio G, Escudero J. Complexity analysis of spontaneous brain activity in mood disorders: A magnetoencephalography study of bipolar disorder and major depression. *Comprehensive Psychiatry*. 2018; **84**: 112–117.

60. Brookes MJ, Woolrich MW, Barnes GR. Measuring functional connectivity in MEG: A multivariate approach insensitive to linear source leakage. *Neuroimage*. 2012; **63**(2): 910–920.

61. Brookes MJ, Tewarie PK, Hunt BAE, et al. A multi-layer network approach to MEG connectivity analysis. *Neuroimage*. 2016; **132**: 425–438.

62. Colclough GL, Brookes MJ, Smith SM, Woolrich MW. A symmetric multivariate leakage correction for MEG connectomes. *Neuroimage*. 2015; **117**: 439–448.

63. Chen SS, Tu PC, Su TP, et al. Impaired frontal synchronization of spontaneous magnetoencephalographic activity in patients with bipolar disorder. *Neuroscience Letters*. 2008; **445**(2): 174–178.

64. Nugent AC, Robinson SE, Coppola R, Furey ML, Zarate CA, Jr. Group differences in MEG-ICA derived resting state networks: Application to major depressive disorder. *NeuroImage*. 2015; **118**: 1–12.

65. Muthukumaraswamy SD, Shaw AD, Jackson LE, et al. Evidence that subanesthetic doses of ketamine cause sustained disruptions of NMDA and AMPA-mediated frontoparietal connectivity in humans. *Journal of Neuroscience*. 2015; **35**(33): 11694–11706.

66. Zhang S, Tian S, Chattun MR, et al. A supplementary functional connectivity microstate attached to the default mode network in depression revealed by resting-state magnetoencephalography. *Progress in Neuro-Psychopharmacology and Biological Psychiatry*. 2018; **83**: 76–85.

67. Wise T, Marwood L, Perkins AM, et al. Instability of default mode network connectivity in major depression: A two-sample confirmation study. *Transl Psychiatry*. 2017; **7**(4): e1105.

68. Hamilton JP, Farmer M, Fogelman P, Gotlib IH. Depressive rumination, the default-mode network, and the dark matter of clinical neuroscience. *Biol Psychiatry*. 2015; **78**(4): 224–230.

69. Zhu X, Zhu Q, Shen H, Liao W, Yuan F. Rumination and default mode network subsystems connectivity in first-episode, drug-naive young patients with major depressive disorder. *Sci Rep*. 2017; **7**: 43105.

70. Perera T, George MS, Grammer G, et al. The clinical TMS society consensus review and treatment recommendations for TMS therapy for major depressive disorder. *Brain Stimul*. 2016; **9**(3): 336–346.

71. Pathak Y, Salami O, Baillet S, Li Z, Butson CR. Longitudinal changes in depressive circuitry in response to neuromodulation therapy. *Frontiers in Neural Circuits*. 2016; **10**(July 2016).

72. Li CT, Chen LF, Tu PC, et al. Impaired prefronto-thalamic functional connectivity as a key feature of treatment-resistant depression: A combined MEG, PET and rTMS study. *PLoS ONE*. 2013; **8**(8).

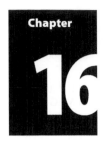

Chapter 16

An Overview of Machine Learning Applications in Mood Disorders

Natasha Topolski, Su Hyun Jeong, and Benson Mwangi

16.1 Machine Learning: An Answer to Historic Challenges in Psychiatry?

Advances in our understanding of the human body and technology have revolutionized modern medicine, allowing us to easily treat many conditions that were once considered a death sentence. The use of an improved understanding of biological processes and the development of disease biomarkers has led to the growth of "precision medicine" – which enables the ability to produce more objective diagnoses through individualized treatments that are more efficient and effective. The core concept of integrating precision medicine into the diagnosis and treatment of disease is now a commonplace and growing in many areas of medicine, notably the use of genomics in oncology. However, diagnosis and treatment in psychiatry remains largely dependent on observable subjective symptoms and without objective biomarkers (1, 2). In addition, individual variability among patients contributes to a wide variation in patient responses to psychiatric treatment. For example, after initial treatment, over 50% of patients with major depressive disorder do not reach remission (3–5). Psychiatric research studies have suggested that there are biologically defined "subgroups" or "bio-types" of mental disorders, an observation that has pushed for a shift to classify psychiatric conditions as "brain disorders" (2). In order to elucidate these subgroups, the National Institute of Mental Health developed the Research Domain Criteria (RDoC) that aims to determine the mechanisms that result in dysfunction through basic science rather than symptomatology. The RDoC framework calls for research that integrates behavioral, biological, and environmental factors to facilitate the development of objective measures of psychopathology (6). Most noticeably though, such an undertaking requires massive data collection and data analysis methods that go beyond the abilities of traditional statistical and data analysis methods. Consequently, machine learning (ML) techniques have provided a promising avenue to analyze large datasets acquired in psychiatric research and support new discoveries. Briefly, ML is a branch of computer science and artificial intelligence that involves developing and validating algorithms that can learn from patterns gleaned from large datasets and subsequently allow predictions on previously "unseen" observations (7). Therefore, due to their ability to handle high-dimensional and large datasets, ML techniques and algorithms are well suited to be a key player in the redefinition of clinical tools used in the diagnosis and treatment of mood disorders (7). In this chapter, we will briefly discuss key concepts used in ML and explore how such concepts and ensuing tools are used in the study and treatment of mood disorders.

16.2 Machine Learning Techniques

ML techniques can be classified into three broad categories, namely supervised ML, unsupervised ML, and reinforcement learning. In this section, we briefly explore these broad categorizations and introduce specific use cases for such methods in the context of research in mood disorders.

16.2.1 Supervised ML

In supervised learning, a ML algorithm is developed and "trained" using a set of observations with corresponding labels. For example, in the context of a mood disorders study, a set of observations may represent neuroimaging scan data from healthy controls and bipolar disorder (BD) patients coupled with corresponding labels (BD +1, healthy controls −1) (Figure 16.1). These observations are subsequently used to "train" an algorithm to recognize characteristics in data, in this case, the neuroimaging scans that differentiate the target groups (e.g., healthy control vs. BD patients). The resulting "trained" algorithm is evaluated using a subset of "novel" labeled observations not included in the algorithm "training" process (8),(9). The most commonly used supervised ML techniques in the mood disorders domain include support vector machines (SVMs), relevance vector machines (RVMs), Elastic Net, and Least Absolute Shrinkage Selection Operator (LASSO) among others as highlighted in Table 16.1. Typical clinical and research applications of supervised ML currently include disease predictive classification (e.g., healthy vs. bipolar disorder (10)) and decoding of continuous clinical scales (e.g., Beck Depression Inventory (11)) using biological data such as neuroimaging scans.

16.2.2 Unsupervised Learning

Unlike supervised ML, where the input data are labeled (e.g., disease +1 vs. healthy −1), in unsupervised ML, the input data are not labeled, and the main goal is to find hidden patterns within a dataset. Therefore, unsupervised ML techniques largely utilize data dimensionality reduction methods (e.g., principal component analysis) coupled with data clustering techniques (e.g., K-means) to identify hidden patterns and clusters

within a dataset. Unsupervised ML techniques have recently been used to identify unique biological groupings or clusters in mood disorders – also known as "biotypes" (12).

16.2.3 Reinforcement Learning

Reinforcement learning entails "training" an algorithm that is able to take specific actions that maximize cumulative rewards. Notably, these algorithms mimic the human decision-making process where there are often an arbitrary number of actions to choose from and eventually learn from positive outcomes (i.e., reward) or negative outcomes (i.e., punishment). Typical examples of reinforcement learning applications have included mapping of positive and negative prediction errors to the firing of dopaminergic neurons in mood and affective disorders (13),(14). Most recently, reinforcement learning algorithms are increasingly being used to select optimal treatments (e.g., antidepressants) as they mimic the trial and error process used in selecting treatments during clinical practice.

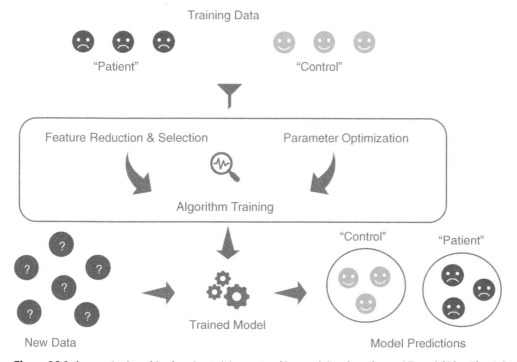

Figure 16.1 A supervised machine learning training protocol in mood disorders where a ML model/algorithm is "trained" to separate patients with mood disorders from healthy controls.

However, despite the three categories of ML algorithms highlighted earlier (i.e., supervised, unsupervised, and reinforcement learning), below we highlight three overarching concepts used in ML to practitioners in establishing and validating ML algorithms before they are reported in research products or deployed for clinical purposes. Here we introduce these concepts.

16.2.4 Selection of Algorithm Training and Validation Samples

An "objective" ML algorithm is the one that is able to "generalize" results to a novel or new sample that it was not previously exposed to. Therefore, in order to develop an "objective" ML algorithm in a ML-related project, the first step entails splitting a dataset into independent "training" and "validation" sets. The "training" set is used in "training" the algorithm by identifying the best algorithm parameters whilst the "validation" set is used to establish whether the final algorithm/model is generalizable by making accurate and objective predictions. Consequently, it is a common practice to separate a dataset into two groups (i.e., training and validation sets) before embarking on a ML project.

16.2.5 Feature and Data Dimensionality Reduction

Raw data, particularly in specific psychiatric research domains such as neuroimaging and genomics are often acquired in high dimensions (e.g., >100,000 voxels) and may also contain measurement noise. In the context of ML, this problem is also referred to as the *"curse-of-dimensionality"* or *"small-n-large-p"* problem where there are significantly large number of predictors (e.g., neuroimaging voxels) as compared to a low number of observations (i.e., subjects) (15) . This may greatly hamper a ML algorithm as it's not able to identify a *best-fit* solution – a problem also known as *overfitting* (15). Therefore, to circumvent this problem, data dimensionality reduction and feature reduction tools such as principal component analysis (PCA) or univariate *t*-test among other techniques are often employed to extract a subset of features or predictors (e.g., neuroimaging voxels) that are meaningful to the ML task at hand. The subset of features or predictors extracted using the data dimensionality or feature reduction techniques are subsequently used to "train" a ML model instead of the original raw data. Previous research studies on this domain have shown that these feature reduction techniques lead to ML models with higher accuracy and better generalization ability by being able to make accurate predictions from previously "unseen" observations in a validation sample.

16.2.6 Model Training and Parameter Optimization

Training a ML algorithm entails establishing parameters that can maximize prediction accuracy and promote model generalizability to a novel or previously "unseen" sample. Therefore, to achieve this goal, it is common practice to use cross-validation methods that support selection of "best-fit" parameters. Therefore, *N-fold* cross-validation (e.g., 10-fold or 5-fold) is often used by randomly separating the data into N subgroups while the algorithm is "trained" on $N - 1$ subgroups and tested on the left-out group. This is repeated so that each group is left out to estimate model prediction errors and accuracy across the N trials. Upon completion, the model and model parameters with the highest accuracy or least errors are selected to establish the final model. The final accuracy on a validation sample determines the generalizability of the model. In Table 16.1, we have briefly outlined key ML techniques and their categorizations.

16.3 Applications of Machine Learning Techniques to Neuroimaging and Clinical Data in Mood Disorders

16.3.1 Diagnostic Classification of Mood Disorders, Decoding Clinical Variables, Identification of Unique Disease Subtypes and Supporting Mechanistic Understanding

Despite recent progress, our understanding of the mechanistic pathophysiology of major mood disorders such as BD and major depressive disorder

Table 16.1 Common methods used in machine learning pipelines

Methods	Model details and categorization (e.g., supervised or unsupervised)
Linear regression models	Regression analysis is a branch of classical statistics where a model formula is developed that characterizes the relationship between a set of independent variables (predictors) and dependent variables (outcomes) that can be plotted as a line. In machine learning, regression can be utilized as an element of the most basic form of supervised learning where regression models developed from training data can be used to predict outcomes of new input data **Common models:** General linear regression, regularized regression (e.g., least absolute shrinkage and selection operator (LASSO) or Elastic Net) **For more information**: Statistical learning with sparsity: the LASSO and generalizations (16) **Categorization:** Supervised
Linear and nonlinear kernel-based models	Kernel-learning ML algorithms use a "kernel function" to convert the selected input predictors or features into a similarity matrix known as a "kernel" that is used to develop classification rules. Kernel functions can vary depending on the data and may include both linear and nonlinear functions (e.g., polynomial or Gaussian) **Common models**: Support Vector Machine (SVM), Relevance Vector Machine (RVM) **For more information**: An introduction to support vector machines and other kernel-based learning methods (17) **Categorization:** Supervised
Decision trees	Decision trees are models that learn through simple heuristics or decision rules. Therefore, deeper decision trees lead to more complex decision rules and result into better ML models **Common models**: Random Forest, Adaboost **For more information**: *The Elements of Statistical Learning* (18) **Categorization:** Supervised
Additive models	Additive models are flexible statistical models often used to characterize nonlinear data. In additive models, multiple functions are added together to create a smoother model that fits the data better than any of the individual functions. Each function in the model retains its form, allowing for relatively simple interpretability (18) **Common models**: Generalized Additive Model **For more information**: *The Elements of Statistical Learning* (18) **Categorization:** Supervised
Artificial neural networks and deep learning	Artificial neural networks (ANNs) are designed to recognize nonlinear patterns in a dataset and make appropriate predictions (e.g., disease vs. healthy control classification) by mimicking how the human brain processes information. These artificial neurons are arranged into multiple layers, where the layer that receives input data is referred to as the input layer while the output layer returns predicted results. It is common practice to have many layers between the input and output layers with those in between referred to as the hidden layers. The most recent category of ANNs, which we refer to as deep learning neural networks, involves utilizing multiple hidden layers (i.e., thousands or millions) of neural networks. **Common models**: Feedforward Neural Networks, Convolutional Neural Networks **For more information**: Deep learning for neuroimaging: a validation study (19) **Categorization:** Supervised
Multivariate data dimensionality reduction	There are many multivariate data dimensionality reduction techniques used in mood disorders and in particular neuroimaging such as; principal component analysis (PCA (20)), independent component analysis (ICA (21)), multidimensional scaling (MDS (22)), local linear embedding (LLE (23)), nonnegative matrix factorization (NNMF (24)) and t-distributed stochastic neighbor embedding (t-SNE (25)). We briefly explore the most common multivariate dimensionality reduction techniques used in neuroimaging and mood disorders research (i.e., ICA and PCA). Specifically, ICA is a multivariate data-driven dimensionality technique, which belongs to the broader

Table 16.1 (cont.)

Methods	Model details and categorization (e.g., supervised or unsupervised)
	category of blind-source separation methods (21, 26) that are used to separate data into underlying independent information components. ICA separates a set of "mixed signals" (e.g., raw data from an fMRI scan) into a set of independent and relevant features (e.g., behavioral paradigm-related signals in fMRI). On the other hand, PCA is a dimensionality reduction technique, which transforms correlated variables into a smaller subset of variables that are not correlated also referred to as principal components. The resulting principal components can capture most of the variance in the data and are often linear combinations of the original or raw data (27). In summary, these techniques are commonly used to separate relevant signal from noise (i.e., denoising) as well as overcome the "curse-of-dimensionality" or "small-n-large-p" problems highlighted earlier in this chapter **Common models:** principal component analysis, independent component analysis **For more information:** A review of feature reduction techniques in neuroimaging (15) **Categorization:** Unsupervised
Multidimensional data clustering	Multidimensional data clustering is a form of unsupervised ML, which entails grouping observations that are "similar" in a higher dimensional space (e.g., >3 dimensions) into clusters or groups. The characteristics that determine group similarities may include distance measures such as the Euclidean distances among observations or statistical distributions. There are several data clustering algorithms such as K-means (28), mean shift (29), and hierarchical clustering (30). However, K-means is by far the most commonly used data clustering algorithm in this field. However, it is common practice to perform data dimensionality reduction using PCA, ICA, t-SNE, or other techniques before implementing data clustering. **Common models**: K-Means, Mean-Shift, Hierarchical Clustering **For more information**: Phenomapping: Methods and measures for deconstructing diagnosis in psychiatry (31) **Categorization:** Unsupervised
Model evaluation metrics	Machine learning algorithms are often evaluated using multiple metrics largely depending on the use case. Briefly, in a supervised predictive classification ML application (e.g., predicting MDD patients from healthy controls), it is common practice to use prediction accuracy, specificity, sensitivity, positive predictive value (PPV), negative predictive value (NPV), receiver-operating characteristic curves (ROC), and area under the ROC (AUROC). These evaluation metrics are also commonly used in biostatistics and diagnostic medicine as described elsewhere (32). On the other hand, supervised predictive regression ML applications that are used to predict or decode continuous variables or outcomes (e.g., Beck Depression Inventory) use other classical statistical measures such as the Pearson correlation coefficient, coefficient of determination, mean absolute error (MAE), and root mean square error (RMSE) (28). In a nutshell, these metrics compare the statistical relationship between "actual" continuous variables against the supervised ML predicted variables. However, the evaluation metrics used in unsupervised ML are comparatively different as they do not have a "ground truth" (e.g., comparisons between actual vs. predicted variables). Therefore, in unsupervised data clustering, the silhouette index value (SIV) (33) is by far the most popular metric used to quantify the number of clusters in a dataset as well as cluster validity. Briefly, the SIV quantifies the similarity of a data point to other points within its own cluster as compared to data points in other data clusters. Recent unsupervised ML studies in mood disorders have largely used this metric to evaluate ML model outcomes (34–37). Other data clustering metrics include, Dunn's cluster validity index [38], Davies–Bouldin index (38, 39), gap statistic (40), and the C-index (41). For a review on unsupervised ML evaluation metrics the reader is pointed to (42). **Common metrics**: Prediction accuracy, Specificity, Sensitivity, ROC, AUROC, Silhouette Index Value **For more information:** Pattern recognition and machine learning (43)

(MDD) still remains limited. Early neuroimaging studies used mass-univariate statistical methods coupled with neuroimaging scan data to elucidate critical insights on brain structural and functional differences between patients with mood disorders and comparative healthy controls. For example, through these studies, fronto-limbic structural abnormalities in BD patients were reported (44). In addition, volumetric and structural connectivity in the anterior cingulate cortex (ACC) in patients with MDD have also been reported (45). More recently, neuroimaging studies have leveraged ML techniques to classify or distinguish individual patients with mood disorders from healthy controls. For example, through a systematic review with fifty-one research studies, Librenza-Garcia and colleagues observed that ML coupled with structural and functional neuroimaging scans can accurately differentiate BD patients from healthy controls and other psychiatric diagnosis such as MDD (10). Another recent systematic review observed gray matter volume reductions in bilateral insula, right superior temporal gyrus, bilateral anterior cingulate cortex, and left superior medial frontal cortex in MDD and BD patients as compared to healthy controls (44). Predictive white matter abnormalities in the genu of the corpus callosum were also observed in both MDD and BD patient groups (44). Other studies have attempted to predict or decode continuous clinical rating scales from neuroimaging scans. This is followed by a subsequent examination of brain regions involved in predicting such clinical rating scales. For example, Mwangi and colleagues (11) reported prediction of the self-reported Beck Depression Inventory (BDI) using structural neuroimaging scans coupled with a kernel-based relevance vector regression ML algorithm in patients with MDD. This study reported correlation between actual BDI scores and predicted BDI scores at Pearson correlation coefficient = 0.694 and significant at $p < 0.0001$. Furthermore, the medial frontal, superior temporal gyrus, and parahippocampal gyrus were heavily involved in decoding the BDI scores in patients with MDD. In another study (46), BDI and Snaith-Hamilton Pleasure Scale (SHAPS) were accurately predicted in a cohort of fifty-eight patients with MDD using a supervised linear regression ML technique and functional connectivity data and identified several functional networks associated with anhedonia and negative

mood as the main contributors. Another study predicted Functioning Assessment Short Test (FAST) (47) from a cohort of thirty-five patients with BD type I using a supervised support vector regression ML algorithm and structural neuroimaging scan data (48). The FAST score is used to measure functional impairment in BD and was predicted by volumetric reductions in the left superior and left rostral medial frontal cortex as well as right lateral brain ventricular enlargements. This indicates that a supervised ML algorithm together with structural neuroimaging scans can predict functional impairment in BD patients. In a similar pattern, multinational studies from the Enhancing NeuroImaging Genetics through Meta-Analysis (ENIGMA) consortium have also reported successful diagnostic classification of MDD (49) and BD (48, 50) patients as compared to healthy controls using neuroimaging scans from thousands of patients acquired from multiple centers around the world.

Recently, there has been a shift in psychiatric research toward identification of data-driven disease subtypes also referred to as phenomapping, which has partly been inspired by the NIMH's RDOC criteria (6). Therefore, researchers have leveraged unsupervised ML techniques such as multivariate data-dimensionality reduction coupled with high-dimensional data clustering algorithms capable of identifying unique disease subtypes in BD and MDD. For instance, Wu and colleagues (37) used an unsupervised ML approach to cluster neurocognitive data derived from BD-I and BD-II patients into two distinct subtypes. Subsequently, the data derived subtypes were validated using a linear regression Elastic Net ML algorithm coupled with fractional anisotropy (FA) and mean diffusivity (MD) measures of brain diffusion tensor imaging (DTI) with 92% and 75.9% accuracy, respectively. Abnormalities in the inferior fronto-occipital fasciculus and minor forceps of the corpus callosum white matter tracts of patients with BD were found to be major contributors in separating the two data-derived subtypes of BD from healthy controls. In another study (51), a data-driven approach was used to identify transdiagnostic subtypes of mood disorders that span multiple clinical diagnoses. This study applied a hierarchical data clustering algorithm to identify unique subgroups that were subsequently validated using an independent sample. However, although there are promising results from the phenomapping literature, we still need to remain cautiously optimistic as attempts to replicate such disease subtypes in independent samples have in some cases not been successful (52).

16.3.2 Prediction of Treatment Response

Prediction of treatment response, such as being able to identify individual patients with MDD that are likely to have a positive response to a particular antidepressant is a well-documented problem in psychiatry (53),(54). Therefore, in the past decade, a plethora of studies in mood disorders have employed ML techniques to predict individual patients' likelihood of responding to antidepressants or mood stabilizers. For instance, Webb and colleagues (55) examined whether a ML technique can recommend individualized treatment in a eight-week trial of sertraline versus placebo with a cohort of 216 depressed individuals. This study observed that a ML technique can identify a subset of MDD patients that are optimally suited for sertraline primarily based on a few clinical and demographic variables. Another study using the Sequenced Treatment Alternatives to Relieve Depression (STAR*D) dataset (56) developed a supervised gradient boosting ML algorithm to predict patients who may benefit from citalopram following a twelve-week course of treatment. The ML algorithm achieved an accuracy of 64.6% and twenty-five clinical variables were selected by the Elastic Net ML algorithm as the top contributors to the observed accuracy. Numerous other studies have used a similar supervised ML approach to predict patients likelihood of response to antidepressants in MDD (57–60), electroconvulsive therapy in MDD (61, 62), and lithium in BD (63) using structural/functional neuroimaging scans, electroencephalogram (EEG), and clinical/demographic data. Although it's not a common practice in psychiatry, recent studies in oncology are beginning to use reinforcement learning algorithms to implement automated radiation adaptive protocols in treating lung cancer (64). The reinforcement learning approach may be particularly well suited for adaptive protocols in MDD as it mimics the current gold standard of selecting optimal antidepressants through a "trial and error" process (65). Lastly, although there is significant progress in optimizing treatments for

patients with mood disorders using ML techniques, the majority of studies have largely used retrospective data and resulting ML models have not been translated into actual clinical practice.

16.3.3 Prediction of Other Clinical Outcomes Such As Suicide, Medication Side Effects and Clinical Staging

ML techniques have also been a powerful asset at assessing and predicting other clinical outcomes such as suicidality and medication side effects, and, to some extent, recent studies have been successful at establishing disease stages. Two recent studies used large electronic medical records (EMR) datasets as input predictors with a number of supervised ML algorithms (e.g., Elastic Net, Random Forest and LASSO) and managed to predict suicide risk among patients in a psychiatric hospital or emergency department with specificity and sensitivity greater than 0.7 (66, 67). Interestingly, Passos and colleagues (68) reported accurate predictions (accuracy = 72%, sensitivity = 72.1%, and specificity = 71.3%) at predicting individual suicide attempters in a preliminary study with a cohort of 144 patients with BD and MDD. The kernel-based relevance vector ML technique used in this study identified previous hospitalizations for depression, a history of psychosis, cocaine dependence, and posttraumatic stress disorder (PTSD) comorbidity as the most relevant predictors of suicide attempt in mood disorders. This further highlights that ML techniques can not only aid in prediction of psychiatric patients at risk of attempting suicide but can also guide researchers to clinical factors that contribute to such events and open novel avenues for clinical interventions. Prediction of medication side effects has also shown promise as a prime application for ML techniques. For example, although lithium is a first-line form of treatment in BD, its risk for developing renal insufficiency reportedly discourages its use in treating BD (69). A study of 5,700 patients receiving treatment with lithium reported a regression ML technique-powered EMR data that was able to predict renal insufficiency risk with an area under the curve (AUC) of 0.81 (69). The authors observed that older age, female sex, history of smoking, history of hypertension, overall burden of medical comorbidity, and diagnosis of schizophrenia or schizoaffective disorder were the major contributing factors in predicting renal insufficiency among those receiving lithium treatment. This highlights that such ML tools can support clinicians to make informed decisions and facilitate the development of strategies that reduce negative outcomes such as side effects. Lastly, we highlight the use of ML techniques in predicting and validating disease stages in mood disorders. A recent study showed that structural brain scans can not only distinguish BD patients from healthy controls but also found that a subgroup of patients characterized by higher lifetime manic episodes including psychiatric hospitalizations had markedly higher gray and white matter density loss (70). The authors concluded ML coupled with structural neuroimaging scans is able to stratify BD patients into clinical stages (e.g., early stage vs. late stage BD) in line with the recently proposed clinical staging model of BD (71–74).

16.4 Conclusion

In this chapter, we have reviewed the core concepts used in ML applications in mood disorders and introduced exemplar studies in this domain. These studies have proposed extensive solutions ranging from diagnostic predictive classification, prediction of clinical variables, as well as prediction of treatment response, side effects, and suicidality. In addition, a wide range of biological (e.g., neuroimaging scans, genomics), clinical, and demographic variables have leveraged ML techniques to predict these clinical outcomes. Most importantly, as ML algorithms are multivariate in nature, they increasingly support integration of data from multiple sources such as joint combination of neuroimaging, genetics, and clinical data to improve prediction power by leveraging variance from multiple biological layers (e.g., brain, genetics, and clinical). A detailed and technical exploration of multimodal data integration or fusion methods is given elsewhere (75). Nevertheless, we predict that such multimodal data integration studies and applications will become a common place in mood disorders research and subsequent clinical applications. In summary, although a tremendous amount of progress has been made in applying these novel technological tools to solve major clinical problems, there are a number of challenges for

the field to overcome to fully utilize these tools in improving outcomes for patients with mood disorders. Whilst not exhaustive, here we briefly discuss some of these challenges.

16.4.1 Interpretability of Machine Learning Models and Variability in Implementations

As highlighted in Table 16.1, ML techniques extend from "simple" linear regression algorithms (e.g., LASSO or Elastic Net) that perform calculations in the same "input space" as the original data to more "complex" nonlinear algorithms (e.g., kernel-based SVMs or ANNs). Noticeably, in the context of this chapter, we refer to "complexity" as instances where the method transforms input data (e.g., neuroimaging or clinical) from their original format into another space (e.g., Gaussian space) as well as other methods such as ANNs with multiple layers. The linear methods are highly interpretable as they do not transform the data into "nonlinear spaces" such as kernel-based methods or ANNs. In other words, the data are not input into a "black box" that lends itself uninterpretable. However, it has also been shown that in some ML use cases, particularly in high-dimensional data (e.g., neuroimaging scans), nonlinear ML methods may provide superior prediction results and therefore necessitating their use. Therefore, interpretability of ML models particularly in kernel-based and deep learning methods still remains a major concern but also an active area of research in ML (76, 77). In short, better interpretable models would allow researchers or clinicians to understand why the algorithm is making certain predictions or recommendations and therefore an informed decision-making process. Variability on how ML algorithms are implemented in the literature still remains a concern. For instance, it is not unusual for ML studies to use different model validation techniques (e.g., 5-fold vs. 10-fold cross-validation or leave-one-out cross-validation), a problem that is compounded by small study sample sizes. A recent empirical study (78) highlighted this shortcoming, which could potentially be resolved by leveraging large datasets and when it's not possible to acquire large cohorts from a single research facility pooling or sharing standardized datasets from multiple centers. For example, the ENIGMA consortium (79) has recently accomplished this goal by implementing several ML models through pooling of datasets from dozens of research centers from around the world in both MDD (80) and BD (50).

16.4.2 Lack of Standards and Other Issues Around Ethics

Applications leveraging ML as a clinical decision support tool are relatively new and therefore without proper regulations and standards. For example, in the United States (US), medical devices and other therapeutics have to undergo regulatory certifications through the US Food and Drug Administration (FDA) agency. Noticeably, in the past it has been unclear if digital health products, which include ML models, need any regulatory approvals. However, in the past year, the US FDA has initiated a precertification pilot program to assess medical software such as ML models using several excellence criteria such as quality (81). Indeed, beyond certifications and standards, data-sharing protocols that facilitate the sharing of sensitive clinical data without compromising patients' privacy will also need to be addressed but there are ongoing global efforts to establish systems able to capture and learn from health-related datasets whilst maintaining a high level of privacy (82–84). Indeed, this is an issue also explored in the most recent positional paper on "big data and machine learning" from a panel of experts representing the International Society of Bipolar Disorders (ISBD) (85).

Model bias where the input data may represent inequities by not being epidemiologically representative has also been highlighted as a major ethical concern (86). Therefore, it is imperative for practitioners involved in implementing and deploying of ML supported tools to ensure that ML training data are truly representative of target populations based on gender, age, race/ethnicity, socioeconomic status among other social factors – without amplifying existing health and social disparities as detailed elsewhere (87, 88). Overall, ML techniques hold great promise for psychiatric research and clinical practice – particularly in mood disorders and we predict that we will continue to witness more of such applications in research studies with some translating into the "real world" or clinics.

References

1. Collins FS, Varmus H. A new initiative on precision medicine. *New England Journal of Medicine.* 2015; **372**(9): 793–795.

2. Insel TR, Cuthbert BN. Brain disorders? precisely. *Science.* 2015; **348**(6234): 499–500.

3. Mrazek DA, Hornberger JC, Anthony Altar C, Degtiar I. A Review of the clinical, economic, and societal burden of treatment-resistant depression: 1996–2013. *Psychiatric Services.* 2014; **65**(8): 977–987.

4. Wong EHF, Yocca F, Smith MA, Lee C-M. Challenges and opportunities for drug discovery in psychiatric disorders: The drug hunters' perspective. *Int J Neuropsychopharmacol.* 2010 October; **13**(9): 1269–1284.

5. Hofmann SG, Asnaani A, Vonk IJJ, Sawyer AT, Fang A. The efficacy of cognitive behavioral therapy: A review of meta-analyses. *Cognitive Therapy and Research.* 2012; **36**(5): 427–440.

6. Cuthbert BN, Insel TR. Toward the future of psychiatric diagnosis: The seven pillars of RDoC. *BMC Med.* 2013 May 14; **11**: 126.

7. Bzdok D, Meyer-Lindenberg A. Machine learning for precision psychiatry: Opportunities and challenges. *Biol Psychiatry Cogn Neurosci Neuroimaging.* 2018 March; **3**(3): 223–30.

8. Iniesta R, Stahl D, McGuffin P. Machine learning, statistical learning and the future of biological research in psychiatry. *Psychol Med.* 2016 September; **46**(12): 2455–2465.

9. Varoquaux G, Thirion B. How machine learning is shaping cognitive neuroimaging. *Gigascience.* 2014 November 17; **3**: 28.

10. Librenza-Garcia D, Kotzian BJ, Yang J, et al. The impact of machine learning techniques in the study of bipolar disorder: A systematic review. *Neuroscience & Biobehavioral Reviews.* 2017; **80**: 538–554.

11. Mwangi B, Matthews K, Douglas Steele J. Prediction of illness severity in patients with major depression using structural MR brain scans. *Journal of Magnetic Resonance Imaging.* 2012; **35**(1): 64–71.

12. Williams LM. Defining biotypes for depression and anxiety based on large-scale circuit dysfunction: A theoretical review of the evidence and future directions for clinical translation. *Depress Anxiety.* 2017 January; **34**(1): 9–24.

13. Maia TV, Frank MJ. From reinforcement learning models to psychiatric and neurological disorders. *Nat Neurosci.* 2011 February; **14**(2): 154–162.

14. Huys QJ, Pizzagalli DA, Bogdan R, Dayan P. Mapping anhedonia onto reinforcement learning: a behavioural meta-analysis. *Biol Mood Anxiety Disord.* 2013 June 19; **3**(1): 12.

15. Mwangi B, Tian TS, Soares JC. A review of feature reduction techniques in neuroimaging. *Neuroinformatics.* 2014 April; **12**(2): 229–244.

16. Hastie T, Tibshirani R, Wainwright M. *Statistical Learning with Sparsity: The Lasso and Generalizations.* CRC Press; 2015. 367.

17. Cristianini N, Shawe-Taylor J. *An Introduction to Support Vector Machines and Other Kernel-based Learning Methods.* Cambridge University Press; 2000. 189.

18. Hastie T, Tibshirani R, Friedman J. *The Elements of Statistical Learning: Data Mining, Inference, and Prediction.* Springer; 2009.

19. Plis SM, Hjelm DR, Salakhutdinov R, et al. Deep learning for neuroimaging: A validation study. *Front Neurosci.* 2014 August 20; **8**: 229.

20. Deutsch H-P. Principle component analysis. In: *Derivatives and Internal Models.* Palgrave Macmillan, London; 2002. pp. 539–547. (Finance and Capital Markets Series).

21. Stone JV. *Independent Component Analysis: A Tutorial Introduction.* MIT Press; 2004.

22. Kruskal JB. Multidimensional scaling by optimizing goodness of fit to a nonmetric hypothesis. *Psychometrika.* 1964; **29**(1): 1–27.

23. Roweis ST. Nonlinear dimensionality reduction by locally linear embedding. *Science.* 2000; **290**(5500): 2323–2326.

24. Lee DD, Seung HS. Learning the parts of objects by non-negative matrix factorization. *Nature.* 1999 October 21; **401**(6755): 788–791.

25. van der Maaten L, Hinton G. Visualizing data using t-SNE. *J Mach Learn Res.* 2008 November 8; **9**: 2579–2605.

26. Calhoun VD, Liu J, Adali T. A review of group ICA for fMRI data and ICA for joint inference of imaging, genetic, and ERP data. *NeuroImage.* 2009; **45**(1): S163–S172.

27. Jolliffe IT. *Principal Component Analysis.* Springer; 2002. (Springer Series in Statistics).

28. Hartigan JA, Wong MA. Algorithm AS 136: A K-means clustering algorithm. *Applied Statistics.* 1979; **28**(1): 100.

29. Cheng Y. Mean shift, mode seeking, and clustering. *IEEE Transactions on Pattern Analysis and Machine Intelligence.* 1995; **17**(8): 790–799.

30. Johnson SC. Hierarchical clustering schemes. *Psychometrika.* 1967; **32**(3): 241–254.

31. Marquand AF, Wolfers T, Dinga R. Phenomapping: Methods and measures for deconstructing diagnosis in psychiatry. *Personalized Psychiatry.* 2019; 119–134.

32. Zhou X-H, Obuchowski NA, McClish DK. *Statistical Methods in Diagnostic Medicine.* Wiley; 2011. (Wiley Series in Probability and Statistics).

33. Rousseeuw PJ. Silhouettes: A graphical aid to the interpretation and validation of cluster analysis. *Journal of Computational and Applied Mathematics.* 1987; **20**: 53–65.

34. Mwangi B, Soares JC, Hasan KM. Visualization and unsupervised predictive clustering of high-dimensional multimodal neuroimaging data. *J Neurosci Methods.* 2014 October 30; **236**: 19–25.

35. Zhang W, Xiao Y, Sun H, et al. Discrete patterns of cortical thickness in youth with bipolar disorder differentially predict treatment response to quetiapine but not lithium. *Neuropsychopharmacology.* 2018; **43**(11): 2256–2263.

36. Marquand AF, Wolfers T, Mennes M, Buitelaar J, Beckmann CF. Beyond lumping and splitting: A review of computational approaches for stratifying psychiatric disorders. *Biol Psychiatry Cogn Neurosci Neuroimaging.* 2016 September; **1**(5): 433–447.

37. Wu M-J, Mwangi B, Bauer IE, et al. Identification and individualized prediction of clinical phenotypes in bipolar disorders using neurocognitive data, neuroimaging scans and machine learning. *Neuroimage.* 2017 January 15; **145**(Pt B): 254–264.

38. Dunn JC. Well-separated clusters and optimal fuzzy partitions. *Journal of Cybernetics.* 1974; **4**(1): 95–104.

39. Davies DL, Bouldin DW. A cluster separation measure. *IEEE Transactions on Pattern Analysis and Machine Intelligence.* 1979; PAMI-**1**(2): 224–227.

40. Tibshirani R, Walther G, Hastie T. Estimating the number of clusters in a data set via the gap statistic. *Journal of the Royal Statistical Society: Series B (Statistical Methodology).* 2001; **63**(2): 411–423.

41. Hubert L, Schultz J. Quadratic assignment as a general data analysis strategy. *British Journal of Mathematical and Statistical Psychology.* 1976; **29**(2): 190–241.

42. Günter S, Bunke H. Validation indices for graph clustering. *Pattern Recognition Letters*. 2003; **24**(8): 1107–1113.

43. Bishop CM. *Pattern Recognition and Machine Learning*. Springer Verlag; 2006.

44. Kim Y-K, Na K-S. Application of machine learning classification for structural brain MRI in mood disorders: Critical review from a clinical perspective. *Prog Neuropsychopharmacol Biol Psychiatry*. 2018 January 3; **80**(Pt B): 71–80.

45. Dusi N, De Carlo V, Delvecchio G, Bellani M, Soares JC, Brambilla P. MRI features of clinical outcome in bipolar disorder: A selected review. *Journal of Affective Disorders*. 2019; **243**: 559–563.

46. Yoshida K, Shimizu Y, Yoshimoto J, et al. Prediction of clinical depression scores and detection of changes in whole-brain using resting-state functional MRI data with partial least squares regression. *PLoS One*. 2017 July 12; **12**(7): e0179638.

47. Rosa AR, Sánchez-Moreno J, Martínez-Aran A, et al. Validity and reliability of the Functioning Assessment Short Test (FAST) in bipolar disorder. *Clinical Practice and Epidemiology in Mental Health*. 2007; **3**(1): 5.

48. Sartori JM, Reckziegel R, Passos IC, et al. Volumetric brain magnetic resonance imaging predicts functioning in bipolar disorder: A machine learning approach. *J Psychiatr Res*. 2018 August; **103**: 237–243.

49. Han LKM, Dinga R, Hahn T, et al. Brain Aging in Major Depressive Disorder: Results from the ENIGMA Major Depressive Disorder working group [Internet]. bioRxiv. 2019 [cited 2019 Sep 5]. p. 560623. Available from: http://dx.doi.org/10.1101/560623

50. Nunes A, for the ENIGMA Bipolar Disorders Working Group, Schnack HG, Ching CRK, Agartz I, Akudjedu TN, et al. Using structural MRI to identify bipolar disorders – 13 site machine learning study in 3020 individuals from the ENIGMA Bipolar Disorders Working Group. Molecular Psychiatry [Internet]. 2018; Available from: http://dx.doi.org/10.1038/s41380-018-0228-9

51. Grisanzio KA, Goldstein-Piekarski AN, Wang MY, et al. Transdiagnostic symptom clusters and associations with brain, behavior, and daily function in mood, anxiety, and trauma disorders. *JAMA Psychiatry*. 2018; **75**(2): 201.

52. Dinga R, Schmaal L, Penninx BWJH, et al. Evaluating the evidence for biotypes of depression: Methodological replication and extension of. *Neuroimage Clin*. 2019 March 27; 22: 101796.

53. Harmer CJ, Duman RS, Cowen PJ. How do antidepressants work? New perspectives for refining future treatment approaches. *Lancet Psychiatry*. 2017 May; **4**(5): 409–418.

54. Rutledge RB, Chekroud AM, Huys QJ. Machine learning and big data in psychiatry: toward clinical applications. *Curr Opin Neurobiol*. 2019 April; **55**: 152–159.

55. Webb CA, Trivedi MH, Cohen ZD, et al. Personalized prediction of antidepressant v. placebo response: Evidence from the EMBARC study. *Psychol Med*. 2019 May; **49**(7): 1118–1127.

56. Rush AJ, John Rush A, Fava M, et al. Sequenced treatment alternatives to relieve depression (STAR*D): Rationale and design. *Controlled Clinical Trials*. 2004; **25**(1): 119–142.

57. Paul R, Andlauer TFM, Czamara D, et al. Treatment response classes in major depressive disorder identified by model-based clustering and validated by clinical prediction models. *Translational Psychiatry* [Internet]. 2019; **9**(1). Available from: http://dx.doi.org/10.1038/s41398-019-0524-4

58. Khodayari-Rostamabad A, Reilly JP, Hasey GM, de Bruin H, MacCrimmon DJ. A machine learning approach using EEG data to predict response to SSRI treatment for major depressive disorder. *Clinical Neurophysiology*. 2013; **124**(10): 1975–1985.

59. Iniesta R, Malki K, Maier W, et al. Combining clinical variables to optimize prediction of antidepressant treatment outcomes. *J Psychiatr Res*. 2016 July; **78**: 94–102.

60. Kautzky A, Dold M, Bartova L, et al. Refining prediction in treatment-resistant depression: Results of machine learning analyses in the TRD III sample. *J Clin Psychiatry* [Internet]. 2018; **79**(1). Available from: http://dx.doi.org/10.4088/JCP.16m11385

61. Cao B, Luo Q, Fu Y, et al. Predicting individual responses to the electroconvulsive therapy with hippocampal subfield volumes in major depression disorder. *Sci Rep*. 2018 April 3; **8**(1): 5434.

62. Redlich R, Opel N, Grotegerd D, et al. Prediction of individual response to electroconvulsive therapy via machine learning on structural magnetic resonance imaging data. *JAMA Psychiatry*. 2016; **73**(6): 557.

63. Fleck DE, Ernest N, Adler CM, et al. Prediction of lithium response in first-episode mania using the LITHium Intelligent Agent (LITHIA): Pilot data

and proof-of-concept. *Bipolar Disord*. 2017 June; **19**(4): 259–272.

64. Tseng H-H, Luo Y, Cui S, et al. Deep reinforcement learning for automated radiation adaptation in lung cancer. *Med Phys*. 2017 December; **44**(12): 6690–6705.

65. Schofield P, Crosland A, Waheed W, et al. Patients' views of antidepressants: From first experiences to becoming expert. *Br J Gen Pract*. 2011 April; **61**(585): 142–148.

66. Kessler RC, Warner CH, Ivany C, et al. Predicting suicides after psychiatric hospitalization in US army soldiers: the army study to assess risk and rEsilience in servicemembers (Army STARRS). *JAMA Psychiatry*. 2015 January; **72**(1): 49–57.

67. Tran T, Luo W, Phung D, et al. Risk stratification using data from electronic medical records better predicts suicide risks than clinician assessments. *BMC Psychiatry*. 2014 Mar 14; **14**: 76.

68. Passos IC, Mwangi B, Cao B, et al. Identifying a clinical signature of suicidality among patients with mood disorders: A pilot study using a machine learning approach. *Journal of Affective Disorders*. 2016; **193**: 109–116.

69. Castro VM, Roberson AM, McCoy TH, Wiste A, Cagan A, Smoller JW, et al. Stratifying risk for renal insufficiency among lithium-treated patients: An electronic health record study. *Neuropsychopharmacology*. 2016 March; **41**(4): 1138–1143.

70. Mwangi B, Wu M-J, Cao B, et al. Individualized prediction and clinical staging of bipolar disorders using neuroanatomical biomarkers. *Biol Psychiatry Cogn Neurosci Neuroimaging*. 2016 March 1; **1**(2): 186–194.

71. Cao B, Passos IC, Mwangi B, et al. Hippocampal volume and verbal memory performance in late-stage bipolar disorder. *J Psychiatr Res*. 2016 February; **73**: 102–107.

72. Lavagnino L, Cao B, Mwangi B, -J. et al. Changes in the corpus callosum in women with late-stage bipolar disorder. *Acta Psychiatrica Scandinavica*. 2015; **131**(6): 458–464.

73. Passos IC, Mwangi B, Vieta E, Berk M, Kapczinski F. Areas of controversy in neuroprogression in bipolar disorder. *Acta Psychiatr Scand*. 2016 August; **134**(2): 91–103.

74. Kapczinski NS, Mwangi B, Cassidy RM, et al. Neuroprogression and illness trajectories in bipolar disorder. *Expert Review of Neurotherapeutics*. 2017; **17**(3): 277–285.

75. Silva RF, Plis SM. How to Integrate Data from Multiple Biological Layers in Mental Health? [Internet]. Personalized Psychiatry. 2019. p. 135–59. Available from: http://dx.doi.org/10.1007/978–3-030–03553-2_8

76. Honeine P, Richard C. Solving the pre-image problem in kernel machines: A direct method. 2009 IEEE International Workshop on Machine Learning for Signal Processing [Internet]. 2009; Available from: http://dx.doi.org/10.1109/mlsp.2009.5306204

77. Jobin A, Ienca M, Vayena E. The global landscape of AI ethics guidelines. Nature Machine Intelligence [Internet]. 2019; Available from: http://dx.doi.org/10.1038/s42256-019–0088-2

78. Varoquaux G, Raamana PR, Engemann DA, et al. Assessing and tuning brain decoders: Cross-validation, caveats, and guidelines. *Neuroimage*. 2017 January 15; **145**(Pt B): 166–179.

79. Thompson PM, Stein JL, Medland SE, et al. The ENIGMA Consortium: large-scale collaborative analyses of neuroimaging and genetic data. *Brain Imaging Behav*. 2014; **8**(2): 153.

80. Zhu D, Riedel BC, Jahanshad N, et al. Classification of major depressive disorder via multi-site weighted LASSO model. *Medical Image Computing and Computer Assisted Intervention – MICCAI 2017*. 2017; 159–167.

81. Developing Software Precertification Program: A Working Model [Internet]. FDA U.S. Food & Drug Administration; 2018 June. Available from: www.fda.gov/media/113802/download

82. Horvitz E, Mulligan D. Data, privacy, and the greater good. *Science*. 2015; **349**(6245): 253–255.

83. Ohno-Machado L, Bafna V, Boxwala AA, et al. iDASH: Integrating data for analysis, anonymization, and sharing. *Journal of the American Medical Informatics Association*. 2012; **19**(2): 196–201.

84. Peterson K, Deeduvanu R, Kanjamala P, Boles K. A blockchain-based approach to health information exchange networks. *NIST Workshop Blockchain Healthcare*. 2016 September; **1**: 1–10.

85. Passos IC, Ballester P, Barros RC, et al. Machine learning and big data analytics in bipolar disorder: A Position paper from the International Society for Bipolar Disorders (ISBD) Big Data Task Force. Bipolar Disorders [Internet]. 2019; Available from: http://dx.doi.org/10.1111/bdi.12828

86. Vayena E, Blasimme A, Glenn Cohen I. Machine learning in medicine: Addressing ethical challenges. *PLoS Med.* 2018 November 6; **15**(11): e1002689.

87. Gianfrancesco MA, Tamang S, Yazdany J, Schmajuk G. Potential biases in machine learning algorithms using electronic health record data. *JAMA Internal Medicine.* 2018; **178** (11): 1544.

88. O'Neil C. *Weapons of Math Destruction: How Big Data Increases Inequality and Threatens Democracy.* Crown Books; 2016.

Chapter

17

Effects of Lithium on Brain Structure in Bipolar Disorder

Jasmine Kaur, Vivian Kafantaris, and Philip R. Szeszko

17.1 Introduction

Bipolar disorder is an episodic, highly impairing mood disorder that is estimated to have a prevalence of 2–3% in the general population and is one of the leading causes of years lived with a disability.(1) Lithium is the gold standard for the treatment of bipolar disorder, and although it is a simple element, its effects on the brain are very complex.(2) Lithium's potential neurotrophic and neuroprotective effects raise the intriguing possibility that it can potentially ameliorate abnormalities in brain structure and thus alter the disease trajectory.

Clinically, over 60% of patients experience long-term reduction of mood episodes and improved quality of life with lithium maintenance treatment; 20–30% are excellent responders to lithium monotherapy with full remission for at least five years.(3) The use of lithium in bipolar disorder has been surpassed, however, by the heavily marketed second-generation antipsychotic medications, especially for its acute treatment, although in adults their efficacy is similar.(4) Because treatments that are effective for acute episodes tend to be continued for maintenance therapy, fewer individuals are likely to be prescribed lithium for maintenance treatment. Lithium may exert its strongest beneficial effects including antisuicide properties during maintenance treatment.(5) Therefore, any evidence that lithium has beneficial effects on the brain and on clinical outcome could reassert lithium's importance in the treatment armamentarium for bipolar disorder.

This chapter will critically review the results of studies that have used magnetic resonance (MR) imaging to examine the effects of lithium on brain structure in individuals with bipolar disorder. The focus will be on studies that were designed specifically to assess these effects using either cross-sectional or longitudinal designs. Thus, this selective review does not include studies that considered medication effects in ancillary or secondary analyses, given several literature reviews on this topic have already been conducted.(6) We also discuss the possibility that changes in brain volume assessed using MR imaging may be confounded by the properties of signal changes associated with properties of water osmosis.(7) We then discuss studies that have evaluated the effects of lithium on the brain in postmortem work to gain additional insight into lithium's purported mechanism(s) of action.

Studies that correlate clinical response to lithium with neuroimaging findings such as volume changes suggest a potential mechanism of therapeutic action for lithium. We therefore discuss the role of brain-derived neurotrophic factor (BDNF) in brain development and specifically its role in hippocampal growth. A potential neurotrophic component of lithium's therapeutic action would be supported if significant associations exist between changes in serum BDNF levels, hippocampus volume, and clinical response. Thus, evidence for a relationship among hippocampal structural changes associated with lithium treatment coupled with BDNF activity are discussed. Finally, we provide evidence that the effects of lithium may be most robust within the dentate gyrus of the hippocampus and discuss implications for the neurobiology of bipolar disorder. We conclude with directions for future research.

17.2 Magnetic Resonance Imaging Studies

Lithium treatment is most consistently associated with increases in hippocampus volume in multiple human cross-sectional MR imaging studies, and in the few longitudinal studies that have been published (see Table 17.1). Evidence for regionally specific findings has been inconsistent,

Table 17.1 Studies examining the effects of lithium on brain structure in bipolar disorder

Study and type	Participants	MRI methods/design	Findings
Berk et al. (21) Single-blind randomized controlled clinical trial	Healthy controls vs. patients with first-episode acute mania (YMRS ≥20) stabilized with quetiapine and lithium, and then randomized to monotherapy with lithium (to level of 0.6 mEq/L) or quetiapine (flexibly dosed up to 800 mg/day) (a) 30 healthy controls (mean age = 21.4; SD = 2.46) (b) 19 patients given quetiapine (mean age = 21.47, SD = 2.14) (c) 20 lithium (+) (mean age = 21.45, SD = 2.31)	3 T Siemens Trio Tim scanner (32-channel head coil). Baseline and longitudinal comparisons carried out using statistical parametric mapping Comparison of volume differences done using the diffeomorphic anatomical registration through exponentiated lie algebra (DARTEL) Gray and white matter volumes at baseline and changes over time in response to medication were measured Patients were assessed at baseline, 3, and 12-month follow-up. Healthy controls assessed at baseline and 12-month follow-up	Patients with mania, after stabilization on combination lithium and quetiapine treatment but before initiation of monotherapy, had reduced gray (orbitofrontal cortex, anterior cingulate cortex, inferior frontal gyrus, and cerebellum) and white (bilateral internal capsule) matter volume compared to controls Lithium was more effective than quetiapine in slowing progression of white matter volume (in left internal capsule) in patients between baseline and 12 months (but not after just 3 months) No changes in gray matter were observed in either of the treated groups
Bearden et al. (8) Cross-sectional analysis	Healthy controls vs. Bipolar I or II patients in any mood state. Patients treated with lithium for ≥ 2 weeks or unmedicated (no psychotropic medications for ≥ 2 weeks and at least 1 month off lithium) (a) 62 healthy controls (mean age = 32.7, SD = 10.1) (b) 21 lithium (+) patients (mean age = 32.9, SD = 11) with a mean serum level = 0.79 (c) 12 untreated bipolar patients, mean age = 36.5 (SD = 10.4)	MRI scans acquired with a 1.5 T GE MRI All images were processed with a series of manual and automated procedures developed at the UCLA Laboratory of Neurolmaging Hippocampal volumes measured cross-sectionally for all groups	Hippocampal volume (mostly on right side) in lithium-treated bipolar patients was as follows: • 10.3% greater compared to controls • 13.9% greater compared to untreated bipolar patients No significant relationships seen between hippocampal volume and lithium dosage, lithium blood level, or duration of lithium treatment.
Bearden et al. (17) Cross-sectional analysis	Healthy controls vs. Bipolar I or II patients in any mood state treated with lithium for ≥ 2 weeks or unmedicated (free of all psychotropic medications for ≥ 2 weeks and at least 1 month off lithium if taken previously)	MRI scans acquired with a 1.5 T GE system. All images were processed with a series of manual and automated procedures developed at the UCLA Laboratory of Neurolmaging	Lithium (+) patients had • greater overall gray matter volumes than normal controls (9.06% on left, 8.58% on right) • volumes higher by 9.8% in frontal lobe, 6.6% in temporal lobe, 10.3%

Study	Sample	Methods	Findings
	(a) 28 healthy controls (mean age = 35.9, SD = 8.5) (b) 20 lithium (+) patients (mean age = 35.1, SD = 10.8) (c) 8 lithium (−) patients (mean age = 38.6, SD 10.0) with 1 taking citalopram (20 mg)	Cortical white and gray matter density was measured cross-sectionally for all groups using MRI	• in parietal lobe (value of 8.1% in occipital lobe was nonsignificant by $p = 0.14$) • smaller cerebrospinal fluid volumes than controls and lithium (−) patients, so overall cerebral volumes were similar across the three groups Lithium (−) patients had similar gray matter volumes as controls White matter volumes did not significantly differ between lithium (+), lithium (−), and control subjects
Foland et al. (9) Cross-sectional analysis	No healthy controls included Bipolar I disorder patients: (a) 12 lithium (+) patients (mean age = 37.5, SD = 10.7) (b) 37 lithium-free patients (mean age = 42.0, SD = 9.1 years) – one patient was taking benzodiazepines and four were taking anticonvulsants	MRI scans performed on a 3 T scanner. Automated extraction of brain tissue was performed using the Brainsuite software package; manual corrections were made by an image analyst blind to patient characteristics Tensor-based morphometry was used to measure amygdala and hippocampal volumes	Global scaling factors were not significantly different among groups Lithium (+) patients showed greater total amygdala and hippocampal volumes compared to lithium (−) patients, especially on the left side: • left amygdala: 3.72% greater • right amygdala: 1.72% greater • left hippocampus: 3.45% greater • right hippocampus: 2.73% greater No significant correlations were found between volumes and illness duration, prior number of manic episodes or prior number of depressive episodes
Giakoumatos et al. (15) Cross-sectional analysis	Healthy controls vs. psychotic bipolar disorder (PBD) patients (a) 342 healthy controls (mean age = 37.1, SD 12.4) (b) 51 lithium (+) PBD patients (mean age = 35.1, SD = 13.8) (c) 135 lithium (−) PBD patients (mean age = 36.2, SD = 13.1)	Subjects were scanned at six sites, using high-resolution isotropic T1-weighted MPRAGE scans Images were run through a first-level auto-reconstruction in FreeSurfer and edited manually by trained raters Automated hippocampal subfield (HSF) segmentation was conducted through a separate FreeSurfer processing pipeline	Lithium (+) treated patients had • thicker cortices compared to lithium (−) patients • significantly greater hippocampal subfield (HSF) volumes than lithium (−) patients • similar HSF volumes compared to controls

Table 17.1 (cont.)

Study and type	Participants	MRI methods/design	Findings
Germana et al. (18) Cross-sectional analysis	No healthy controls. Patients with bipolar I, meeting criteria for remission for 6 months (a) 74 BD I patients (mean age = 43.4, SD = 11.9) with a mean duration of illness = 18.6 years (SD = 11.1 years) (b) Lithium (+): 28 patients (37.8%), mean dose = 856.7 mg (SD = 239) and mean duration of treatment = 43 months (c) On valproate: 8 patients (10.8%) with a mean dose = 1050 mg (SD = 396.4 mg) and mean duration of treatment = 65 months (d) On carbamazepine: 10 patients (13.5%), mean duration of treatment = 65 months (e) On other/combined anticonvulsants: 10 patients (13.5%) (f) On antipsychotics: 18 patients (24.3%) – 11 on olanzapine, 4 on risperidone, 3 on quetiapine	Regional gray matter thickness and hippocampal subfield (HSF) volume was extracted from MR images MRI scans were conducted using a 1.5 T GE system. Each MR image was normalized and segmented into gray matter, white matter, and CSF using unified segmentation in SPM5 using voxel-based morphometry	Lithium (+) treated patients had • increased gray matter volumes in the right subgenual anterior cingulate extending into the hypothalamus, the left postcentral gyrus, the hippocampus/amygdala complex and left insula Gray matter and total intracranial volumes were comparable between lithium (+) patients and those in other treatment groups White matter volumes were lowest in valproate patients, highest in carbamazepine patients CSF volumes lowest in antipsychotic patients, highest in valproate patients Valproate (+) patients had less white matter and higher CSF fractional volumes compared to all other groups
Hajek et al. (10) Cross-sectional analysis	Healthy controls vs. Bipolar I or II patients. Lithium (+) group must have had adequate Li treatment for ≥2 years with Li levels 0.5 to 1.2 mmol/L or every blood test taken at least twice a year Lithium (−) group must have <3 months of lithium exposure, with no lithium at least 24 months prior to scan (a) 50 healthy controls (mean age = 44.66, SD = 9.04)	MRI scans performed with available scanners at various participating sites A single rater blind to diagnostic status and lithium treatment history measured hippocampal volumes with manual mensuration	Lithium (+) patients had • significantly larger hippocampal volumes compared to lithium (−) patients • comparable hippocampal volumes as controls Among lithium (+) patients, volumes were similar regardless of the number of mood episodes while on lithium treatment. Left hippocampus was larger than right in all groups

Study	Sample	Methods	Findings
	(b) 37 lithium (+) patients (mean age = 48.08, SD = 11.17) (c) 19 lithium (−) patients (mean age = 43.16, SD = 11.68)		Lithium (+) patients had • significant association between lithium treatment duration and increased left amygdala volume • trend for an association with the right amygdala, but not for hippocampal volumes • global brain volumes comparable to lithium (−) patients and healthy controls
Hartberg et al. (16) Cross-sectional analysis	Healthy controls vs. bipolar spectrum patients (a) 300 healthy controls (mean age = 35.0, SD = 9.6) (b) 34 lithium (+) bipolar patients (mean age = 34.7, SD = 10.8) (c) 147 lithium (−) bipolar patients (mean age = 35.3, SD = 11.8)	MRI scans acquired on a 1.5 T Siemens scanner FreeSurfer (v5.2) was used to compute volumes of the hippocampal subfields, total hippocampal volume, amygdala volume, and intracranial volume (ICV)	Lithium (−) patients had • smaller volumes compared to healthy controls in the right CA1 and subiculum subfields, bilateral CA2/3, CA4/DG subfields, total hippocampal volumes, and left amygdala volumes • patients with >6 affective episodes had significantly smaller left CA1 and CA2/3 volumes compared to both the Li (+) patients and healthy controls
Lopez-Jaramillo et al. (19) Cross-sectional analysis	Healthy controls vs. euthymic bipolar I patients (a) 20 healthy controls (mean age = 39.55, SD 10.25) (b) 16 lithium (+) patients (mean age = 40.87, SD = 7.10) with a median lithium level = 0.76 mEq/L (c) 16 untreated patients (mean age = 41.81, SD = 9.70)	MRI scans acquired on a 1.5 T Phillips scanner and segmented to generate volumetric measures of cortical and subcortical brain areas, ventricles, and global brain, using Freesurfer	Lithium (+) patients compared to untreated patients had • significantly larger volumes in bilateral amygdala and bilateral thalamus • significantly smaller volumes in central and anterior half of the corpus callosum • no differences in global brain volume, volume of hippocampus, or other brain structures under study

Table 17.1 (cont.)

Study and type	Participants	MRI methods/design	Findings
			Compared to controls, lithium (+) patients had • significantly larger volumes for bilateral amygdala, bilateral thalami, and left hippocampus • more white matter hypointensities • no differences in volume of corpus callosum or global brain volume • no differences in global brain volume, basal ganglia, or other brain structures
Lyoo et al. (24) Longitudinal study	Healthy controls vs. bipolar patients randomly assigned to either lithium or valproate (VPA) treatment for 16 weeks (a) 14 healthy controls (mean age = 33.5, SD = 9.5) (b) 13 lithium (+) bipolar patients (mean age = 31.3, SD = 9.3) with a mean serum level = 0.65 mEq/L, SD = 0.19 (c) 9 VPA-treated bipolar patients (mean age = 28.5, SD = 8.5) with a mean serum level = 56.3 ng/mL, SD = 24.5	Participants underwent MRI scanning on a 1.5 T SIGNA whole-body scanner All image analyses were performed under blinded conditions Segmentations of baseline and aligned follow-up scans into images of GM, WM, and CSF were performed based on voxel intensity and spatial information using SPM	Lithium (+) patients had • increased gray matter volumes compared to both VPA-treated patients and healthy controls; this peaked at 11.5 weeks and was corresponding to an increase of 2.56% and equivalent to 17.6 cm^3 • no significant changes in white matter volumes over time VPA-treated patients had • no significant changes in gray or white matter volumes compared to healthy controls
Monkul et al. (27) Longitudinal study	13 Healthy volunteers with no DSM-IV diagnosis were given lithium over 4 weeks, titrated to lithium level of at least 0.6 mEq/L. No controls. MRI scans performed at baseline and at the end of 4 weeks Lithium doses 600–1,500 mg/day, mean dose 1,281 mg/day Mean age = 25.9, SD = 10 Mean lithium levels: (a) 1st week: 0.34 mEq/L (b) 2nd week: 0.53 mEq/L (c) 3rd week: 0.67 mEq/L (d) 4th week: 0.83 mEq/L	MRIs were performed on a 1.5 T GE scanner Voxel-based morphometry was performed using SPM2 This study defined the cingulate, dorsolateral prefrontal cortex (DLPFC), amygdala, and hippocampus bilaterally as regions of interest (ROIs)	At the end of 4 weeks of lithium administration: • total white matter volumes were increased by 2% • total brain volume and total gray matter volume remained unchanged • left DLPFC (Brodmann's area 46) gray matter volume was significantly increased • left anterior cingulate gray matter volume was significantly increased • no ROIs showed significant change in white matter

Study	Sample	Methods	Results
			- no other ROIs (other than listed above) showed significant change in gray matter - mean lithium blood levels were not significantly correlated with changes
Moore et al. (25) Longitudinal study	No healthy controls. Bipolar I patients included (all in depressed state) Patients on psychotropic medications first had a minimum 2-week washout period (depending on half-life of the medication taken) 10 Lithium (+) bipolar patients (mean age = 33.0, SD = 15.1) with lithium level about 0.8 mEq/L	MRI scans conducted on 1.5 T system. Image formatting and volumetric measurements were made using image-processing software Medx and National Institutes of Health (NIH) Image software MRi scans were done at baseline (medication-free, after a >2-week medication washout) and after 4 weeks of lithium treatment	Compared to lithium (−) treated patients, lithium (+) patients had - significantly increased total gray matter volume (8 of 10 patients) - mean change was 3%, about a 24 cm³ increase in total gray matter volume - no significant changes in white matter volume or cerebral water content
Moore et al. (26) Longitudinal study	No healthy controls. Bipolar I or II patients, all in depressed or euthymic state Minimum 2-week med washout period (depending on half-life of the medication taken) (a) 28 Lithium (+) bipolar patients; 10 patients participated in Moore et al (25) study (mean age = 33, SD = 11) with lithium level about 0.8 mEq/L after first week of treatment	MRI scans conducted on 1.5 T Signa scanner. Image formatting and volumetric measurements were made using image-processing software Medx and National Institutes of Health (NIH) Image software MRI scans were done at baseline (medication-free, after a >2-week medication washout) and after 4 weeks of lithium treatment	Lithium (+) treated patients had - no changes in total brain volume or white matter volume - an increase in total gray matter volume in 20 patients (including both treatment responders and nonresponders) - trend for a correlation between clinical improvement and change in gray matter volume Among lithium treatment responders: - 8% increase in the left subgenual prefrontal cortex GM volume
Sassi et al. (20) Cross-sectional analysis	Healthy controls vs. lithium (+) bipolar patients vs. untreated bipolar patients off all psychotropic meds for at least 2 weeks (usually due to noncompliance) (a) 46 Healthy controls (mean age = 35.5, SD = 10.3) (b) 17 Lithium (+) bipolar patients (mean age = 31.1, SD = 8.8) of whom 14 were euthymic and 3	3D MRI images were obtained with a 1.5 T-GE scanner. Gray matter, white matter, and intracranial volumes (ICV) were measured by a trained rater, blind to patient's identity or group assignment, using a semiautomated method and following standardized procedures, after having achieved intra-class	Lithium (+) patients had - larger intracranial and total gray matter volumes than both untreated patients and healthy controls - no correlation between lithium dose and volumes

Table 17.1 (cont.)

Study and type	Participants	MRI methods/design	Findings
	were depressed. Mean dosage = 1,111.8 mg/day, SD = 356) and mean length of treatment was 131 weeks, SD = 250 (c) 12 Untreated bipolar patients (mean age = 37.7, SD = 10.6) of whom 4 were euthymic, 7 depressed, and 1 hypomanic	correlation coefficients for each of these measures of 0.90	
Selek et al. (23) Longitudinal study	Healthy controls vs. bipolar I patients in various states (euthymic, depressed, manic, hypomanic) Participants were required to be drug-free for at least 2 weeks prior to study (a) 11 healthy controls (mean age = 35.57, SD = 14.74) (b) 24 lithium (+) bipolar patients (mean age = 31.75, SD = 8.12) with a mean serum level = 0.67 mEq/L	MRI scans performed on 1.5 T GE scanner Cortical reconstruction and volumetric segmentation were performed with the Freesurfer image analysis suite. Prefrontal cortex, dorsolateral prefrontal cortex, anterior cingulate cortex, hippocampus, and amygdala volumes were obtained MRI scans were completed at baseline and 4 weeks after lithium treatment	Lithium (+) who were clinical responders had • increased volumes of the left prefrontal cortex, especially left dorsolateral prefrontal cortex after treatment. Lithium (+) who were clinical nonresponders had • decreased left hippocampal and right anterior cingulate cortex volumes after treatment compared to baseline

however. Bearden and colleagues (8) reported that (mainly right) hippocampal volume in lithium-treated patients with bipolar disorder was 10.3% greater compared to non-medicated healthy controls and 13.9% greater compared to bipolar patients not treated with lithium. In that study, there were no significant associations between hippocampal volume and lithium dosage, blood level, or treatment duration. Similarly, Foland and colleagues (9) reported that patients with bipolar disorder treated with lithium demonstrated greater volume compared to bipolar patients not taking lithium including the (% in parentheses) left amygdala (3.72%), right amygdala (1.72%), left hippocampus (3.45%), and right hippocampus (2.73%). There were no significant associations between brain volume and illness duration, and prior number of manic or depressive episodes. Along these lines, Hajek et al. (10) reported that patients with bipolar disorder treated with lithium had significantly larger hippocampal volume compared to patients with bipolar disorder not treated with lithium and healthy controls. In addition, volumes were comparable among patients treated with lithium regardless of the number of prior mood episodes. In one of the few pediatric studies conducted to date, Baykara et al. (11) reported that right hippocampal volume was enlarged in patients with bipolar disorder treated with lithium, relative to untreated controls.

A few cross-sectional studies investigated the effects of lithium on hippocampal volume in patients with bipolar disorder who had either very short- or long-term treatment. Hajek et al. (12) studied 17 patients with bipolar disorder who had at least 2 years of regularly monitored lithium treatment, 12 bipolar patients with less than 3 months of total lifetime lithium treatment and no lithium treatment prior to 2 years before an MR imaging scan and 11 healthy controls. Voxel-based morphometry indicated that the non-lithium treatment group had smaller left hippocampal volume compared to controls with a trend for lower volumes than the lithium-treated group who did not differ from controls, consistent with meta-analysis (13). At the other end of the spectrum, Yucel et al. (14) compared hippocampal volume among three groups of patients with bipolar disorder including those treated with lithium between one and eight weeks, patients who were unmedicated at the time of scan, and patients treated with either valproic acid or lamotrigine. Results indicated a bilateral increase in hippocampal volume that was evident in the head of the hippocampus among patients treated with lithium, even after a brief period of treatment. These findings suggest that the effects of lithium on the brain may be evident even within weeks of treatment initiation.

Several studies examined the relationship between lithium treatment and hippocampal subfield volumes using MR imaging. In one of the largest cross-sectional studies to date Giakoumatos et al. (15) reported that 51 patients with psychotic bipolar disorder treated with lithium had thicker cortical volume and greater hippocampal subfield volumes compared to 135 patients with psychotic bipolar disorder not being treated with lithium and 342 healthy controls. Patients being treated with lithium had comparable hippocampal subregion volumes as healthy controls. In a study by Hartberg et al. (16), investigation of hippocampal subfield volumes revealed smaller total hippocampal volume, including the right CA1 and subiculum subfields, and bilateral CA2/3, CA4/DG subfields among the patients not being treated with lithium compared to healthy controls. Interestingly, in that study there was a significant positive association between lithium treatment duration and larger amygdala volume.

Other cross-sectional studies provide evidence that the effects of lithium may be more widespread in the brain. For example, Bearden et al. (17) reported that patients with bipolar disorder treated with lithium ($n = 20$) had greater volume in the frontal (9.8%), temporal (6.6%), and parietal (10.3%) lobes compared to eight patients with bipolar disorder of whom only one was taking psychotropic medication (i.e., citalopram). In addition, patients with bipolar disorder not treated with lithium had gray matter volumes comparable to healthy controls ($n = 28$). Also, in that study no differences in white matter volume were observed between patients treated with lithium and patients not receiving lithium. Germana et al. (18) reported that patients with bipolar disorder treated with lithium had more gray matter in the right subgenual anterior cingulate, left postcentral gyrus, hippocampus/amygdala complex, and left insula. In a study by Lopez-Jaramillo et al. (19), patients treated with lithium had significantly larger bilateral amygdala and thalamic volume (but no differences in hippocampal volume) compared to patients with bipolar disorder not treated with lithium. Moreover, compared to controls, patients treated with lithium had significantly larger bilateral amygdala, bilateral thalamus, and left hippocampus volume. Lastly, Sassi et al. (20) reported that patients with bipolar disorder treated with lithium had greater total brain gray matter volume compared to patients not currently receiving psychotropic treatment and healthy controls.

Results from longitudinal neuroimaging studies in patients with bipolar disorder treated with lithium provide stronger support compared to cross-sectional studies for the hypothesis that enhancement of neuroplasticity is a component of lithium's therapeutic mechanism. Such studies have demonstrated brain changes in both the gray and white matter. In a single-blind randomized controlled clinical trial, Berk and colleagues (21) reported that lithium was more effective than quetiapine in slowing progression of white matter volume loss within the left internal capsule between baseline and twelve months without associated gray matter changes. In a study by Yucel et al. (22), patients were rescanned twice after baseline: approximately two years and then again four years following initiation of lithium maintenance therapy. They found increases of 4–5% in hippocampal volume after two years and these increases were maintained at the four-year scan and associated with improvements in cognitive functioning.

Several controlled trials investigated the effects of lithium on brain imaging measures prior to and then following controlled treatment. In a longitudinal study of twenty-four patients with bipolar disorder, Selek et al. (23) conducted MR imaging scans at baseline and then again following four weeks of lithium treatment. Participants were required to be drug-free for at least two weeks prior to study entry. Patients with bipolar disorder categorized as clinical responders to lithium had increased left prefrontal volume (and in particular the dorsolateral prefrontal cortex) following treatment. In contrast, patients with bipolar disorder categorized as clinical nonresponders to lithium had decreased left hippocampal and right anterior cingulate cortex volume following treatment. Lyoo et al. (24) conducted longitudinal MR imaging and evaluated clinical response to treatment in twenty-two patients with bipolar disorder

who were psychotropic drug naive to mood stabilizers and antipsychotics. Patients were randomly assigned to receive either valproic acid or lithium and followed for sixteen weeks. Patients treated with lithium had greater gray matter volume (corresponding to an increase of 2.56%), which peaked at approximately ten to twelve weeks of treatment compared to both patients treated with valproic acid and healthy controls.

Two studies by Moore et al. (25) (26) examined the effects of lithium treatment on MR imaging measures in the context of a controlled clinical trial. In both studies, patients had a two-week medication washout period and were scanned prior to and then again following four weeks of blinded lithium treatment. In the first study (25), eight of the ten patients treated with lithium demonstrated an increase of approximately 3% in total gray matter volume without associated changes in white matter volume or cerebral water content. In the second study (26), these investigators reported an increase in total gray matter volume in twenty patients, which included both treatment responders and nonresponders. There was a trend for a correlation between clinical improvement and change in gray matter volume and increases were most prominent in the prefrontal cortex. Notably, there was an 8% increase in the left subgenual prefrontal cortex gray matter volume without any observed changes in total brain or white matter volume among patients treated with lithium.

One longitudinal study should be noted given that it investigated the effects of lithium on the brain in thirteen right-handed healthy volunteers (27). These individuals received MR imaging exams prior to and then following four weeks of lithium treatment at therapeutically relevant dosages. Using optimized voxel-based morphometry results indicated that both right and left dorsolateral prefrontal cortex and left anterior cingulate gray matter volume increased following lithium treatment. In addition, total white matter volume increased in contrast to total brain volume and total gray matter volume, which demonstrated no changes after lithium treatment. These data thus highlight brain changes associated with lithium treatment in the absence of a psychiatric illness confound.

17.3 Mechanisms of Brain Changes Associated with Lithium Treatment

Some data suggest that the effects of lithium on the brain may be a function of changes in osmosis that affect the MR signal. In a study by Phatak and colleagues (28), they sought to investigate whether lithium administration alters brain water home-ostasis and possible purported mechanisms invol-ving changes in inositol concentration. Lithium chloride was administered to rats for either eleven days or five weeks. Brains were assayed for tissue water and for inositol using chromatography-mass spectrometry. These investigators found that lithium administration for five weeks was associated with a 3.1% increase in tissue water content within the frontal cortex and hippocam-pus. The white matter in the brain was not inves-tigated and effects were not observed in rats fed lithium chloride for eleven days. The findings appeared to be unrelated to both changes in brain inositol concentration and/or blood sodium concentration.

Cousins et al. (7) acquired MR imaging scans in thirty-one healthy males prior to and then following administration of lithium or placebo for eleven days. They used two techniques to quantify brain structure including voxel-based morphometry, which segments tissue into differ-ent classes using signal intensity and structural image evaluation (using normalization of atro-phy), which provides information regarding changes in the position of boundaries within the brain. They reported that voxel-based morpho-metry was associated with an increase in gray matter volume that was not evident with placebo. In contrast, the use of structural image evaluation, using normalization of atrophy revealed no dif-ference between lithium and placebo. These results were interpreted to suggest that lithium might influence the intensity of the magnetic reso-nance signal producing artifactual volumetric findings related to alterations in image contrast. Moreover, administration of lithium was asso-ciated with a reduction in the T1 relaxation of the gray matter only. More recently, Necus et al. (29) used multinuclear 3D lithium magnetic reso-nance imaging (7Li-MRI) to identify lithium's location in the brain and possible mechanisms of action focusing on the white matter.

Postmortem animal studies investigating the effects of lithium on brain morphology may shed additional light on the underlying neurobiological processes contributing to volume changes. For example, studies that show increased neuronal or synaptic functioning following lithium expo-sure could further refute the osmotic etiology of the increased volumes associated with lithium treatment. Several animal studies reported an association between lithium dose and serum level, duration of lithium exposure and changes in brain morphology. Riadh et al. (30) examined the relationship between lithium dose (1 g/kg vs. 2 g/kg) and duration of exposure (one month vs. three months) on changes in brain volume. The low-dose 1 g/kg/day lithium group with clinically subtherapeutic serum levels (0.3–0.42 mEq/L) exhibited no change in brain weight or regional changes at either time point. In contrast, the higher-dose lithium group (2 g/kg/day; levels 0.75–0.8 mEq/L), which is considered mid-therapeutic in humans, demonstrated an increase in brain weight after one month. Notably, histo-logical changes were only observed after three months and only in the group that achieved serum levels in the therapeutic range. In particu-lar, the entorhinal cortex demonstrated increased myelination density after three months in the 2 g/kg/day dose group while the CA3 area of the hippocampus had increased neurite growth and axon diameter.

A rodent study by Vernon et al. (31) used MR imaging and autopsy findings to compare the effects of chronic treatment with haloperidol, or lithium or vehicle control on whole and regional brain volumes in adolescent rats. Haloperidol was associated with reductions in whole brain volume (−4%) and cortical gray matter (−6%) that appeared concomitant with an increase in the corpus striatum (+14%). In contrast, chronic lithium treatment was associated with increases in whole-brain volume (+5%) and cortical gray mat-ter (+3%) without associated changes in striatal volume. Particularly noteworthy was that follow-ing eight weeks of drug withdrawal, the changes associated with haloperidol administration nor-malized in contrast to the lithium-treated animals that retained significantly greater total brain volumes, which was confirmed postmortem. Shim et al. (32) demonstrated enhanced cell firing of granule cells in the dentate gyrus of rats treated with 2 mEq/L/kg/day of lithium for two weeks that were associated with mid-therapeutic levels of lithium (0.51–0.78 mEq/L). Taken together, these studies suggest that administration of lithium is associated with cellular changes in rodent studies at therapeutically relevant levels and are consistent with results of MR imaging studies.

17.4 Brain-Derived Neurotrophic Factor

BDNF is regulated by the BDNF gene located on chromosome 11 and plays a major role in brain development, including canonical nerve growth factor. It is known to be instrumental in the central nervous system, and especially the hippocampus, to support existing neurons and to facilitate new growth of neurons. BDNF has several known single nucleotide polymorphisms that have been demonstrated to have functional effects in the brain. BDNF protein readily crosses the blood–brain barrier (33) and the high correlation between peripheral and cerebrospinal fluid levels indicates that peripheral BDNF levels may indeed reflect central BDNF activity.(34) Changes in serum BDNF levels may be a useful biomarker of lithium's efficacy that may be mediated by the hippocampus.

Cross-sectional studies consistently report strong correlations between peripheral BDNF levels and hippocampal volumes.(35)(36) One longitudinal study assessed both BDNF and hippocampal volume concurrently in relation to outcome.(37) That study involved a nonpsychiatric sample of healthy older adults who were randomly assigned to receive training in aerobic exercise or stretching exercises for one year. Following the aerobic exercise training, but not the stretching intervention, the volume of the anterior hippocampus increased bilaterally by 2%. Participants with the greatest increases in anterior hippocampal volume also had the largest increases in serum BDNF levels. The observed increases in hippocampal volume following exercise training were associated with improvements in memory, indicating that the increased volume confers functional benefits.

A meta-regression analysis of cross-sectional data from over 1,100 adult participants confirmed that serum BDNF levels are significantly lower in patients with mania or bipolar depression than in healthy controls.(38) It is well established that lithium upregulates BDNF gene expression in rodent studies.(39)(40) Moreover, acute lithium response in bipolar patients is associated with increased BDNF levels.(41)

In an adult longitudinal study in mania, a significant increase (ranging from 25% to 46%) in plasma BDNF level was observed following twenty-eight days of monotherapy with lithium compared to pretreatment.(42) One longitudinal treatment study of children with bipolar disorder included a peripheral BDNF protein level assessment. In that study (43), peripheral BDNF mRNA levels, a measure of BDNF gene expression, were assessed before and after eight weeks of treatment of whom the majority were receiving lithium. Moreover, increases in BDNF mRNA levels significantly correlated with reductions in mania severity.

Support for the possibility that early increases in serum BDNF levels may prove to be a useful biomarker of lithium's long-term efficacy is provided by a cross-sectional study of euthymic adult bipolar patients receiving lithium prophylaxis for at least five years.(3) Even during euthymic periods, patients differed in BDNF levels according to their long-term course of illness. Mean BDNF levels were highest in the group of excellent responders to lithium monotherapy (n = 30; 21.3%) who were in full remission without a recurrence for at least five years, followed by partial responders to adjunctive lithium (n = 61; 43.3%) in whom recurrence rates decreased by at least 50% following lithium initiation. The remaining patients who were euthymic, but had less than a 50% decline in recurrences since lithium initiation had significantly lower mean BDNF levels than the responder groups and were the only patient group that had lower BDNF levels than healthy controls.

In an early two-phase study of lithium vs. valproic acid in a chemically induced animal model of mania, Frey et al. (44) administered saline vs. lithium vs. valproic acid following seven days of treatment with amphetamine in an acute treatment model. There was no change in BDNF within the hippocampus with either saline or valproic acid, but a significant increase in BDNF concentration was observed following seven days of lithium treatment. It is noteworthy that this effect was observed only among amphetamine-treated animals, suggesting that it is not simply the presence of lithium that increases

BDNF levels. In a prophylaxis model, animals were pretreated for seven days with saline vs. lithium vs. valproic acid. When challenged with amphetamine vs. saline for seven days (to induce hyperactivity) only the rats pretreated with saline exhibited the behavior and decreased BDNF levels. The lithium pretreated rats showed no increase in movement and had increased BDNF levels following amphetamine.

The robust neuroprotective effects of lithium and its relation to BDNF are further supported by studies that utilized chemically induced animal models of mania. In one study, rats given the chemical ouabain exhibited hyperlocomotion, which was associated with reduced BDNF levels in the hippocampus.(40) This study compared the effects of lithium vs. valproic acid on hippocampal BDNF. Although both treatments were effective in reducing manic-like behavior, lithium, but not valproic acid administration reversed the chemically induced decreases in hippocampal BDNF, thus supporting its neurotrophic properties. Moreover, the lithium-induced increases in hippocampal BDNF were associated with a reduction in manic-like behavior after seven days of lithium treatment. Notably, in further support of lithium's prophylactic efficacy, pretreatment with lithium, but not valproic acid prevented the chemically induced decrease in BDNF levels observed in this study.

17.5 Hippocampal Subregion Neuroplasticity

Because the dentate gyrus is one of the most neuroplastic areas of the brain and contains the highest concentration of neurotrophic factors, early changes in volume may be detected there more readily compared to other brain regions. Therefore, early changes detected in the dentate gyrus may serve as a proxy for changes occurring in other parts of the brain that may be clinically relevant to bipolar disorder. This is supported from the results of several animal studies. Immunohistochemical analyses indicated that lithium produced a significant 25% increase in the BrdU-labeled cells in the dentate gyrus of the rodent hippocampus.(45) In addition, lithium's more robust neurotrophic properties are supported by the significantly increased cell proliferation in the dentate gyrus of the adult rat after lithium exposure, but not after exposure to fluoxetine or an investigational agent.(46) Hammonds and Shim (39) reported that four weeks of lithium treatment was associated with upregulation of BDNF and Shim et al. (47) reported that lithium treatment increased the amount and distribution of dendritic branches within the dentate gyrus. Lithium's neurotrophic effects in the dentate gyrus may therefore be mediated, at least in part, by BDNF.

In a four-week comparison with olanzapine treatment, Hammonds and Shim (39) demonstrated that rats receiving lithium demonstrated a significantly greater upregulation of BDNF in the dentate gyrus compared to rats receiving olanzapine. Neither medication produced significant changes in BDNF in hippocampal subregions other than the dentate gyrus, supporting the hypothesis that lithium may exert neurotrophic effects on specific subregions of the hippocampus. Earlier work by this group investigating the effects of two weeks of lithium exposure vs. vehicle on rat hippocampus found no effect on BDNF levels in DG or CA1. This lack of effect of lithium on hippocampal BDNF is consistent with Frey et al. (44), where rats treated for fourteen days with saline and lithium demonstrated no change in BDNF, but those treated with amphetamine and lithium did. In an earlier study from that group Shim et al. (32) reported a functional effect on synaptic signaling in the dentate gyrus among lithium-treated rats as demonstrated by increased cell firing in granule cells. Although regional volume changes in areas other than the hippocampus may also correlate with changes in serum BDNF, the investigation of the dentate gyrus can be readily accomplished at 3 T and its boundaries can be delineated, thereby facilitating replication by other investigators.(48)

17.6 Summary and Future Directions

Although its exact therapeutic mechanism of action is still unknown, there is emerging support for lithium's hypothesized neurotrophic and neuroprotective effects in adults with bipolar disorder from both cross-sectional and longitudinal MR imaging studies. In addition, the magnitude of volume changes reported following lithium initiation may suggest a possible contribution from changes in white matter architecture, especially increases in myelin and myelin-producing oligo-dendrocytes.(49)

Several studies indicate a relationship between increases in gray matter volume and lithium treatment that may be evident soon after initiating treatment. Increases in hippocampus volume and serum BDNF protein levels are associated with treatment response across a variety of disorders and both can be measured reliably using clinically available tools. BDNF plays an important role in regulating hippocampal neurogenesis and protecting neuronal viability.(50)

Taken together, an association between volume changes in the dentate gyrus subregion of the hippocampus and changes in serum BDNF levels would corroborate that lithium has a central neurotrophic effect and that peripheral BDNF levels may reflect neurotrophic changes in the brain. If confirmed in larger studies, serum BDNF levels would have clinical applicability as an early treatment biomarker of lithium response. Currently, it is unknown if hippocampal volume changes in humans are due to an increased number of neurons and/or neuronal connections and whether they directly contribute to lithium's therapeutic efficacy. A focus on changes within the dentate gyrus subregion of the hippocampus, where neurotrophic changes may be the most pronounced could make it easier for other groups to localize and replicate findings using highly reliable MR imaging approaches.(48)

Future studies could examine whether the presence of early biomarkers correlate with long-term prophylactic response to lithium maintenance treatment and assess whether lithium treatment during adolescence could ameliorate neurodevelopmental abnormalities that are believed to play a role in bipolar pathogenesis. In addition, future work can examine whether early increases in serum BDNF protein levels can be used to predict longer-term lithium response. Specifically, the use of a within-subjects design that measures change in BDNF levels and dentate gyrus volume relative to baseline over differing amounts of time in lithium-naive patients will enable investigators to capture the specific treatment effects of lithium in each subject.

Significant associations between increases in hippocampal volume with lithium response could open new opportunities to potentially correct neurodevelopmental abnormalities in pediatric patients. This has the potential to change disease trajectory for a significant proportion of young patients suffering from this common and devastating brain disorder. Confirmation of the clinical utility of these potential BDNF biomarkers could have a great impact on maintenance treatment selection for patients who may not have been offered an early lithium trial. In addition, confirmation of a beneficial effect on neuroplasticity will also advance our understanding of lithium's mechanism of therapeutic action in bipolar disorder and help elucidate the underlying pathophysiology of the disease itself.

We also acknowledge the contribution of BDNF gene polymorphisms to lithium's prophylactic efficacy may have clinical applications in the future.(51) The degree of early change in serum BDNF level within an individual patient is likely to be a more sensitive and accurate biomarker of treatment response, given the multiple environmental factors that may affect clinical response. We therefore conclude that the association between lithium-related changes in serum BDNF protein levels, changes in hippocampal (and dentate gyrus) morphology, and improvement in mood state warrants further study in bipolar disorder.

References

1. Ferrari AJ, Stockings E, Khoo JP, Erskine HE, Degenhardt L, Vos T, Whiteford HA. The prevalence and burden of bipolar disorder: findings from the Global Burden of Disease Study 2013. *Bipolar Disord*. 2016 August; **18**(5): 440–450. DOI 10.1111/bdi.12423. PubMed PMID: 27566286.

2. Machado-Vieira R, Manji HK, Zarate CA Jr: The role of lithium in the treatment of bipolar disorder: convergent evidence for neurotrophic effects as a unifying hypothesis. *Bipolar Disord*. 2009 June; **11** Suppl 2 : 92–109.PMCID: 2800957.

3. Suwalska A, Sobieska M, Rybakowski JK. Serum brain-derived neurotrophic factor in euthymic bipolar patients on prophylactic lithium therapy. *Neuropsychobiology*. 2010; **62**(4): 229–234. Epub 2010 August 14. PMID: 20714172.

4. Baldessarini RJ, Tondo L, Vázquez GH. Pharmacological treatment of adult bipolar disorder. *Mol Psychiatry*. 2018 April 20. DOI 10.1038/s41380-018-0044-2. [Epub ahead of print] Review. PubMed PMID: 29679069.

5. Schaffer A, Isometsä ET, Tondo L, et al. Epidemiology, neurobiology and pharmacological interventions related to suicide deaths and suicide attempts in bipolar disorder: Part I of a report of the

International Society for Bipolar Disorders Task Force on Suicide in Bipolar Disorder. *Aust N Z J Psychiatry.* 2015 September; **49**(9): 785–802. DOI 10.1177/0004867415594427. Epub 2015 July 16. Review. PubMed PMID: 26185269; PubMed Central PMCID: PMC5116383.

6. Hafeman DM, Chang KD, Garrett AS, Sanders EM, Phillips ML. Effects of medication on neuroimaging findings in bipolar disorder: an updated review. *Bipolar Disord.* 2012 June;**14**(4): 375–410. DOI 10.1111/j.1399-5618.2012.01023.x. Review. PubMed PMID: 22631621.

7. Cousins DA, Aribisala B, Ferrier IN, Blamire AM. Lithium, gray matter, and magnetic resonance imaging signal. *Biol Psychiatry.* 2013; **73**: 652–657.

8. Bearden CE, Thompson PM, Dutton RA, et al. Three-dimensional mapping of hippocampal anatomy in unmedicated and lithium-treated patients with bipolar disorder. *Neuropsychopharmacology.* 2008 May; **33**(6): 1229–1238. Epub 2007 August 8. PubMed PMID: 17687266.

9. Foland LC, Altshuler LL, Sugar CA, et al. Increased volume of the amygdala and hippocampus in bipolar patients treated with lithium. *Neuroreport.* 2008 January 22; **19**(2): 221–224. DOI 10.1097/WNR.0b013e3282f48108. PubMed PMID: 18185112; PubMed Central PMCID: PMC3299336.

10. Hajek T, Bauer M, Simhandl C, et al. Neuroprotective effect of lithium on hippocampal volumes in bipolar disorder independent of long-term treatment response. *Psychol Med.* 2014 February; **44**(3): 507–517. DOI 10.1017/S0033291713001165. Epub 2013 May 31. PubMed PMID: 23721695.

11. Baykara B, Inal-Emiroglu N, Karabay N, et.al Increased hippocampal volumes in lithium treated adolescents with bipolar disorders: A structural MRI study. *J Affect Disord.* 2012 May; **138**(3): 433–439. DOI 10.1016/j.jad.2011.12.047. Epub 2012 February 9.

12. Hajek T, Cullis J, Novak T, et al. Hippocampal volumes in bipolar disorders: Opposing effects of illness burden and lithium treatment. *Bipolar Disord.* 2012 May; **14**(3): 261–270. DOI 10.1111/j.1399-5618.2012.01013.x.

13. Hajek T, Kopecek M, Höschl C, Alda M. Smaller hippocampal volumes in patients with bipolar disorder are masked by exposure to lithium: a meta-analysis. *J Psychiatry Neurosci.* 2012 September; **37**(5): 333–343. DOI:10.1503/jpn.110143.

14. Yucel K, Taylor VH, McKinnon MC, et al. Bilateral hippocampal volume increase in patients with bipolar disorder and short-term lithium treatment. *Neuropsychopharmacology.* 2008 January; **33**(2): 361–367. Epub 2007 April 4. PubMed PMID: 17406649.

15. Giakoumatos CI, Nanda P, Mathew IT, et al. Effects of lithium on cortical thickness and hippocampal subfield volumes in psychotic bipolar disorder. *J Psychiatr Res.* 2015 February; **61**: 180–187. DOI 10.1016/j.jpsychires.2014.12.008. Epub 2014 December 23. PubMed PMID: 25563516; PubMed Central PMCID: PMC4859940.

16. Hartberg CB, Jørgensen KN, Haukvik UK, et al. Lithium treatment and hippocampal subfields and amygdala volumes in bipolar disorder. *Bipolar Disord.* 2015 August; **17**(5): 496–506. DOI:10.1111/bdi.12295. Epub 2015 March 24. PubMed PMID: 25809287.

17. Bearden CE, Thompson PM, Dalwani M, et al. Greater cortical gray matter density in lithium-treated patients with bipolar disorder. *Biol Psychiatry.* 2007 July 1; **62**(1): 7–16. Epub 2007 January 19. PubMed PMID: 17240360; PubMed Central PMCID: PMC3586797.

18. Germaná C, Kempton MJ, Sarnicola A, et al. The effects of lithium and anticonvulsants on brain structure in bipolar disorder. *Acta Psychiatr Scand.* 2010 December; **122**(6): 481–487. DOI 10.1111/j.1600-0447.2010.01582.x. PubMed PMID: 20560901.

19. López-Jaramillo C, Vargas C, Díaz-Zuluaga AM, et al. Increased hippocampal, thalamus and amygdala volume in long-term lithium-treated bipolar I disorder patients compared with unmedicated patients and healthy subjects. *Bipolar Disord.* 2017 February; **19**(1): 41–49. DOI 10.1111/bdi.12467. Epub 2017 Feb 27. PubMed PMID: 28239952.

20. Sassi RB, Nicoletti M, Brambilla P, et al. Increased gray matter volume in lithium-treated bipolar disorder patients. *Neurosci Lett.* 2002 August 30; **329**(2):243–245. PubMed PMID: 12165422.

21. Berk M, Dandash O, Daglas R, et al. Neuroprotection after a first episode of mania: a randomized controlled maintenance trial comparing the effects of lithium and quetiapine on grey and white matter volume. *Transl Psychiatry.* 2017 January 24; **7**(1): e1011. DOI 10.1038/tp.2016.281. Erratum in: *Transl Psychiatry.* 2017 February 21;**7**(2):e1041. PubMed PMID: 28117843; PubMed Central PMCID: PMC5545739.

22. Yucel K, McKinnon MC, Taylor VH, et al. Bilateral hippocampal volume increases after long-term lithium treatment in patients with bipolar disorder: A longitudinal MRI study. *Psychopharmacology (Berl).* 2007 December; **195**

(3): 357–367. Epub 2007 August 20. PubMed PMID: 17705060.

23. Selek S, Nicoletti M, Zunta-Soares GB, et al. A longitudinal study of fronto-limbic brain structures in patients with bipolar I disorder during lithium treatment. *J Affect Disord.* 2013 September 5; **150**(2): 629–633. DOI 10.1016/j.jad.2013.04.020. Epub 2013 June 10. PubMed PMID: 23764385.

24. Lyoo IK, Dager SR, Kim JE, et al. Lithium-induced gray matter volume increase as a neural correlate of treatment response in bipolar disorder: A longitudinal brain imaging study. *Neuropsychopharmacology.* 2010 July; **35**(8): 1743–1750. DOI 10.1038/npp.2010.41. Epub 2010 March 31. PubMed PMID: 20357761; PubMed Central PMCID: PMC3055479.

25. Moore GJ, Bebchuk JM, Wilds IB, Chen G, Manji HK. Lithium-induced increase in human brain grey matter. *Lancet.* 2000 Oct 7;356 (9237):1241–2. Erratum in: *Lancet* 2000 December 16;356(9247):2104.Menji HK [corrected to Manji HK]. PubMed PMID: 11072948.

26. Moore GJ, Cortese BM, Glitz DA, et al. A longitudinal study of the effects of lithium treatment on prefrontal and subgenual prefrontal gray matter volume in treatment-responsive bipolar disorder patients. *J Clin Psychiatry.* 2009 April 21; **70**(5): 699–705. DOI:10.4088/JCP.07m03745. PubMed PMID: 19389332.

27. Monkul ES, Matsuo K, Nicoletti MA, et al. Prefrontal gray matter increases in healthy individuals after lithium treatment: A voxel-based morphometry study. *Neurosci Lett.* 2007 December 11; **429**(1): 7–11. Epub 2007 October 10. PubMed PMID: 17996370; PubMed Central PMCID: PMC2693231.

28. Phatak P, Shaldivin A, King LS, Shapiro P, Regenold WT. Lithium and inositol: effects on brain water homeostasis in the rat, *Psychopharmacology (Berl).* 2006; **186**: 41–47.

29. Necus JM, Sinha N, Smith FE, et al. White matter microstructural properties in bipolar disorder and its relationship to the spatial distribution of lithium in the brain. Submitted doi:http://dx.doi.org/10.1101/346528 bioRxiv preprint first posted online Jun. 13, 2018.

30. Riadh N, Allagui MS, Bourogaa E, et al. Neuroprotective and neurotrophic effects of long term lithium treatment in mouse brain. *Biometals.* 2011; **24**: 747–757. DOI 10.1007/s10534-011-9433-6.

31. Vernon AC, Natesan S, Crum WR, et al. Contrasting effects of haloperidol and lithium on

rodent brain structure: A magnetic resonance imaging study with postmortem confirmation. *Biol Psychiatry.* 2012 May 15; **71**(10): 855–863. DOI 10.1016/j.biopsych.2011.12.004. Epub 2012 January 15. PubMed PMID: 22244831.

32. Shim SS, Hammonds MD, Ganocy SJ, Calabrese JR. Effects of sub-chronic lithium treatment on synaptic plasticity in the dentate gyrus of rat hippocampal slices. *Prog Neuropsychopharmacol Biol Psychiatry.* 2007 March 30; **31**(2): 343–347.Epub 2006 November 9. PubMed PMID: 17097205.

33. Pan W, Banks WA, Fasold MB, Bluth J, Kastin AJ. Transport of brain-derived neurotrophic factor across the blood-brain barrier. *Neuropharmacology.* 1998 December; **37**(12): 1553–1561. PubMed PMID: 9886678.

34. Pillai A, Kale A, Joshi S, et al. Decreased BDNF levels in CSF of drug-naive first-episode psychotic subjects: correlation with plasma BDNF and psychopathology. *Int J Neuropsychopharmacol.* 2010 May; **13**(4): 535–539. Epub 2009 November 27. PubMed PMID: 19941699.

35. Eker C, Kitis O, Taneli F, et al. Correlation of serum BDNF levels with hippocampal volumes in first episode, medication-free depressed patients. *Eur Arch Psychiatry Clin Neurosci.* 2010 October; **260**(7): 527–533.DOI 10.1007/s00406-010-0110-5. Epub 2010 March 20.

36. Rizos E, Papathanasiou M, Michalopoulou P, et al. Association of serum BDNF levels with hippocampal volumes in first psychotic episode drug-naïve schizophrenic patients. *Schizophr Res.* 2011 July; **129**(2–3): 201–204.

37. Erickson KI, Voss MW, Prakash RS, et al. Exercise training increases size of hippocampus and improves memory. *Proc Natl Acad Sci U S A.* 2011 February 15; **108**(7): 3017–3022. DOI 10.1073/pnas.1015950108. Epub 2011 January 31. PubMed PMID: 21282661; PubMed Central PMCID: PMC3041121.

38. Fernandes BS, Gama CS, Ceresér KM, et al. Brain-derived neurotrophic factor (BDNF) as a state-marker of mood episodes in bipolar disorders: a systematic review and meta-regression analysis. *J Psychiatr Res.* 2011 August; **45**(8): 995–1004. Epub 2011 May 6. Review. PubMed PMID: 21550050.

39. Hammonds MD, Shim SS. Effects of 4-week treatment with lithium and olanzapine on levels of brain- derived neurotrophic factor (BDNF), B-cell CLL/lymphoma 2 and phosphorylated cyclic adenosine monophosphate response element-binding protein in the sub-regions of the hippocampus. *Basic Clin Pharmacol Toxicol.* 2009

August; **105**(2): 113–119. Epub 2009 April 17. PubMed PMID: 19486334.

40. Jornada LK, Moretti M, Valvassori SS, et al. Effects of mood stabilizers on hippocampus and amygdala BDNF levels in an animal model of mania induced by ouabain. *J Psychiatr Res*. 2010 un; **44**(8): 506–510. Epub 2009 December 1. PubMed PMID: 19954800.

41. de Sousa R, van de Bilt M, Diniz B, et al. Lithium increases plasma brain-derived neurotrophic factor in acute bipolar mania: A preliminary 4-week study. *Neurosci Lett*. 2011 April 20; **494**(1): 54–56.

42. Tramontina JF, Andreazza AC, Kauer-Sant'anna M, et al. Brain-derived neurotrophic factor serum levels before and after treatment for acute mania. *Neurosci Lett*. 2009 March 13; **452**(2):111–113. Epub 2009 January 15.

43. Pandey GN, Rizavi HS, Dwivedi Y, Pavuluri MN. Brain-derived neurotrophic factor gene expression in pediatric bipolar disorder: Effects of treatment and clinical response. *J Am Acad Child Adolesc Psychiatry*. 2008 September; **47**(9): 1077–1085. PubMed PMID: 18664999.

44. Frey BN, Andreazza AC, Cereсér KM, et al. Effects of mood stabilizers on hippocampus BDNF levels in an animal model of mania. *Life Sci*. 2006 June 13; **79**(3): 281–286. Epub 2006 February 7. PubMed PMID: 16460767.

45. Chen G, Rajkowska G, Du F, Seraji-Bozorgzad, N., Manji HK. Enhancement of hippocampal neurogenesis by lithium. *J. Neurochem*. 2000; **75**: 1729–1734.

46. Hanson ND, Nemeroff CB, Owens MJ. Lithium, but not fluoxetine or the corticotropin-releasing factor receptor 1 receptor antagonist R121919, increases cell proliferation in the adult dentate gyrus. *J Pharmacol Exp Ther*. 2011 April; **337**(1): 180–186. DOI 10.1124/jpet.110.175372. Epub 2011 January 10. PubMed PMID: 21220416; PubMed Central PMCID: PMC3063735.

47. Shim SS, Hammonds MD, Mervis RF. Four weeks lithium treatment alters neuronal dendrites in the rat hippocampus. *Int J Neuropsychopharmacol*. 2013 July; **16**(6): 1373–1382. DOI 10.1017/S1461145712001423. Epub 2013 January 18.

48. Rhindress K, Ikuta T, Wellington R, Malhotra AK, Szeszko PR. Delineation of hippocampal subregions using T1-weighted magnetic resonance images at 3 Tesla. *Brain Struct Funct*. 2015 November; **220**(6): 3259–3272. DOI 10.1007/s00429-014-0854-1. Epub 2014 August 1.

49. Kafantaris V, Spritzer L, Doshi V, Saito E, Szeszko PR. Changes in white matter microstructure predict lithium response in adolescents with bipolar disorder. *Bipolar Disord*. 2017 November; **19**(7): 587–594. DOI 10.1111/bdi.12544. Epub 2017 October 9. PubMed PMID: 28992395.

50. Markham A, Cameron I, Bains R, et al. Brain-derived neurotrophic factor-mediated effects on mitochondrial respiratory coupling and neuroprotection share the same molecular signaling pathways. *Eur J Neurosci*. 2012 February; **35**(3): 366–374. PubMed PMID: 22288477.

51. Rybakowski JK, Czerski P, Dmitrzak-Weglarz M, et al. Clinical and pathogenic aspects of candidate genes for lithium prophylactic efficacy. *J Psychopharmacol*. 2012 March; **26**(3): 368–373. Epub 2011 Sep 2.

Chapter 18

Molecular Imaging of Dopamine and Antipsychotics in Bipolar Disorder

Sameer Jauhar

18.1 Introduction

There is a curious disparity between the body of literature linking the dopamine system to schizophrenia/psychosis and bipolar disorder. This is surprising, given the similarities between the tenets of the dopamine hypothesis and schizophrenia and some states observed in bipolar disorder.

In this chapter, the author will present the evidence for a link between changes in the dopamine system and facets of bipolar disorder, the use of antipsychotics in bipolar disorder, and the possible integration of this knowledge in studying antipsychotic response and the dopamine system in bipolar disorder.

18.2 Dopamine and Bipolar Disorder

Attempts to link the dopamine system to bipolar disorder date back to catecholamine hypotheses of affective disorders (1), where a relative deficit was linked to depression, and increase or potentiation related to elation, though the focus at that time was predominantly on noradrenaline, as opposed to dopamine. This hypothesis has adapted over the years, taking into account data from animal, behavioral pharmacology, clinical trials, and molecular imaging (2). Unlike the dopamine hypothesis of schizophrenia/psychosis, dopamine's role is thought to be more fluid and specific for differing states of the illness.

The main animal models have included hyperlocomotion, seen as a phenotype of manic behavior, induced by amphetamines (3) and also seen in mice with a mutation in a circadian clock gene (ClockΔ19 mice). Behaviorally, these mice demonstrate altered sleep patterns, with less immobility in the forced swim test and increased preference for rewarding stimuli such as sucrose and less depression-like behavior (4). This model

has been linked to increased dopamine synthesis, tyrosine hydroxylase activity, and a daytime spike in daytime dopamine (5).

To this should be added modulation of behavior in animal models of depression, a bidirectional (induction or relief of depressive symptoms caused by mild stress) caused by modulating (inhibition/excitation) optogenetic recruitment of dopamine neurons in freely moving rodents (6). Linking both states in the same mice, using the association between seasonality and mood (i.e., mania and summer, depression and winter), Young et al. showed that mice with reduced dopamine transporter (DAT) expression exhibited hypersensitivity to summer-like and winter-like photoperiods, including more extreme mania-relevant and depression-relevant behaviors (7).

Pharmacological evidence for dopamine's role in inducing hypomania/mania comes from studies with L-dihydroxyphenylalanine (L-DOPA) (8), bromocriptine (9), amphetamine (10), and antimanic effects of dietary tyrosine depletion (11) and alpha-methyl-*p*-tyrosine (AMPT) administration, a dopamine depleting agent (12).

The clearest evidence for the role of dopamine in bipolar disorder comes from clinical antipsychotic trials (see later).

In essence, the current model proposes a dysregulation of the dopamine system, switching of mood states being associated with relative excess (elevation) and reduction (depression) in the dopamine system. It is acknowledged that this does not adequately cover mixed states, though these could signify more flux within the system.

18.3 The Use of Antipsychotics in Bipolar Disorder

The first study of antipsychotics in bipolar disorder was in the acute phase of mania; the first study the author is aware of occurring in 1952, Delay and Deniker showing effects of chlorpromazine in manic states (13), a subsequent placebo-controlled study showing chlorpromazine to have greater efficacy in mania, compared to placebo (14). This is reflected in the antipsychotics licensed by the United States Food and Drug Administration (FDA) for use in treatment of bipolar disorder, which include aripiprazole (mania/mixed features and maintenance), asenapine (mania/mixed features), cariprazine (mania/mixed features, depression), chlorpromazine (mania/mixed features), lurasidone (depression), olanzapine (mania/mixed features/maintenance), olanzapine-fluoxetine (depression), quetiapine (immediate-release; mania/mixed features, depression, maintenance), quetiapine extended-release (mania/mixed features, depression, not maintenance), risperidone (mania/mixed features), ziprasidone (mania/mixed features, maintenance).

18.3.1 Acute Treatment of Mania

A recent synthesis of trials for mania found antipsychotics remain the most effective treatments, using response rate as an outcome measure, thirty-seven trials demonstrating a response rate of 49.7%, compared to seven trials showing response rate of 49.1% for lithium and eight trials indicating a response rate of 48.4% for anticonvulsants (15). Most trials are brief (around three weeks and response were broadly defined as <50% in ratings on a mania scale). This is broadly similar to a 2011 meta-analysis that measured change in scale, with haloperidol, the archetypal D_2 blocker, showing the greatest effect size (16).

18.3.2 Acute Treatment of Depression

Examination of antipsychotics licensed for acute depression indicates heterogeneity among compounds (17), most of which do not have direct effects on the dopamine system (olanzapine plus fluoxetine, lurasidone, quetiapine). A recent trial of cariprazine showed some effects on depression symptoms, using the Montgomery Asperg Depression Rating Scale (MADRS), with a least-square reduction of 2.5 versus placebo at 1.5 mg and 3 for 3 mg daily (18). It is also worth noting lack of efficacy at 3 mg in a prior trial (though difference of 4 on MADRS for 1.5 mg) (19), and contrasting these differences to those for other licensed antipsychotics, for example, quetiapine, where the mean difference in MADRS was approximately 15 for 300 mg/day (allowing for effects on sedation and weight gain, this difference is striking (20).) The findings with cariprazine can be contrasted with those of aripiprazole (see later), which may be a result of cariprazine having more agonistic properties (21).

18.3.3 Maintenance Treatment

A 2017 systematic review and meta-analysis of SGAs in maintenance treatment included fifteen RCTs, lasting from six months to two years, and one observational study lasting four years (22). This examined monotherapy and adjunctive therapy to lithium, sodium valproate, or lamotrigine. Antipsychotics included olanzapine (four trials), quetiapine (four trials), aripiprazole (three trials), risperidone (three trials), and ziprasidone (one trial). Meta-analyses demonstrated antipsychotic monotherapy superior to placebo, reducing overall relapse risk (olanzapine: RR 0.52 (95% CI 0.-38–0.71), two studies; quetiapine: HR 0.37 95% CI 0.31–0.45), two studies; risperidone: RR 0.61 (95% CI 0.47–0.80), two studies). It should be acknowledged that the quality of the studies was inferior. As adjunct to mood stabilizers (lithium/valproate/lamotrigine), given to people who had responded to acute treatment, efficacy was seen for aripiprazole (RR 0.65, 95% CI 0.50–0.85; two studies), olanzapine (RR 0.49 (95% CI 0.27–0.91; one study), quetiapine (RR 0.38, 95% CI 0.32–0.46; two studies), and ziprasidone (RR 0.62, 95% CI 0.40–0.96; one study). One trial with risperidone long-acting injection (LAI) in people with bipolar 1 disorder and four or more episodes in the prior year, was not statistically significant in the meta-analysis for relapse to any mood episode, though did show benefit in a fifty-two-week follow-up compared to placebo as an adjunct to treatment as usual, with a 2.3-fold decreased risk of relapse to any mood episode (22, 23). Adjunctive quetiapine was the only drug that reduced manic (RR 0.39, 95% CI 0.30–0.52; two studies) and depressive (RR 0.38, 95% CI 0.29--0.49; two studies) episodes. All but one study had an enriched design, that is, patients were taking the drug prior to randomization. (A form of selection bias.) Two of the RCTs included people with bipolar 2 disorder. Accounting for side effects, discontinuation rates as adjunct varied from a hazard ratio of 0.66 (ziprasidone) to 0.89 (aripiprazole), with weight gain (defined as an increase of >7%) noted when meta-analyzing all antipsychotics.

Lurasidone was not examined in this review. This has an FDA license as monotherapy and adjunctive treatment to lithium and divalproex for acute treatment of bipolar depression. Following a six-week double-blind placebo-controlled RCT of lurasidone monotherapy or adjunctive treatment with lithium or divalproex, participants were randomized to an extended six-month trial of lurasidone as monotherapy or adjunct. Though not the primary outcome, treatment-emergent mania occurred in 1.3% in the monotherapy group, and in 3.8% in the adjunctive group. Among extension study baseline responders, 10.2% met post hoc criteria for depression relapse during six months of treatment in the monotherapy group, 10.2% meeting relapse criteria in the adjunctive therapy group. The nature of the trial makes it challenging to compare depression and mania relapse to other treatments, though the low incidence of manic relapse should be noted (23, 24). A recent twenty-six-week double-blind placebo-controlled trial of asenapine maintenance therapy in 253 people with bipolar disorder found a statistically significantly longer time to recurrence of any mood episode (manic or depression), HR 0.16 for manic episode, HR 0.35 for depressive episode, though not for mixed episodes (the study may have been underpowered for this, these being post hoc analyses)(24, 25). RCTs of LAIs should be added to this literature. A randomized placebo-controlled fifty-two-week trial of aripiprazole depot showed a beneficial effect in bipolar 1 illness, with a hazard ratio of 0.45 in recurrence of any mood episode, with a signal predominantly for preventing manic episodes, mirroring the evidence for oral aripiprazole (25, 26). Similar efficacy is also seen for risperidone LAI, versus placebo, from two trials, of eighteen and twenty-four months' duration (26–28), in relapse prevention, with a combined risk ratio of 0.42 for manic, hypomanic, or mixed symptoms, though not for depression relapse. A review summarizing three trials of LAI versus oral antipsychotics found no difference in relapse rates, though sensitivity analysis showed benefit in people with rapid cycling illness (29).

18.4 Dopamine Synthesis and Metabolism

To enable a clear understanding of the role of dopamine in molecular imaging, it is worth summarizing the process of dopamine synthesis and metabolism (Figure 18.1).

As stated by Cumming, "the life history of a dopamine molecule begins in the liver", where its precursor tyrosine is synthesized, and ends in the kidney, where it is excreted in urine (29, 30). Tyrosine is formed from the amino acid phenylalanine or obtained through dietary intake. Tyrosine is then transported in blood plasma, to cross the blood–brain barrier, where facilitated diffusion allows entry. In the brain, tyrosine is either incorporated into other proteins or used as a precursor for the synthesis of DOPA by catecholamine neurons. In the latter process, tyrosine is converted to L-DOPA by tyrosine hydroxylase, considered the rate-limiting enzyme in dopamine synthesis (it is almost completely saturated by tyrosine). Tyrosine activity can be modulated by a number of amines acting on the catalyst site. The majority of L-DOPA is then converted to dopamine by the enzyme aromatic acid decarboxylase (AADC). Other fates for L-DOPA include being exported out of the brain or being used as a substrate for catechol-O-methyltransferase (COMT), resulting in the production of O-methyldopa (OMD). It has therefore been pointed out that AADC can also contribute to dopamine synthesis (31). After being formed within the cytoplasm or intracellular space of the dopamine neuron, dopamine is then actively transported to synaptic vesicles by vesicular monoamine transporter 2 (VMAT 2), where it is stored and subsequently released. Reuptake of

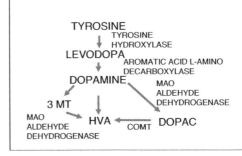

Figure 18.1 Pathway of dopamine synthesis and metabolism

dopamine into presynaptic terminals is regulated by the DAT (in the striatum). Unbound dopamine is then metabolized by monoamine oxidase (MAO) and COMT. The main branch of catabolism then follows the deamination of dihydroxyphenylacetic acid (DOPAC), which is then O-methylated to homovanillic acid (HVA). In a separate process, a small amount of brain dopamine is O-methylated to produce 3-methoxytyramine (3-MT), which is then deaminated by MAO to produce HVA. Both DOPAC and HVA leave the brain via facilitated diffusion, either directly to the bloodstream or via cerebrospinal fluid (CSF).

18.5 Molecular Imaging of the Dopamine System

Wagner and colleagues, in 1983, were the first to show visualization of dopamine receptors in the human brain, with [^{11}C]-*N*- methylspiperone (31, 32). The resolution of early studies (10–12 mm) only enabled visualization of large areas, such as striatum (33). Molecular imaging of dopamine in the human brain can be split into the presynaptic (which can be grouped together into dopamine synthesis capacity, dopamine release, and synaptic dopamine, which can be assessed using pharmacological challenge with dopamine depleting or releasing agents (34)), dopamine transporter availability, and dopamine receptor availability (Figure 18.2).

Common tracers and methods are given below, in Table 18.1 (PET tracers unless otherwise specified).

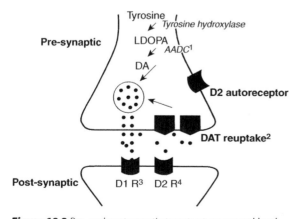

Figure 18.2 Pre- and postsynaptic targets at a neuronal level
Figure adapted from Cropley et al., Biological Psychiatry, 2006 (35)

18.5.1 Presynaptic System

Dopamine synthesis capacity is measured by quantifying the uptake of the enzyme AADC, a precursor to dopamine, though this is acknowledged as not being the rate-limiting step in dopamine production (this being tyrosine hydroxylase)(55).

The endogenous production of dopamine can also be assessed indirectly, using amphetamine challenge.

As recognized for tracers such as raclopride, endogenous dopamine competes with some tracers for binding at $D_{2/3}$ receptors. At a simplified level, D_2 receptors exist in low- and high-affinity states for agonists such as dopamine, with D_2 high the functional state in the striatum. Antagonists will bind at both D_2 high and low states, and agonists will compete for D_2 high states with endogenous dopamine, are therefore more vulnerable to competition by endogenous DA, and therefore more sensitive. This led to the development of D_2 agonist radiotracers, as listed earlier. These are more sensitive to the effects of amphetamine challenge on binding potential (BP) of D_2 receptors than raclopride. For example, Narendran et al. demonstrated 1.5 times the effect of amphetamine on BP in striatum relative to raclopride, using [^{11}C] NPA (56), and Shotbolt et al. showed a similarly large change in BP with PHNO (in healthy volunteers) (57).

18.5.2 Extra-Striatal Imaging of the Dopamine System

While F-DOPA PET has a very good signal-to-noise ratio in the striatum (Figure 18.3), it is poorer at quantifying dopamine synthesis capacity in extra-striatal regions, the same test–retest study that showed good intraclass coefficients (ICC) for striatum showing poorer ICC in extra-striatal regions (75). Specific regions of poor reliability (ICC<0.5) were hippocampus, amygdala, and medial frontal gyrus. Ki^{cer} in the thalamus, posterior cingulate cortex, anterior orbital gyrus, and medial frontal gyrus was equal or less than that of adjacent white matter, which raises doubts regarding the validity of measuring Ki^{cer} in these regions. Partial volume correction for the white matter for F-DOPA PET in extra-striatal regions has been suggested, based on finding greater Ki^{cer} in white matter compared to gray matter, despite no evidence to suggest appreciable AADC in white matter (58).

Table 18.1 Common tracers used to image the dopamine system in vivo

Component of DA system	Tracer	Technical notes
Dopamine synthesis capacity (presynaptic)		
	[^{18}F]-DOPA (36)	Indexes AADC
	[β-^{11}C]L-DOPA ([^{11}C]-DOPA) (31)	Indexes AADC
	6-[^{18}F]-l-*meta*- tyrosine (FMT) (37)	Tenfold greater affinity for AADC than F-DOPA, not substrate for COMT
	3-[^{18}F]fluoro-α- fluoromethyl-*p*-tyrosine (FMT) (38)	Substrate for tyrosine hydroxylase activity
Dopamine transporter		
	[^{123}I] Beta-CIT (SPECT) (39)	
	[^{11}C]-nomifensine (40)	
	[^{11}C]WIN35428 (41)	
	[^{11}C]d-threo-methylphenidate (42)	
	[^{99}mTc]TRODAT-1 (43)	
D$_1$ receptor family		
Antagonists	[^{11}C]SCH-23390 (44)	
	[^{11}C]NNC 112 (45)	Also binds to 5HT$_{2A}$ receptors
Agonists		
	(+)-Dinapsoline (46)	
D$_2$ receptor family		
Antagonists		
	[^{11}C]3-*N*-methyl-spiperone (47)	
	[^{11}C]raclopride (48)	
	(S)-*N*-[(1-ethyl-2-pyrrolidinyl)] methyl-2-hydroxy-3-iodo-6-methoxybenzamide ([^{123}I]IBZM) (49)	
	[^{18}F]fallypride (50)	
	[^{11}C]FLB457 (51)	
Agonists		
	[^{11}C]-(+)-4-propyl-3,4,4a,5,6,10*b*-hexahydro-2 *H*-naphtho[1,2-*b*][1,4]oxazin-9-ol ([^{11}C]PHNO) (52)	D$_3$ selective
	(-)-*N*-[^{11}C]propyl-norapomorphine (NPA) (53)	Full D$_2$/D$_3$ (predominantly D$_2$ high) agonist
	[*O-methyl*-^{11}C]2-methoxy-*N*-propylnorapomorphine). [^{11}C]MNPA (54)	

Given that extra-striatal regions such as the limbic and cortical dopamine systems have lower density populations of D$_2$ receptors, tracers such as [^{11}C] raclopride and [^{123}I] IBZM have less utility here, due to signal-to-noise ratio, with low-affinity or high nonspecific binding, respectively. Therefore high-affinity tracers such as [^{18}F] fallypride and [^{11}C] FLB457 were developed, the former used in striatal and extra-striatal regions, the latter used only in extra-striatal regions, due to its ultra-high affinity.

These tracers are used in dopamine release paradigms, and problems that limit their use in stimulant paradigms include the fact that stimulant effects on the prefrontal cortex occur outwith the dopamine synapse and therefore the process of displacement is dependent on diffusion, as well as effects of COMT in the cortex. While the stimulant challenge has shown a difference between fallypride and FLB 457 (56), task-based paradigms have failed to show a difference (59). The agonist tracer PHNO has

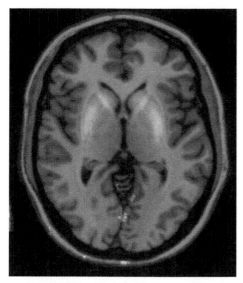

Dopamine Synthesis Capacity

Ki^{cer} (1/min)

0.00   0.03

Figure 18.3 A normative map of dopamine synthesis capacity as measured with FDOPA PET. A black and white version of this figure will appear in some formats. For the colour version, refer to the plate section.

been used in extra-striatal regions such as the substantia nigra, where D_3 receptors predominate (PHNO has a high affinity for these receptors) though it has limited utility in cortical regions (60).

18.6 Molecular Imaging of the Dopamine System in Bipolar Disorder

All known published molecular imaging studies of the dopamine system in bipolar disorder are presented in Table 18.2. In keeping with the hypothesis that dopamine may have a state component in bipolar disorder, the phase of bipolar disorder and patient characteristics are included.

As can be seen from Table 18.2, the molecular imaging literature on dopamine function in bipolar psychosis is sparse, and most of the literature relates to mania, euthymia, and depression without psychosis.

There are too few studies to make any clear inferences, and of the available studies, most are underpowered and present conflicting findings.

The findings can be summarized, according to disease state as given in subsequent sections.

18.6.1 Euthymic States

An amphetamine challenge SPECT study, giving an indirect measurement of synaptic DA showed no difference between patients and controls (64).

Studies examining the dopamine transporter have shown conflicting findings, of higher availability of DAT in seventeen people who were drug-free for two months (67), decrease availability in a group of eleven euthymic and depressed patients with bipolar disorder, free of medication for two weeks (65).

The Suhara study, examining D_1 density, is difficult to interpret, as the ligand (11 C-SCH23390) has poor specificity in extra-striatal areas (69).

18.6.2 Bipolar Depression

Both studies examining dopamine transporters in bipolar depression have found conflicting results, with decreased and increased availability (65, 66).

18.6.3 Mania

Yatham et al. found no difference in dopamine synthesis capacity in nonpsychotic mania, compared to controls, and no difference in $D_{2/3}$ density in this same cohort (62, 68).

18.6.4 Bipolar Psychosis

Two papers covering the same sample measured D_2 receptor density in bipolar psychosis, calculating B_{max} after administration of haloperidol lactate. The authors found increased density in antipsychotic-free people with bipolar psychosis, compared to people with bipolar disorder without psychosis, and a correlation between psychotic symptoms (measured using the present state examination) and receptor density in this group (70). It should be acknowledged that the tracer in this study had nonspecific binding, the B_{max} of the ligand for 5HT$_{2A}$ being 30% (71). A recent PET study of dopamine synthesis capacity in first-episode bipolar psychosis found elevated Ki in the striatum, and a correlation with positive psychotic symptoms (63).

18.7 What is the Mechanism of Antipsychotic Response in Bipolar Disorder?

What appears clear from the evidence initially presented, and the trial evidence is that response to

241

Table 18.2 Molecular imaging studies of the dopamine system in bipolar disorder

Author (year)	Component of DA system (tracer)	Phase of BD	Patients; controls (n)	Patient characteristics	Main finding
Zubieta et al, 2000 (61)	• Vesicular monoamine transporter protein (presynaptic system) (+)[^{11}C] dihydrotetrabenazine (DTBZ)	Euthymic	16;16	Prior psychotic mania, on various medications (carbamezepine, lamotrigine, valproic acid, lithium)	Increased uptake brainstem and thalamus, correlation between brainstem and executive function
Yatham et al 2002 (62)	Pre-synaptic (F-DOPA)	Nonpsychotic mania	13;13	AP and MS naive, first episode	No difference in Ki
Jauhar et al 2017 (63)	Pre-synaptic ^{18}F-DOPA	Psychosis (n = 16 of 22)	22;22	First-episode antipsychotic naive (n=10), antipsychotic free (n=8), currently psychotic (n=16)	Elevation in whole sample, compared to controls, correlation with positive psychotic symptoms
Anand et al 2000 (64)	$D_{2/3}$ density 123I-IBZM SPECT, amphetamine challenge, i.e, measurement of synaptic DA	Euthymic	13;13	Drug free (n = 7)	No difference, no correlation in patients of post amphetamine binding and YMRS
Anand et al 2011 (65)	DA transporter [(11) C]CFT	Euthymic/ depressed phase	11;13	Unmedicated for at least two weeks Depressed (n = 6), euthymic (n = 5)	Lower DAT availability in bipolar patients in bilateral dorsal caudate
Amsterdam and Newberg, 2007 (66)	Dopamine transporter [^{99}mTc] TRODAT-1 (SPECT)	Depression	5;46	Drug free for one week	Increased binding potential in posterior putamen and left caudate
Chang et al, 2010I (67)	Dopamine transporter [^{99}mTc] TRODAT-1 (SPECT)	Euthymic	17;7	Drug free for 2 months, euthymic 4 months	Increased striatal DAT, compared to controls.
Yatham et al, 2002 (68)	$D_{2/3}$ density [(11)C]raclopride	Non-psychotic mania	13;14	Antipsychotic and mood-stabiliser naive	No significant difference in binding potential
Wong et al, 1997 (69)	$D_{2/3}$ density [^{11}C]N-methylspiperone	Mania-11 (7 psychotic) Depression-3	14;24	Drug naive (n-11), drug-free (n-3)	Increased $D_{2/3}$ density in caudate

Pearlson et al, 1995 (70)	$D_{2/3}$ density [^{11}C]N-methylspiperone before and after haloperidol lactate	14;12 *3 depressed, 11 manic)	Antipsychotic naïve or antipsychotic free>6 months, psychotic bipolar disorder ($n = 7$ of 14)	Higher B_{max} for people with psychosis (bipolar and schizophrenia) compared to controls, correlation with psychotic symptoms
Suhara et al, 1992 (69)	D_1 density [^{11}C]-SCH23390	10;21 Depressed, $n = 3$, euthymic $n = 6$, mania, $n = 1$	Drug free for one week, $n = 9$	↓ D_1 in frontal cortex

antipsychotics is variable and also phase-specific. The DA system, and by extension, primarily dopamine blocking antipsychotics appear to exert acute effects on mania and prevention of mania. The acute response to bipolar depression is not so clear and, unlike in schizophrenia (72, 73), the molecular imaging, as it exists, is unable to shed further light on this. With the exception of cariprazine, all other licensed treatments for bipolar depression most probably exert their effects through other receptor targets, or at best in addition to effects on dopamine.

Molecular imaging studies of the DA system in bipolar depression would, therefore, appear warranted, and enable a more mechanistic approach to be developed.

18.8 Future Directions

Future molecular imaging studies of the DA system in bipolar disorder should attempt to unpick mechanisms across phases of illness, in the same individuals, ideally in the first episode of illness, where services do exist (74). Linking response (and nonresponse) of differing antipsychotics, with different receptor affinities, would answer a lot of the etiological questions brought up in this chapter. Use of tracers targeting other neurotransmitter systems, for example, the $5HT_{2A}$ receptor agonist, $[^{11}C]$ Cimbi-36, measuring serotonin release, in longitudinal studies, may help to elucidate mechanisms underlying phase-specific changes in bipolar disorder.

Acknowledgments

The author would like to thank Dr. Abhishekh Ashok, who gave valuable comments on this manuscript and Mattia Veronese, who helped with Figure 18.3.

The author would also like to acknowledge Professor Oliver Howes, without whom none of the knowledge gained in molecular imaging would have taken place, and Professor Allan Young, whose input regarding the clinical relevance of antipaychotics in bipolar disorder has been 9 and continues to be) invaluable.

References

1. Schildkraut JJ. The catecholamine hypothesis of affective disorders: A review of supporting evidence. *Am J Psychiatry*. 1965 November 1; **122**(5): 509–522.

2. Ashok AH, Marques TAR, Jauhar S, et al. The dopamine hypothesis of bipolar affective disorder: The state of the art and implications for treatment. *Mol Psychiatry*. 2017 May; **22**(5): 666–679.

3. Beyer DKE, Freund N. Animal models for bipolar disorder: From bedside to the cage. *Int J Bipolar Disord* [Internet]. 2017 October **13**:

4. Mania-like behavior induced by disruption of CLOCK | PNAS [Internet]. [cited 2019 Jul 19]. Available from: www.pnas.org/content/104/15/6406.

5. Sidor MM, Spencer SM, Dzirasa K, et al. Daytime spikes in dopaminergic activity drive rapid mood-cycling in mice. *Mol Psychiatry*. 2015 November; **20**(11): 1406–1419.

6. Tye KM, Mirzabekov JJ, Warden MR, et al. Dopamine neurons modulate neural encoding and expression of depression-related behaviour. *Nature*. 2013 January 24; **493**(7433): 537–541.

7. Young JW, Cope ZA, Romoli B, et al. Mice with reduced DAT levels recreate seasonal-induced switching between states in bipolar disorder. *Neuropsychopharmacol Off Publ Am Coll Neuropsychopharmacol*. 2018; **43**(8):1721–1731.

8. Murphy DL, Brodie HKH, Goodwin FK, Bunney WE. Regular induction of hypomania by L -dopa in "bipolar" manic-depressive patients. *Nature*. 1971 January; **229**(5280): 135.

9. Vlissides DN, Gill D, Castelow J. Bromocriptine-induced mania? *Br Med J* 1978 February 25; **1**(6111): 510–510.

10. Jacobs D, Silverstone T. Dextroamphetamine-induced arousal in human subjects as a model for mania. *Psychol Med*. 1986 May; **16**(2): 323–329.

11. McTavish SF, McPherson MH, Harmer CJ, et al. Antidopaminergic effects of dietary tyrosine depletion in healthy subjects and patients with manic illness. *Br J Psychiatry J Ment Sci*. 2001 October; **179**: 356–360.

12. Anand A, Darnell A, Miller HL, et al. Effect of catecholamine depletion on lithium-induced long-term remission of bipolar disorder. *Biol Psychiatry*. 1999 April 15; **45**(8): 972–978.

13. Delay J, Deniker P. 38 cas de psychoses traites par la cure prolong&. et continue de 4560 RP. *Ann Med Psychol*. 1952; **110**: 364–396.

14. Klein DF, Oaks G. Importance of psychiatric diagnosis in prediction of clinical drug effects. *Arch Gen Psychiatry*. 1967 January 1; **16**(1): 118–126.

15. Baldessarini RJ, Tondo L, Vázquez GH. Pharmacological treatment of adult bipolar disorder. *Mol Psychiatry*. 2019 February; **24**(2): 198–217.

16. Cipriani A, Barbui C, Salanti G, et al. Comparative efficacy and acceptability of antimanic drugs in acute mania: A multiple-treatments meta-analysis. *Lancet Lond Engl*. 2011 October 8; **378**(9799): 1306–1315.

17. Jauhar S, Young AH. Controversies in bipolar disorder; role of second-generation antipsychotic for maintenance therapy. *Int J Bipolar Disord*. 2019 March 27; **7**(1): 10.

18. Cariprazine Treatment of Bipolar Depression: A Randomized Double-Blind Placebo-Controlled Phase 3 Study | American Journal of Psychiatry [Internet]. [cited 2019 Jun 26].

19. Durgam S, Earley W, Lipschitz A, et al. An 8-week randomized, double-blind, placebo-controlled evaluation of the safety and efficacy of cariprazine in patients with bipolar I depression. *Am J Psychiatry*. 2016 March 1; **173**(3): 271–281.

20. Young AH, McElroy SL, Bauer M, et al. A double-blind, placebo-controlled study of quetiapine and lithium monotherapy in adults in the acute phase of bipolar depression (EMBOLDEN I). *J Clin Psychiatry*. 2010 February; **71**(2): 150–62.

21. Veselinović T, Paulzen M, Gründer G. Cariprazine, a new, orally active dopamine D2/3 receptor partial agonist for the treatment of schizophrenia, bipolar mania and depression. *Expert Rev Neurother*. 2013 November; **13**(11): 1141–1159.

22. Lindström L, Lindström E, Nilsson M, Höistad M. Maintenance therapy with second generation antipsychotics for bipolar disorder – A systematic review and meta-analysis. *J Affect Disord*. 2017; **15**(213): 138–150.

23. Macfadden W, Alphs L, Haskins JT, et al. A randomized, double-blind, placebo-controlled study of maintenance treatment with adjunctive risperidone long-acting therapy in patients with bipolar I disorder who relapse frequently. *Bipolar Disord*. 2009 December; **11**(8): 827–839.

24. Ketter TA, Sarma K, Silva R, et al. Lurasidone in the long-term treatment of patients with bipolar disorder: A 24-week open-label extension study. *Depress Anxiety*. 2016 May 1; **33**(5): 424–434.

25. Szegedi A, Durgam S, Mackle M, et al. Randomized, double-blind, placebo-controlled trial of asenapine maintenance therapy in adults with an acute manic or mixed episode associated with bipolar I disorder. *Am J Psychiatry*. 2018 01; **175**(1): 71–79.

26. Calabrese JR, Sanchez R, Jin N, et al. Efficacy and safety of aripiprazole once-monthly in the maintenance treatment of bipolar I disorder: A double-blind, placebo-controlled, 52-week randomized withdrawal study. *J Clin Psychiatry*. 2017; **78**(3): 324–331.

27. Quiroz JA, Yatham LN, Palumbo JM, et al. Risperidone long-acting injectable monotherapy in the maintenance treatment of bipolar I disorder. *Biol Psychiatry*. 2010 July 15; **68**(2): 156–162.

28. Vieta E, Montgomery S, Sulaiman AH, et al. A randomized, double-blind, placebo-controlled trial to assess prevention of mood episodes with risperidone long-acting injectable in patients with bipolar I disorder. *Eur Neuropsychopharmacol J Eur Coll Neuropsychopharmacol*. 2012 November; **22**(11): 825–835.

29. Kishi T, Oya K, Iwata N. Long-acting injectable antipsychotics for prevention of relapse in bipolar disorder: A systematic review and meta-analyses of randomized controlled trials. *Int J Neuropsychopharmacol* [Internet]. 2016 September 21; **19**(9): pyw038. DOI:10.1093/ijnp/pyw038.

30. Cumming Paul. *Imaging Dopamine*. Cambridge University Press; 2009.

31. Cumming Paul. *Imaging Dopamine*. Cambridge University Press. 2009.

32. Wagner HN, Burns HD, Dannals RF, et al. Imaging dopamine receptors in the human brain by positron tomography. *Science*. 1983 September 23; **221**(4617): 1264–1266.

33. Nord M, Farde L. Antipsychotic occupancy of dopamine receptors in schizophrenia. *CNS Neurosci Ther*. 2011 April 1; **17**(2): 97–103.

34. Piccini P, Pavese N, Brooks DJ. Endogenous dopamine release after pharmacological challenges in Parkinson's disease. *Ann Neurol*. 2003 May; **53**(5): 647–653.

35. Cropley VL, Fujita M, Innis RB, Nathan PJ. Molecular imaging of the dopaminergic system and its association with human cognitive function. *Biol Psychiatry*. 2006 May 15; **59**(10): 898–907.

36. Garnett ES, Firnau G, Nahmias C. Dopamine visualized in the basal ganglia of living man. *Nature*. 1983 September 8; **305**(5930): 137–138.

37. Barrio JR, Huang SC, Yu DC, et al. Radiofluorinated L-m-tyrosines: New in-vivo probes for central dopamine biochemistry. *J Cereb Blood Flow Metab Off J Int Soc Cereb Blood Flow Metab*. 1996 July; **16**(4): 667–678.

38. DeJesus OT, Murali D, Kitchen R, et al. Evaluation of 3-[18 F]fluoro-alpha-fluoromethyl-p-tyrosine as a tracer for striatal tyrosine hydroxylase activity. *Nucl Med Biol*. 1994 May; **21**(4): 663–667.

39. Innis R, Baldwin R, Sybirska E, et al. Single photon emission computed tomography imaging of monoamine reuptake sites in primate brain with

[123I]CIT. *Eur J Pharmacol.* 1991 August 6; **200** (2–3): 369–370.

40. Aquilonius S-M, Bertröm K, Eckernäs S-Å, et al. In vivo evaluation of striatal dopamine reuptake sites using 11 C-nomifensine and positron emission tomography. *Acta Neurol Scand.* 1987 October 1; **76**(4): 283–287.

41. Wong DF, Yung B, Dannals RF, et al. In vivo imaging of baboon and human dopamine transporters by positron emission tomography using [11 C]WIN 35,428. *Synapse.* 1993 October 1; **15**(2): 130–142.

42. Volkow ND, Ding YS, Fowler JS, et al. A new PET ligand for the dopamine transporter: Studies in the human brain. *J Nucl Med Off Publ Soc Nucl Med.* 1995 December; **36**(12): 2162–2168.

43. Mozley PD, Stubbs JB, Plössl K, et al. Biodistribution and dosimetry of TRODAT-1: a technetium-99 m tropane for imaging dopamine transporters. *J Nucl Med Off Publ Soc Nucl Med.* 1998 December; **39**(12): 2069–2076.

44. Halldin C, Stone-Elander S, Farde L, et al. Preparation of 11 C-labelled SCH 23390 for the in vivo study of dopamine D-1 receptors using positron emission tomography. *Int J Rad Appl Instrum [A].* 1986; **37**(10): 1039–1043.

45. Halldin C, Foged C, Chou YH, et al. Carbon-11-NNC 112: a radioligand for PET examination of striatal and neocortical D1-dopamine receptors. *J Nucl Med Off Publ Soc Nucl Med.* 1998 December; **39**(12): 2061–2068.

46. Sit S-Y, Xie K, Jacutin-Porte S, et al. (+)-Dinapsoline: An efficient synthesis and pharmacological profile of a novel dopamine agonist. *J Med Chem.* 2002 August 1; **45**(17): 3660–3668.

47. Leysen JE, Gommeren W, Laduron PM. Spiperone: A ligand of choice for neuroleptic receptors. 1. Kinetics and characteristics of in vitro binding. *Biochem Pharmacol.* 1978 February 1; **27** (3): 307–316.

48. Köhler C, Hall H, Ogren SO, Gawell L. Specific in vitro and in vivo binding of 3 H-raclopride. A potent substituted benzamide drug with high affinity for dopamine D-2 receptors in the rat brain. *Biochem Pharmacol.* 1985 July 1; **34** (13):2251–229.

49. Kung HF, Pan S, Kung MP, et al. In vitro and in vivo evaluation of [123I]IBZM: A potential CNS D-2 dopamine receptor imaging agent. *J Nucl Med Off Publ Soc Nucl Med.* 1989 January; **30**(1): 88–92.

50. Mukherjee J, Christian BT, Dunigan KA, et al. Brain imaging of 18 F-fallypride in normal volunteers: blood analysis, distribution, test-retest studies, and preliminary assessment of sensitivity

to aging effects on dopamine D-2/D-3 receptors. *Synap N Y N.* 2002 December 1; **46**(3): 170–88.

51. Olsson H, Halldin C, Swahn CG, Farde L. Quantification of [11 C]FLB 457 binding to extrastriatal dopamine receptors in the human brain. *J Cereb Blood Flow Metab Off J Int Soc Cereb Blood Flow Metab.* 1999 October; **19**(10): 1164–1173.

52. Seeman P, Ko F, Willeit M, McCormick P, Ginovart N. Antiparkinson concentrations of pramipexole and PHNO occupy dopamine D2high and D3high receptors. *Synapse.* 2005 November 1; **58**(2): 122–128.

53. Hwang DR, Kegeles LS, Laruelle M. (-)-N-[(11)C] propyl-norapomorphine: A positron-labeled dopamine agonist for PET imaging of D(2) receptors. *Nucl Med Biol.* 2000 August; **27**(6): 533–539.

54. Finnema SJ, Seneca N, Farde L, et al. A preliminary PET evaluation of the new dopamine D2 receptor agonist [11 C]MNPA in cynomolgus monkey. *Nucl Med Biol.* 2005 May; **32**(4): 353–360.

55. Jauhar S, Veronese M, Rogdaki M, et al. Regulation of dopaminergic function: An [18 F]-DOPA PET apomorphine challenge study in humans. *Transl Psychiatry.* 2017 February 7; **7**(2): e1027.

56. Narendran R, Frankle WG, Mason NS, et al. Positron emission tomography imaging of amphetamine-induced dopamine release in the human cortex: A comparative evaluation of the high affinity dopamine D2/3 radiotracers [11C] FLB 457 and [11C]fallypride. *Synap N Y N.* 2009 June; **63**(6): 447–461.

57. Shotbolt P, Tziortzi AC, Searle GE, et al. Within-subject comparison of [11C]-(+)-PHNO and [11C]raclopride sensitivity to acute amphetamine challenge in healthy humans. *J Cereb Blood Flow Metab.* 2012 January; **32**(1): 127–136.

58. Cropley VL, Fujita M, Bara-Jimenez W, et al. Pre- and post-synaptic dopamine imaging and its relation with frontostriatal cognitive function in Parkinson disease: PET studies with [11C]NNC 112 and [18F]FDOPA. *Psychiatry Res.* 2008 July 15; **163**(2): 171–82.

59. Hernaus D, Mehta MA. Prefrontal cortex dopamine release measured in vivo with positron emission tomography: Implications for the stimulant paradigm. *NeuroImage.* 2016 November 15; **142**: 663–667.

60. Laruelle, Marc. Measuring dopamine synaptic transmission with molecular imaging and pharmacological challenges: The state of the art. In: Gerhard Gründer, editors. *Molecular Imaging in the Clinical Neurosciences.* New York: Springer; 2012, pp. 163–203.

61. Zubieta J-K, Huguelet P, Ohl LE, et al. High vesicular monoamine transporter binding in asymptomatic bipolar I disorder: Sex differences and cognitive correlates. *Am J Psychiatry*. 2000 October 1; **157**(10): 1619–1628.

62. Yatham LN, Liddle PF, Shiah I-S, et al. PET study of [(18)F]6-fluoro-L-dopa uptake in neuroleptic- and mood-stabilizer-naive first-episode nonpsychotic mania: Effects of treatment with divalproex sodium. *Am J Psychiatry*. 2002 May; **159**(5): 768–774.

63. Jauhar S, Nour MM, Veronese M, et al. A test of the transdiagnostic dopamine hypothesis of psychosis using positron emission tomographic imaging in bipolar affective disorder and schizophrenia. *JAMA Psychiatry*. 2017 October 11; **74**(12): 1206–1213.

64. Anand A, Verhoeff P, Seneca N, et al. Brain SPECT imaging of amphetamine-induced dopamine release in euthymic bipolar disorder patients. *Am J Psychiatry*. 2000 July; **157**(7): 1108–1114.

65. Anand A, Barkay G, Dzemidzic M, et al. Striatal dopamine transporter availability in unmedicated bipolar disorder. *Bipolar Disord*. 2011; **13**(4): 406–413.

66. Amsterdam JD, Newberg AB. A preliminary study of dopamine transporter binding in bipolar and unipolar depressed patients and healthy controls. Neuropsychobiology. 2007; **55**(3–4): 167–170.

67. Chang TT, Yeh TL, Chiu NT, et al. Higher striatal dopamine transporters in euthymic patients with bipolar disorder: A SPECT study with [99mTc]TRODAT-1. *Bipolar Disord*. 2010 February 1; **12**(1): 102–106.

68. Yatham LN, Liddle PF, Lam RW, et al. PET study of the effects of valproate on dopamine D2 receptors in neuroleptic- and mood-stabilizer-naive patients with nonpsychotic mania. *Am J Psychiatry*. 2002 October 1; **159**(10): 1718–1723.

69. Suhara T, Nakayama K, Inoue O, et al. D1 dopamine receptor binding in mood disorders measured by positron emission tomography. *Psychopharmacology (Berl)*. 1992; **106**(1): 14–18.

70. Pearlson GD, Wong DF, Tune LE, et al. In vivo D2 dopamine receptor density in psychotic and nonpsychotic patients with bipolar disorder. *Arch Gen Psychiatry*. 1995 June; **52**(6): 471–477.

71. Leung K. 3-N-[11C]methylspiperone. In: *Molecular Imaging and Contrast Agent Database (MICAD)* [Internet]. Bethesda (MD): National Center for Biotechnology Information (US); 2004 [cited 2019 July 20].

72. Jauhar S, Howes OD. Understanding and predicting variability in response to treatment in psychotic disorders: In vivo findings. *Clin Pharmacol Ther*. 2019 May; **105**(5): 1079–1081.

73. Jauhar S, Veronese M, Nour MM, et al. Determinants of treatment response in first-episode psychosis: An 18 F-DOPA PET study. *Mol Psychiatry*. 2019 October; **24**(10): 1502–1512.

74. Jauhar S, Ratheesh A, Davey C, et al. The case for improved care and provision of treatment for people with first-episode mania. *Lancet Psychiatry* [Internet]. 2019 October 01; **6**(10): P869–876.

75. Egerton A, Demjaha A, McGuire P, Mehta MA, Howes OD. The test-retest reliability of 18F-DOPA PET in assessing striatal and extrastriatal presynaptic dopaminergic function. Neuroimage. 2010 Apr 1;50(2):524–31.

Chapter 19

Brain Imaging and the Mechanisms of Antidepressant Action

Beata R. Godlewska, Sudhakar Selvaraj, and Philip J. Cowen

19.1 Introduction

The history of pharmacological treatments for depression began in the 1950s, with the serendipitous discovery of the antidepressant potential of drugs like the tricyclic antidepressant, imipramine. Since then, many new, safer, and better tolerated, antidepressant drugs have appeared on the market (1), and now depression can be treated widely in primary care. However, finding a treatment effective for an individual patient is not a trivial task, with only around 30% of patients responding to their first antidepressant (AD) medication, most requiring multiple changes, and about one-third not responding at all (2). With about 20% of the population worldwide suffering from depression at least once in their lifetime (3), there is a great need for new treatments as well as better targeting of available medications.

Knowledge of how effective ADs work is the key to the successful development of new treatments. The development of imaging technology allowing in vivo exploration of the human brain has substantially accelerated research on this subject. Neuroimaging methods, presented in detail in an earlier chapter, quickly became basic tools for exploring complex relationships between brain structure and function and clinical aspects of depression. Most knowledge regarding neural mechanisms of antidepressant drug action was gained through functional and structural magnetic resonance imaging (fMRI, sMRI), although other methods, such as positron emission tomography (PET), electroencephalography (EEG), magnetoencephalography (MEG), single-photon emission computed tomography (SPECT), and diffusion tensor imaging (DTI) have also been employed. The focus, initially on individual brain regions, more recently shifted toward an exploration of brain networks, during rest and activity.

This chapter will present the current state of knowledge about neural mechanisms of AD action.

19.2 Treatments in Context: A Short Account of the Neural Basis for Depression

Therapeutic mechanisms of drug action must modify the dysfunction underlying a health condition for which they are prescribed. At a simple level, it is hoped that appropriate medications will correct abnormalities leading to the development of symptoms. At the same time, by exploring how medications affect the neurobiology of disorders, more knowledge about this pathology can be gained.

Neuroimaging has greatly contributed to the understanding of pathomechanisms of depression and provided a framework to understand AD mechanisms of action. The past three decades of research provided good insight into the role of intrinsic brain networks, within- and between-network connectivity, and the role of individual structures in the development of depressive symptoms. Although research is ongoing, some widely acknowledged theories have been developed.

The first and well-supported formulation of depression, the fronto-limbic model, focuses on dysfunction in reactivity to emotionally valenced information and regulation of emotional responses. The model proposes that limbic structures responsible for the rapid automatic processing of salient emotional stimuli (such as amygdala, anterior cingulate cortex (ACC), insula, medial prefrontal cortex (mPFC), and orbito-frontal cortex (OFC)) are overreactive, in particular to negatively valenced affective stimuli, while other frontal structures (in particular dorsolateral prefrontal cortex (dlPFC)) are hypoactive and unable to exert necessary regulatory control (4–6). This results in mood-congruent negative bias in the processing of emotionally salient information and forms the basis for the development and maintenance of low mood. At the behavioral

248

level, this bias is expressed as, for example, classification of neutral or ambiguous faces as negative, better memory for information with negative emotional content, increased attention to negative material, and deficits in executive control and working memory tasks (7). Dysfunction in the fronto-limbic circuit has been proposed to be particularly important for symptoms such as low mood, hopelessness, and negative perceptions and memories.

Further hypotheses focused on reward guided learning and decision-making deficits as the basis for another core symptom of depression, anhedonia, and proposed dysfunction in cortico–striatal–thalamic connectivity as a neural scaffolding for these abnormalities (8, 9). This circuitry was also suggested to have a role in emotional regulation and appraisal.

Recently, more focus was directed on the role of dysfunction in connectivity within and between large-scale brain networks, with a particular role for the default mode network (DMN) (10). DMN is linked to internally oriented attention and self-referential thinking. Its hyperactivity and hyperconnectivity (11) and a failure to deactivate during the performance of external tasks were proposed as a neural basis for increased self-focus and depressive ruminations (12). Other networks of particular importance for depression are central executive network (CEN), involved in high-level cognitive functions, and salience network (SN), important for detection and integration of emotional and sensory stimuli, and the switch between DMN and CEN (10). A meta-analysis of experimental studies provided support for all three models (13).

19.3 An Impact of AD on the Brain

Neuroimaging, in particular, fMRI, has been an invaluable tool in elucidating the mechanisms of AD action at the neural level. Imaging studies provided robust support for the impact of ADs on the circuitry involved in detection and response to emotionally salient stimuli and regulation of emotional responses. This direction of research is inseparably related to another theme of vital significance, the search for treatment response biomarkers. Although this subject will be described in details in another chapter, we will briefly mention some findings in the context of the antidepressant mode of action.

19.3.1 Impact of "Classical" Antidepressant Medications

Studies exploring neural mechanisms of AD action employed a number of drugs typically used in the clinical practice, including sertraline (14–19), fluoxetine (20–26), citalopram (27, 28), escitalopram (17, 19, 29–34), paroxetine (17, 35), venlafaxine (19, 26, 36–40), reboxetine (27), and mirtazapine (39, 40). Most studies focused on affective processing, and only a minority tested cognitive or reward-related processes (22, 30, 41, 42).

The most common paradigm used in sMRI and fMRI studies involved a longitudinal design, with two imaging sessions before ADs were started and after a period of treatment corresponding to a time when the clinical response is usually assessed (4–12 weeks). Due to the fact that dysfunction in affective processing is the core symptomatic domain in depression, most functional studies used visual stimuli with emotional valences, such as viewing emotional faces or pictures with emotional load, for example, from International Affective Picture System. Stimuli presentation varied between the studies, for example, both explicit and implicit paradigms were used; the latter involved an exposure to emotional stimuli while performing an unrelated undemanding cognitive task, for example, gender determination. Emotional stimuli could be overtly presented or masked, that is, shown for a time insufficient for their conscious perception and then replaced by a neutral image. Some studies did not use any tasks and examined resting-state functional connectivity, exploring unconstrained network function in the context of minimal cognitive demands. Importantly, many of these studies investigated a relationship between a change in neural reactivity under AD treatment and clinical improvement. Exploration of differential effects of treatments in responders and nonresponders allowed a finer-grained understanding of the factors important for AD response.

Most studies focused on depressed patients, with healthy volunteers used as comparison groups. However, to understand the effect of the drug without a confounding impact of typical depressive symptoms, such as low mood or anhedonia, studies in healthy volunteers have been valuable (43–45). Usually, ADs were shown to have a similar effect in both depressed and healthy populations, with the strongest convergence in the amygdala, followed by the ACC, insula, and putamen. Differences were, however, also noted and may result, for example, from varying neuropsychological/psychopharmacological mechanisms underlying the AD effect in healthy controls versus depressed patients or from baseline differences between depressed and healthy individuals (46).

Converging evidence from individual studies, supported by a recent meta-analysis (46), showed normalization of brain reactivity to emotional stimuli after a few weeks of AD treatment, with an overall decrease in response to negative emotional stimuli and increase in response to positive ones. This was seen across the network of structures implicated in the processing of salient emotional information. The robust effect of ADs on some – but not all – of the structures in emotional circuitry may indicate that these brain regions are particularly important for AD mechanisms of action. The most robustly supported finding was attenuation of amygdala reactivity; a medication effect was also consistently observed in the ACC, insula, mPFC, putamen, and dlPFC (46).

Normalization of dlPFC reactivity to emotional stimuli reflected the restoration of effective regulation and control over enhanced limbic reactivity. Interestingly, this effect was observed for emotional paradigms, while the opposite effect – attenuation of response – was often seen when cognitive paradigms were used (47). Although dlPFC is a node for emotional and cognitive processing, it is possible that processing of emotional information and cognitive tasks without emotional context poses different demands on dlPFC, which can be reflected by a differential neural response to medication using those paradigms (47).

Another key structure identified as the key site of AD action is the ACC, in particular, the pregenual and subgenual portions (pgACC and sgACC). The data support antidepressant treatment-induced attenuation of the ACC activity across implicit and explicit emotional paradigms and cognitive tasks (48). pgACC has a central position within neural circuits involved in emotional and cognitive processing; it is one of the main nodes in DMN and a crucial hub for the correct top-down regulation of initial limbic responses. It has widespread anatomical and functional connections with the limbic system, ventral

striatum, hypothalamus, and dlPFC and hence plays a role in a number of processes found to be abnormal in depression (49). Increased pretreatment pgACC activity, normalized by AD treatments, may represent enhanced emotional appraisal and hyperreactivity of the salience network to negative stimuli.

Interestingly, this increased reactivity may be an important predictive marker of AD response. Indeed, thus far, increased baseline activity of pgACC has been identified as the most consistent marker of good therapeutic response, across a variety of treatments, including both pharmacological and psychological approaches, and independent of the imaging paradigm used (48, 50, 51). Interestingly, the fast acting antidepressant glutamatergic drug ketamine initially increased pgACC reactivity, which could reflect a shift of the pgACC into a state advantageous for therapeutic response (52). It has also been suggested that increased reactivity may reflect more preserved fronto-cingulate function and adaptive self-referential processing (50).

The insula is a key part of the salience network and a structure involved in emotion regulation and maintaining interoceptive awareness of body states. In depression, both attenuation and enhancement of insula's activity were observed and subsequently shown to normalize over the course of AD treatment. The role of the insula in clinical improvement is, however, still poorly understood, and its interactions with treatments are likely to be complex. This was illustrated by a recent study which suggested that both baseline hypo- and hypermetabolism of the anterior insula can be linked to a positive clinical outcome, but to different types of treatments. Hypometabolism was predictive of a good response to CBT and poor response to escitalopram, while hypermetabolism was associated with a good response to escitalopram but lack of benefit of CBT (53). If replicated, this finding would be of great clinical value, as based on insula activity, some patients might be offered CBT, generally less widely available than pharmacological treatments, as their first treatment.

Regarding other regions, the findings were more variable. Those regions included areas implicated in reward processing and motivation (nucleus accumbens, posterior OFC) and visual processing/attention to emotional stimuli (V1 area of the visual cortex and posterior cingulate cortex) (47). It is possible that these structures are less sensitive to the effect of "typical" ADs, or that changes in their function are secondary to AD effect in other brain regions. For example, the visual cortex is a part of the visual-limbic feedback loop. Some studies showed changes in visual cortex corresponding to changes in the amygdala, with increased responsivity to positive and decreased responsivity to negative stimuli after a few weeks of AD treatment (20, 54).

Given that emotional symptoms are the core symptoms of depression, most studies focused on the effect of AD on affective circuitry. Only a minority of investigations assessed the impact of medications on neural underpinnings of cognitive impairment in depression (27, 41). One such study showed a reduction in dlPFC reactivity to inhibitory "no go" responses in Go/NoGo task after eight weeks of antidepressant treatment in treatment responders only (41). The same effect was seen in healthy controls receiving antidepressant treatment. Moreover, responders had similar dlPFC responses as healthy controls pretreatment, suggesting that intact activation in the frontoparietal network during response inhibition may be a necessary substrate for AD response.

19.3.2 Structural Effects of "Typical" AD Actions

Although neurogenesis is one of the processes triggered by ADs (55), structural changes often remain undetected with neuroimaging during treatment with ADs; this may be related to inadequate sensitivity of these methods to reveal more subtle changes in brain structure. The most common findings related to an increase in volume and attenuation of the shrinkage of the hippocampus, dlPFC, and ACC. This supports laboratory findings, suggesting that AD induced increase in serotonin or 5-hydroxytryptamine (5-HT) (5HT) and noradrenalin (NA) enhances BDNF and other neurotropic factors, resulting in neurogenesis and structural remodeling, in healthy and depressed individuals alike (56).

DTI studies suggested the importance of white matter integrity for AD effect. For example, impaired integrity of the tracts connecting the ACC, dlPFC, and hippocampus was linked to poor treatment outcome (57). Another DTI study showed that integrity of the stria terminalis

and cingulate portion of the cingulum bundle was good predictors of remission to AD medications (58). The same authors proposed an algorithm based on an assessment of left middle frontal and right angular gyrus volumes and integrity of the left cingulum bundle, right superior fronto-occipital fasciculus, and right superior longitudinal fasciculus, which allowed identification of nonresponders to AD treatment with 100% accuracy in a small group of patients (59). Clearly replication is needed.

19.3.3 Focus on Brain Connectivity

The brain structures discussed earlier do not act in separation but are integrated into neural networks that interact at a variety of scales. New analytical approaches allowing an assessment of functional (temporal) and effective (directional) connectivity suggest that ADs restore functional integrity and connectivity of brain networks. Although the findings are heterogeneous (10, 60), a general conclusion can be drawn that changes in neural networks support putative mechanisms of AD action based on earlier studies. For example, ADs were shown to increase amygdala connectivity with dlPFC (61), which could translate into greater inhibitory (16).

Attenuation of DMN hyperconnectivity by ADs was suggested, both within DMN and with other regions, such as the limbic system (62). Interestingly, this normalization of activity possibly occurs only in parts of DMN, which was suggested as the basis for future relapse (63). Some studies explored changes in network connectivity in the context of treatment response[e.g., 64]. For example, treatment-resistant patients showed abnormal functional connectivity between anterior and posterior DMN (65), between DMN and CNN, and between DMN and cerebellum (66, 67). In general, in treatment-resistant patients, widespread connectivity abnormalities were observed. What this means for AD efficacy is yet to be understood.

19.3.4 "Bottom-Up" or "Top-Down" Effect?

There is a growing consensus that ADs act primarily in the "bottom-up" direction. ADs effect on limbic structures is robust and consistently shown by neuroimaging studies both in MDD and healthy volunteers. At the same time, it was claimed that the enhancement of dlPFC activity was seen in MDD only, suggesting that "top-down" could not be the direction of change (46).

19.3.5 New Antidepressant Drugs: Ketamine

While much is known about how typical ADs work, neural effects of "new kids on the block," that is fast-acting glutamatergic drugs such as ketamine, are less known. Thus far research seems to indicate that ketamine, unlike classical ADs, may have different – often opposite – neural effect in people with depression and healthy individuals, hence extrapolation of the data from healthy volunteer studies may require some caution (68).

Generally speaking, ketamine was shown to have a robust and consistent widespread effect across frontal, temporal, and occipital regions and was proposed to normalize attention- and emotion-related brain activity (68). Its effects in decreasing connectivity of DMN structures and strengthening executive control circuitry were proposed as potential ways its effects may be exerted (68). An increase in global brain connectivity of prefrontal and striatal regions was correlated with antidepressant effect (69).

As noted earlier, ketamine infusion increased pgACC activity, which may be interpreted as a shift of pgACC into a state of higher responsiveness after the therapeutic intervention (52). Indeed, this activation showed a strong correlation with reduction in MDD symptoms twenty-four hours post infusion. In nonhuman primates, increases in cortical and subcortical connectivity to dlPFC were shown to persist beyond ketamine's clearance, possibly contributing to its AD effect (70). The neural mechanisms of ketamine action need more research, with further exploration of the timeline of the therapeutic response (e.g., shortly after infusion vs. twenty-four hours vs. longer term).

19.3.6 A Note on Ligand PET Studies

Although studies using ligand PET technology are not numerous, they are worth a separate mention due to a unique insight they provide into AD mechanism of action. PET, and earlier SPECT, approaches are the methods allowing in vivo exploration of the phenomena happening at the molecular level, in particular, estimation of the degree of binding in the brain. PET uses radiolabeled ligands, and a choice of targets largely depends on whether a relevant highly selective ligand can be made available. The majority of PET studies investigated the 5-HT transporter (5-HTT) and serotonin type 1A (5-HT1A) receptor. Recently more ligands for the 5-HT2A receptor have been developed, promising an extension of PET investigations on the 5-HT system (71).

Although the effect of ADs on the 5-HT system has long been studied, the use of PET allows a new level of understanding of AD mechanisms. Increased pretreatment binding at 5-HT1A receptors at raphe nuclei was shown to discriminate between responders and nonresponders to escitalopram (72); interestingly, the binding decreased after SSRI treatment, yet this decrease was unrelated to a degree of clinical response (73). In healthy individuals, citalopram infusion enhanced amygdala response to fearful vs. neutral facial expressions, and this enhancement correlated with the availability of 5-HT1A receptors in dorsal raphe nucleus, supporting a role for 5-HT1A receptors in emotional processing (45).

A few weeks of treatment with a number of drugs, including SSRIs, tricyclic antidepressants, and mirtazapine, was shown to produce 70–80% 5-HTT occupancy; however, no correlation with symptomatic improvement was seen (74). On the other hand, some studies have found a relationship between SSRI treatment response and various aspects of pretreatment 5-HTT binding. For example, Miller et al. reported that lower binding in the midbrain, amygdala, and ACC predicted a poor response (75). Others have reported correlations between clinical response to SSRIs and the ratio between binding in projection areas (amygdala and habenula) and the median raphe nucleus (76) or in the ratio of the striatum to midbrain binding (77). This needs more research, but above studies seem to suggest that response to treatment may be linked to the pretreatment level of binding at both 5-HT1A receptor and 5-HT transporter, rather than changes in their occupancy over time. It was also suggested that the relationship in receptor binding between brain regions is more important than absolute levels in individual structures (78). These studies emphasize the potential for PET data to predict treatment response.

PET also helps to explore complex relationships between the dose, receptor occupancy, and clinical improvement, which can lead to improvement of clinical practice. For example, such research was conducted on the binding of venlafaxine (79) and duloxetine (80) to NA transporter, showing that at standard therapeutic doses, duloxetine occupied a significant proportion (about 50%) of NA transporters while with venlafaxine, a dose of at least 150 mg daily was required to achieve this effect.

PET has also been used to assess brain metabolism through the administration of 18 F –fluorodeoxyglucose (FDG). FDG PET studies showed, for example, lower metabolism in the midbrain, basal ganglia, parahippocampal gyrus, and thalamus as predictors of a good AD response, while a study above showed a potential of FDG PET to discriminate between responders to medication and psychotherapy (53).

19.4 Understanding Finer-Grained Aspects of Antidepressant Action

19.4.1 The Role for Negative Bias Attenuation and Cognitive Neuropsychological Model

Attempts at understanding the delay in the therapeutic effect of conventional ADs resulted in a hypothesis focusing on the role of emotional processing bias in AD mechanisms of action. This so-called cognitive-neuropsychological model of antidepressant action proposes that ADs do not have a direct effect on mood but instead induce a number of biological effects that lead to an early positive shift in emotional processing. For mood improvement to happen, this newly formed positive bias needs to interact with the environment to form new positive associations. This process takes time, which was proposed as an explanation for the delay in AD action (81, 82).

The model was validated in healthy and depressed individuals. Attenuation of the negative processing bias was shown at the behavioral and neural levels as early as after a single dose, in the absence of clinically significant mood changes. This was observed across a number of classical antidepressants, including SSRIs, NRIs, atypical drugs – mirtazapine and agomelatine, and a medicinal herb St John's wort. Similar to longer-term studies, neuroimaging data showed changes across a number of structures important for negative bias formation and putative mechanisms of depression, such as the amygdala, ACC, and putamen. The absence of mood improvement in the presence of a clear neural change in reactivity to emotional stimuli suggests that negative bias normalization predates mood change. Studies using placebo suggest that medication effect exceeds that of placebo (31) and is largely independent of the learning effect caused by repeated testing (83).

Critically for model validation, it was necessary to explore whether this early positive shift was indispensable for treatment response. A recent study showed that in subsequent responders to escitalopram, after seven days of treatment, there was a decrease in neural response to fearful versus happy facial expressions in brain regions involved in emotional processing, including the amygdala, insula, ACC, PCC, and thalamus (84) (Figure 19.1). Importantly, at this point, no significant mood improvement was seen. It was, therefore, suggested that an early positive shift in emotional processing plays an important role in the mechanism of action of antidepressant medications and response to treatment.

According to the model, social interactions are necessary for the translation of newly formed positive bias into mood improvement. Thus far, this notion has been only tested by behavioral studies, which showed, for example, the predictive value of early attenuation of negative bias only in those who perceived the level of social support as adequate (85). In this context, it is interesting that training a negative bias seemed to affect mood only in those who faced stressful situations (86).

19.4.2 Different Drugs, Different Patterns of Neural Change?

Once general mechanisms of AD action became conceptualized, it became pertinent to explore the differences between the effects of drugs belonging to separate pharmacological groups, or even individual medications. This understanding could have immense practical value, in particular in the context of individualized treatment approaches.

Although this area of research is in its infancy, some interesting data already emerged. An example of research initiatives in this field is a multicenter project International Study to

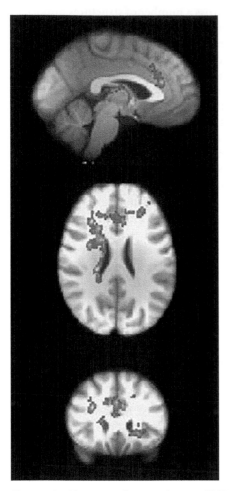

Figure 19.1 This picture illustrates the use of fMRI as a tool in research on treatment response biomarkers. Ths picture presents results of the whole-brain level analysis of response to masked sad vs happy facial expressions (thresholded at Z=2.3 and cluster-corrected with a family wise error (FWE) P<.05). Responders to escitalopram showed increased pre-treatment activation across a number of structures including anterior cingulate cortex, paracingulate gyrus, thalamus and putamen, as compared to non-responders to treatment. For details of the study see Godlewska et al., 2016. A black and white version of this figure will appear in some formats. For the colour version, refer to the plate section.

Predict Optimized Treatment in Depression (iSPOT), a project assessing biomarkers of treatment response to SSRIs sertraline and escitalopram and an SNRI venlafaxine. One of the findings suggested that hyporeactivity, and post-treatment normalization, of amygdala response to subliminal presentations of happy and fearful facial expressions, predicted good clinical response to all tested treatments (19). At the same time, baseline hyperreactivity to subliminal

sadness was predictive of the lack of response to venlafaxine treatment, which produced a shift toward hyporeactivity rather than normalization after eight weeks of treatment.

Another iSPOT report suggested increased dlPFC activation to a Go/NoGo task during inhibitory "no go" responses, followed by its reduction over treatment, as a general treatment response predictor, and baseline inferior parietal activation to Go/NoGo task as a differential predictor of response to SSRIs and SNRIs (41). Remission to SSRIs was linked to greater pretreatment activation in this region, while remission to SNRIs was related to baseline attenuation of response.

Studies on resting-state functional connectivity also suggested differential effects of SSRIs and SNRIs on neural networks (64). These findings suggest a possibility that although certain brain regions may play a role in treatment response to medications in general, their baseline activity state may dictate which particular drugs are most likely to produce a good clinical outcome; this differential response may be related to contrasts in the mechanisms of action of pharmacological groups or even individual antidepressant medications.

Neuroimaging also helped to explore how ADs of different pharmacological profile affect neural processing of individual emotions. Research on those above cognitive neuropsychological model suggested that SSRIs tended to attenuate the response to fear (shown as a decrease in fear recognition and amygdala reactivity to fearful faces), while an increase in recognition of happy facial expressions followed NRI treatment. This is particularly interesting in the light of the hypotheses linking the development of negative affect, experienced as sadness, to abnormal 5-HT neurotransmission, and a loss of positive affect and anhedonia – to noradrenergic (NA) and dopaminergic (DA) dysfunction; NA also participates in modulation and enhancement of memories with emotional content (81). These observations may have translational potential. For example, in the process of drug development, even if mechanisms of a new compound are not fully known, its neural effect while performing emotional tasks may suggest its usefulness against certain types of depressive symptoms and thereby inform further work.

19.4.3 Importance of Additional Factors for Antidepressant Action

Additional factors may influence whether a medication will have a therapeutic effect. Although the role of many such factors – such as inflammation or traumatic childhood experiences – has been postulated, little is known about their actual impact on ADs efficacy. The need for such research is illustrated by a finding that increased pretreatment dlPFC reactivity on a working memory task was predictive of the good clinical outcome but only in individuals without a history of childhood abuse (87).

Another neuroimaging study showed a significant increase in the accuracy of remission prediction based on the integrity of the white matter tracts – stria terminalis and a cingulate portion of the cingulum bundle – after including age as a modifying factor. A better understanding of how various factors may affect response to AD treatments may have direct practical relevance. For example, if social interactions are needed for clinical response, as postulated by the abovementioned cognitive neuropsychological model (82), an addition of behavioral or psychological elements to pharmacological treatments may be beneficial (88).

19.4.4 Effect of a Single and Repeated Doses

A meta-analysis (46) has recently shown that the neural effects of repeated dosing were relatively consistent between the studies, while a neural response to a single dose and short-term treatment was more diverse, with both attenuation and enhancement of emotional circuitry activity. Although this finding may be related to differences in designs of the studies, it is also plausible that processing of emotions during AD treatment changes over time and may differ between medication groups (46). For example, a single administration of SSRIs was shown to increase fear recognition and fear processing in the amygdala (89), which was not seen after a week or later in treatment. Interestingly anxiety is a common side-effect early in the course of SSRI treatment. Research in individuals with high neuroticism trait, healthy people with no depressive symptoms who nevertheless show negative neural and cognitive bias in emotional processing – revealed enhanced recognition of positive emotions and shortened gaze maintenance at facial expressions after a single SSRI citalopram dose (90). The same groups of individuals also show enhanced amygdala response to both positive and negative emotions, accompanied by elongated gaze maintenance, after seven days of treatment (91). This was interpreted in relation to the initial anxiogenic effect of SSRIs, abolished through improved engagement with social stimuli after a few days of treatment. More research is needed to understand the timeline of changes induced by ADs and how it relates to the therapeutic effect.

19.5 Final Remarks

Elucidation of the neural mechanisms of AD effects is an ongoing process. With increasing knowledge of these mechanisms, the focus shifts toward translational aspects, in particular establishing individualized treatment approaches and new drug development.

This happens in the context of a change in how mental health disorders are viewed and attempts at moving from clinical diagnoses to dimensional approaches (92). It was proposed that symptomatic domains, defined by current knowledge of biological and behavioral underpinnings of emotion, cognition, motivation, and social behavior, should replace diagnostic labels. This approach is represented in the Research Domain Criteria (93).

Neuroimaging has greatly advanced the understanding of neural mechanisms underlying the therapeutic effects of ADs, and a more consistent picture has slowly emerged, despite practical issues, such as heterogeneity of the samples, differences in study designs, and modest numbers of participants in single studies. In the future, research may be helped by computational approaches. The usefulness of computational methods can be illustrated by a study which, through machine learning algorithms, classified depressed patients into four subtypes based on dysfunctions in functional connectivity between fronto-striatal and limbic networks; these subtypes were characterized by different symptomatic profiles and response to transcranial magnetic stimulation (94). Future research has indeed the potential to produce a step change in treatment-related research. The speed of technological advances and fast-growing knowledge hold a strong promise of translation of scientific findings into clinically relevant applications soon.

References

1. Cipriani A, Furukawa TA, Salanti G, et al. Comparative efficacy and acceptability of 21 antidepressant drugs for the acute treatment of adults with major depressive disorder: a systematic review and network meta-analysis. *Lancet* 2018; **391**: 1357–1366.

2. Warden D, Rush AJ, Trivedi MH, et al. The STAR*D Project results: a comprehensive review of findings. *Curr Psychiatry Rep* 2007; **9**: 449–459.

3. Ferrari AJ, Charlson FJ, Norman RE, et al. Burden of depressive disorders by country, sex, age, and year: findings from the global burden of disease study. *PLoS Med* 2013; **10**: e1001547.

4. Mayberg HS. Limbic-cortical dysregulation: a proposed model of depression. *Journal of Neuropsychiatry & Clinical Neurosciences* 1997; **9**: 471–481.

5. Drevets WC. Neuroimaging and neuropathological studies of depression: implications for the cognitive–emotional features of mood disorders. *Current Opinion in Neurobiology* 2001; **11**: 240–249.

6. Mayberg HS. Modulating dysfunctional limbic-cortical circuits in depression: towards development of brain-based algorithms for diagnosis and optimised treatment. *British Medical Bulletin* 2003; **65**: 193–207.

7. Roiser JP, Elliott R, Sahakian BJ. Cognitive mechanisms of treatment in depression. *Neuropsychopharmacology* 2012; **37**: 117–136.

8. Peters SK, Dunlop K, Downar J. Cortico-striatal-thalamic loop circuits of the salience network: a central pathway in psychiatric disease and treatment. *Front Syst Neurosci* 2016; **27**: 104.

9. Fettes P, Schulze L, Downar J. Cortico-striatal-thalamic loop circuits of the orbitofrontal cortex: promising therapeutic targets in psychiatric illness. *Front Syst Neurosci* 2017; **27**: 25.

10. Brakowski J, Spinelli S, Dörig N, et al. Resting state brain network function in major depression – Depression symptomatology, antidepressant treatment effects, future research. *J Psychiatr Res* 2017; **92**: 147–159.

11. Whitfield-Gabrieli S, Ford JM. Default mode network activity and connectivity in psychopathology. *Annu Rev Clin Psychol* 2015; **8**: 49–76.

12. Wang X, Öngür D, Auerbach RP, et al. Cognitive vulnerability to major depression: view from the intrinsic network and cross-network Interactions. *Harv Rev Psychiatry* 2016; **24**: 188–201.

13. Graham J, Salimi-Khorshidi G, Hagan C, et al. Meta-analytic evidence for neuroimaging models of depression: state or trait? *J Affect Disord* 2013; **151**: 423–431.

14. Sheline YI, Barch DM, Donnelly JM, et al. Increased amygdala response to masked emotional faces in depressed subjects resolves with antidepressant treatment: an fMRI study. *Biol Psychiatry* 2001; **50**: 651–658.

15. Anand A, Li Y, Wang Y, et al. Antidepressant effect on connectivity of the mood-regulating circuit: an fMRI study. *Neuropsychopharmacology* 2005; **30**: 1334–1344.

16. Anand A, Li Y, Wang Y, et al. Reciprocal effects of antidepressant treatment on activity and connectivity of the mood regulating circuit: an fMRI study. *J Neuropsychiatry Clin Neurosci* 2007; **19**: 274–282.

17. Fales CL, Barch DM, Rundle MM, et al. Antidepressant treatment normalizes hypoactivity in dorsolateral prefrontal cortex during emotional interference processing in major depression. *J Affect Disord* 2009; **112**: 206–211.

18. Victor TA, Furey ML, Fromm SJ, et al. Changes in the neural correlates of implicit emotional face processing during antidepressant treatment in major depressive disorder. *Int J Neuropsychopharmacol* 2013; **16**: 2195–2208.

19. Williams LM, Korgaonkar MS, Song YC, et al. Amygdala reactivity to emotional faces in the prediction of general and medication-specific responses to antidepressant treatment in the randomized iSPOT-D trial. *Neuropsychopharmacology* 2015; **40**: 2398–2408.

20. Fu CH, Williams SC, Cleare AJ, et al. Attenuation of the neural response to sad faces in major depression by antidepressant treatment: a prospective, event-related functional magnetic resonance imaging study. *Arch Gen Psychiatry* 2004; **61**: 877–889.

21. Fu CH, Williams SC, Brammer MJ, et al. Neural responses to happy facial expressions in major depression following antidepressant treatment. *Am J Psychiatry* 2007; **164**: 599–607.

22. Walsh ND, Williams SC, Brammer MJ, et al. A longitudinal functional magnetic resonance imaging study of verbal working memory in depression after antidepressant therapy. *Biol Psychiatry* 2007; **62**: 1236–1243.

23. Chen CH, Suckling J, Ooi C, et al. Functional coupling of the amygdala in depressed patients treated with antidepressant medication. *Neuropsychopharmacology* 2008; **33**: 1909–1918.

24. Wang Y, Xu C, Cao X, et al. Effects of an antidepressant on neural correlates of emotional processing in patients with major depression. *Neurosci Lett* 2012; **527**: 55–59.

25. Tao R, Calley CS, Hart J, et al. Brain activity in adolescent major depressive disorder before and after fluoxetine treatment. *Am J Psychiatr* 2012; **169**: 381–388.

26. Heller AS, Johnstone T, Light SN, et al. Relationships between changes in sustained fronto-striatal connectivity and positive affect in major depression resulting from antidepressant treatment. *Am J Psychiatr* 2013; **170**: 197–206.

27. Wagner G, Koch K, Schachtzabel C, et al. Differential effects of serotonergic and noradrenergic antidepressants on brain activity during a cognitive control task and neurofunctional prediction of treatment outcome in patients with depression. *J Psychiat Neurosci* 2010; **35**: 247–257.

28. Arnone D, McKie S, Elliott R, et al. Increased amygdala responses to sad but not fearful faces in major depression: relation to mood state and pharmacological treatment. *Am J Psychiatr* 2012, **169**: 841–850.

29. Jiang W, Yin Z, Pang Y, et al. Brain functional changes in facial expression recognition in patients with major depressive disorder before and after antidepressant treatment: A functional magnetic resonance imaging study. *Neural Regen Res* 2012; **7**: 1151–1157.

30. Stoy M, Schlagenhauf F, Sterzer P, et al. Hyporeactivity of ventral striatum towards incentive stimuli in unmedicated depressed patients normalizes after treatment with escitalopram. *J Psychopharmacol* 2012; **26**: 677–688.

31. Godlewska BR, Norbury R, Cowen PJ, et al. Short-term SSRI treatment normalizes amygdala hyperactivity in depressed patients. *Psych Medicine* 2012; **42**: 2609–2617.

32. Rosenblau G, Sterzer P, Stoy M, et al. Functional neuroanatomy of emotion processing in major depressive disorder is altered after successful antidepressant therapy. *J Psychopharmacol* 2012; **26**: 1424–1433.

33. Miller JM, Schneck N, Siegle GJ, et al. fMRI response to negative words and SSRI treatment outcome in major depressive disorder: a preliminary study. *Psychiat Res* 2013, **214**: 296–305.

34. Wang L, Li K, Zhang Q, et al. Short-term effects of escitalopram on regional brain function in first-episode drug-naive patients with major depressive disorder assessed by resting-state functional magnetic resonance imaging. *Psychol Med* 2014; **44**: 1417–1426.

35. Ruhe HG, Booij J, Veltman DJ, et al. Successful pharmacologic treatment of major depressive disorder attenuates amygdala activation to negative facial expressions: a functional magnetic resonance imaging study. *J Clin Psychiat* 2012; **73**: 451–459.

36. Davidson RJ, Irwin W, Anderle MJ, et al. The neural substrates of affective processing in depressed patients treated with venlafaxine. *Am J Psychiatr* 2003, **160**: 64–75.

37. Schaefer, KM Putnam HS, Benca RM, et al. Event related functional magnetic resonance imaging measures of neural activity to positive social stimuli in pre- and post-treatment depression. *Biol Psychiat* 2006; **60**: 974–986.

38. Benedetti F, Radaelli D, Bernasconi A, et al. Changes in medial prefrontal cortex neural responses parallel successful antidepressant combination of venlafaxine and light therapy. *Arch Ital Biol* 2009; **147**: 83–93.

39. Lisiecka D, Meisenzahl E, Scheuerecker J, et al. Neural correlates of treatment outcome in major depression. *Int J Neuropsychoph* 2011; **14**: 521–534.

40. Samson AC, Meisenzahl E, Scheuerecker J, et al. Brain activation predicts treatment improvement in patients with major depressive disorder. *J Psychiat Res* 2011; **45**: 1214–1222.

41. Gyurak A, Patenaude B, Korgaonkar MS, et al. Frontoparietal activation during response inhibition predicts remission to antidepressants in patients with major depression. *Biol Psychiatry* 2016; **79**: 274–281.

42. Rzepa E, McCabe C. Anhedonia and depression severity dissociated by dmPFC resting-state functional connectivity in adolescents. *J Psychopharmacol* 2018; **32**: 1067–1074.

43. Harmer CJ, Bhagwagar Z, Perrett DI, et al. Acute SSRI administration affects the processing of social cues in healthy volunteers. *Neuropsychopharmacology* 2003; **28**: 148–152.

44. Scheidegger M, Henning A, Walter M, et al. Effects of ketamine on cognition-emotion interaction in the brain. *Neuroimage* 2016; **124**: 8–15.

45. Selvaraj S, Walker C, Arnone D, et al. Effect of citalopram on emotion processing in humans: a combined 5-HT1A [11 C]CUMI-101 PET and functional MRI study. *Neuropsychopharmacology* 2018; **43**: 655–664.

46. Ma Y. Neuropsychological mechanism underlying antidepressant effect: a systematic metaanalysis. *Mol Psychiatry* 2015; **20**: 311–19.

47. Wessa M, Lois G. Brain functional effects of psychopharmacological treatment in major depression: a focus on neural circuitry of affective processing. *Curr Neuropharmacol* 2015; **13**: 466–479.

48. Fu CH, Steiner H, Costafreda SG. Predictive neural biomarkers of clinical response in depression: a meta-analysis of functional and structural neuroimaging studies of pharmacological and psychological therapies. *Neurobiol Dis* 2013; **52**: 75–83.

49. Etkin A, Egner T,. Kalisch R. Emotional processing in anterior cingulate and medial prefrontal cortex. *Trends Cogn Sci* 2011; **15**: 85–93.

50. Pizzagalli DA. Frontocingulate dysfunction in depression: toward biomarkers of treatment response. *Neuropsychopharmacology* 2011; **36**: 183–206.

51. Arnone D. Functional MRI findings, pharmacological treatment in major depression and clinical response. *Prog Neuropsychopharmacol Biol Psychiatry* 2019; **91**: 28–37.

52. Downey D, Dutta A, McKie S, et al. Comparing the actions of lanicemine and ketamine in depression: key role of the anterior cingulate. *Eur Neuropsychopharmacol.* 2016; **26**: 994–1003.

53. McGrath CL, Kelley ME, Holtzheimer PE III, et al. Toward a neuroimaging treatment selection biomarker for major depressive disorder. *JAMA Psychiatry* 2013; **70**: 821–829.

54. Keedwell P, Drapier D, Surguladze S, et al. Neural markers of symptomatic improvement during antidepressant therapy in severe depression: subgenual cingulate and visual cortical responses to sad, but not happy, facial stimuli are correlated with changes in symptom score. *J Psychopharmacol* 2009; **23**: 775–788.

55. Boku S, Nakagawa S, Toda H, et al. Neural basis of major depressive disorder: Beyond monoamine hypothesis. *Psychiatry Clin Neurosci* 2018; **72**: 3–12.

56. Dusi N, Barlati S, Vita A, et al. Brain structural effects of antidepressant treatment in major depression. *Curr Neuropharmacol* 2015; **13**: 458–465.

57. Gunning FM, Cheng J, Murphy CF, et al. Anterior cingulate cortical volumes and treatment remission of geriatric depression. *Int J Geriatr Psychiatry* 2009; **24**: 829–836.

58. Korgaonkar MS, Williams LM, Song YJ, et al. Diffusion tensor imaging predictors of treatment outcomes in major depressive disorder. *Br J Psychiatry* 2014; **205**: 321–328.

59. Korgaonkar MS, Rekshan W, Gordon E, et al. Magnetic resonance imaging measures of brain structure to predict antidepressant treatment outcome in major depressive disorder. *E Bio Medicine* 2014; **2**: 37–45.

60. Dichter GS, Gibbs D, Smoski MJ. A systematic review of relations between resting-state functional-MRI and treatment response in major depressive disorder. *J Affect Disord* 2015; **172**: 8–17.

61. Yang R, Zhang H, Wu X, et al. Hypothalamus-anchored resting brain network changes before and after sertraline treatment in major depression. *Biomed Res Int* 2014; **2014**: 915026.

62. Posner J, Hellerstein DJ, Gat I, et al. Antidepressants normalize the default mode network in patients with dysthymia. *JAMA Psychiatry* 2013; **70**: 373–382.

63. Li B, Liu L, Friston KJ, et al. A treatment-resistant default mode subnetwork in major depression. *Biol Psychiatry* 2013; **74**: 48–54.

64. Wagner G, de la Cruz F, Köhler S, et al. Treatment associated changes of functional connectivity of midbrain/brainstem nuclei in major depressive disorder. *Sci Rep* 2017; **7**: 8675.

65. de Kwaasteniet B, Ruhe E, Caan M, et al. Relation between structural and functional connectivity in major depressive disorder. *Biol Psychiatry* 2013; **74**: 40–47.

66. Guo WB, Liu F, Chen JD, et al. Abnormal neural activity of brain regions in treatment-resistant and treatment-sensitive major depressive disorder: a resting-state fMRI study. *J Psychiatr Res* 2012; **46**: 1366–1373.

67. Guo W, Liu F, Xue Z, et al. Abnormal resting-state cerebellar-cerebral functional connectivity in treatment-resistant depression and treatment sensitive depression. *Prog Neuropsychopharmacol Biol Psychiatry* 2013; **44**: 51–57.

68. Maltbie EA, Kaundinya GS, Howell LL. Ketamine and pharmacological imaging: use of functional magnetic resonance imaging to evaluate mechanisms of action. *Behav Pharmacol* 2017; **28**: 610–622.

69. Abdallah CG, Averill LA, Collins KA, et al. Ketamine treatment and global brain connectivity in major depression. *Neuropsychopharmacology* 2017; **42**:1210–1219.

70. Gopinath K, Maltbie E, Urushino N, et al. Ketamine-induced changes in connectivity of functional brain networks in awake female

nonhuman primates: a translational functional imaging model. *Psychopharmacology (Berl)* 2016; **233**: 3673–3684.

71. da Cunha-Bang S, Ettrup A, Mc Mahon B, et al. Measuring endogenous changes in serotonergic neurotransmission with [11 C]Cimbi-36 positron emission tomography in humans. *Transl Psychiatry* 2019; **9**: 134.

72. Miller JM, Hesselgrave N, Ogden RT, et al. Brain serotonin 1A receptor binding as a predictor of treatment outcome in major depressive disorder. *Biol Psychiatry* 2013, 15; **74**: 760–767.

73. Gray NA, Milak MS, DeLorenzo C, et al. Antidepressant treatment reduces serotonin-1A autoreceptor binding in major depressive disorder. *Biol Psychiatry* 2013; **74**: 26–31.

74. Spies M, Knudsen GM, Lanzenberger R, et al. The serotonin transporter in psychiatric disorders: insights from PET imaging. *Lancet Psychiatry* 2015; **2**: 743–755.

75. Miller JM, Oquendo MA, Ogden RT, et al. Serotonin transporter binding as a possible predictor of one-year remission in major depressive disorder. *J Psychiatr Res* 2008; **42**: 1137–1144.

76. Lanzenberger R, Kranz GS, Haeusler D, et al. Prediction of SSRI treatment response in major depression based on serotonin transporter interplay between median raphe nucleus and projection areas. *Neuroimage* 2012; **63**: 874–871.

77. Yeh YW, Ho PS, Kuo SC, et al. Disproportionate reduction of serotonin transporter may predict the response and adherence to antidepressants in patients with major depressive disorder: a positron emission tomography study with 4-[18 F]-ADAM. *Int J Neuropsychopharmacol.* 2015 Jan 7;18(7): pyu120.

78. James GM, Baldinger-Melich P, Philippe C, et al. Effects of selective serotonin reuptake inhibitors on interregional relation of serotonin transporter availability in major depression. *Front Hum Neurosci* 2017; **11**: 48.

79. Arakawa R, Stenkrona P, Takano A, et al. Venlafaxine ER blocks the norepinephrine transporter in the brain of patients with major depressive disorder: a PET study using [18 F] FMeNER-D2. *Int J Neuropsychopharmacol* 2019; **22**: 278–285.

80. Moriguchi S, Takano H, Kimura Y, et al. Occupancy of norepinephrine transporter by duloxetine in human brains measured by positron

emission tomography with (S,S)-[18 F] FMeNER-D2. *Int J Neuropsychopharmacol* 2017; **20**: 957–962.

81. Pringle A, Harmer CJ. The effects of drugs on human models of emotional processing: an account of antidepressant drug treatment. *Dialogues Clin Neurosci* 2015; **17**: 477–487.

82. Godlewska BR. Cognitive neuropsychological theory: reconciliation of psychological and biological approaches for depression. *Pharmacol Ther* 2018; pii: S0163–7258(**18**)30232–30238.

83. Komulainen E, Heikkilä R, Nummenmaa L, et al. Short-term escitalopram treatment normalizes aberrant self-referential processing in major depressive disorder. *J Affect Disord* 2018; **236**: 222–229.

84. Godlewska BR, Browning M, Norbury R, et al. Early changes in emotional processing as a marker of clinical response to SSRI treatment in depression. *Transl Psych* 2016; **6**: e957.

85. Shiroma PR, Thuras P, Johns B, et al. Emotion recognition processing as early predictor of response to 8-week citalopram treatment in late-life depression. *Int J Geriatr Psychiatry* 2014; **29**: 1132–1139.

86. MacLeod C, Rutherford E, Campbell L, et al. Selective attention and emotional vulnerability: assessing the causal basis of their association through the experimental manipulation of attentional bias. *J Abnorm Psychol* 2002; **111**: 107–123.

87. Miller S, McTeague LM, Gyurak A, et al. Cognition-childhood maltreatment interactions in the prediction of antidepressant outcomes in major depressive disorder patients: results from the iSPOT-D trial. *Depress Anxiety* 2015; **32**: 594–604.

88. Holmes EA, Ghaderi A, Harmer CJ, et al. Commission on psychological treatments research in tomorrow's science. *The Lancet Psychiatry* 2018; **5**: 237–286.

89. Browning M, Reid C, Cowen PJ, Goodwin GM, Harmer CJ. A single dose of citalopram increases fear recognition in healthy subjects. *J Psychopharmacol* 2007; **21**: 684–690.

90. Jonassen R, Chelnokova O, Harmer C, et al. A single dose of antidepressant alters eye-gaze patterns across face stimuli in healthy women. *Psychopharmacology* 2014; **232**: 953–958.

91. Di Simplicio M, Norbury R, Reinecke A, et al. Paradoxical effects of short-term antidepressant treatment in fMRI emotional processing models in

volunteers with high neuroticism. *Psychol Med* 2014; **44**: 241–252.

92. McArthur RA. Aligning physiology with psychology: translational neuroscience in neuropsychiatric drug discovery. *Neuroscience & Biobehavioral Reviews* 2017; **76**: 4–21.

93. Insel TR. The NIMH Research Domain Criteria (RDoC) Project: precision medicine for psychiatry. *Am J Psychiatry* 2014; **171**: 395–397.

94. Drysdale AT, Grosenick L, Downar J, et al. Resting-state Connectivity Biomarkers Define Neurophysiological Subtypes of Depression Nat Med. 2017 Jan;23(1):28–38.

Chapter 20

Neuroimaging Studies of Effects of Psychotherapy in Depression

Isabelle E. Bauer and Thomas D. Meyer

20.1 Introduction

Depression is one of the leading causes of mortality, disability, and loss of productivity. The World Health Organization (WHO) ranks depressive disorders as the eleventh cause of disability and mortality (1, 2). The worldwide lifetime prevalence of depression is around 12% (3). In spite of the considerable burden of depression both in terms of prevalence and public health impact, the search for more effective treatments for depression is still ongoing. Emerging evidence suggests that personalizing treatments based on individuals' biosignature could be the "way forward" (4).

An increasing number of studies have therefore sought to identify potential biological predictors of clinical outcomes that could guide treatment selection. While the majority of these studies have primarily focused on pharmacological treatments (5, 6), few of them have examined potential correlates of psychotherapeutic outcome. Psychotherapy, specifically cognitive behavioral and interpersonal therapies, has been shown to be particularly efficacious in the treatment of depression. A large meta-analysis concluded that following psychotherapy, 62% of depressed patients no longer met criteria for depression. By comparison, only 48% of depressed patients achieved full remission following care-as-usual, which was defined as interventions other than the psychotherapy received as part of the clinical trial (7). While there is not much evidence for differences in effectiveness across psychotherapies when looking at short-term effects (8), the combined treatment with psychotherapy and medication appears to have superior therapeutic benefits when compared with monotherapy (9, 10). Further, a meta-analysis of eleven studies following up patients for approximately fifteen months showed a small-to-moderate effect size favoring psychotherapy

relative to pharmacotherapy (11). These findings indicate that the long-term benefits of psychotherapy may outweigh those of pharmacotherapy. Understanding the neural mechanisms involved in successful psychotherapy has, therefore, substantial clinical relevance for guiding personalized treatments and potentially refining current psychotherapy techniques.

Neuroimaging in psychotherapy is a very new, yet active and growing research area. It holds substantial clinical potential as, in the future, it may provide information on the neural correlates related to the effects of specific therapeutic interventions. To date, studies have integrated psychotherapy and multiple imaging measures by assessing psychotherapy-related brain changes in function of treatment response. Baseline imaging measures have also been examined with the aim of predicting treatment response (12). These studies have provided preliminary insight into the potential neural mechanisms of action of psychotherapy, and may lead to the development of guidelines on how to select treatment for individual patients on the basis of indicators of brain functioning at baseline.

In summary, the application of imaging techniques to study the process and outcome of psychotherapy has the potential to significantly improve our understanding of neural processes underlying changes during psychotherapy and treatment. This review chapter aims to provide up-to-date information on the effects of psychotherapy on the brain and evidence of potential imaging predictors of clinical outcomes.

20.2 Literature Search

In the past decade, an increasing number of studies have integrated imaging techniques into psychotherapy research across psychiatric disorders (13–18). Given that the definition of "psychotherapy" is broad and encompasses a number of therapeutic approaches and techniques, this chapter will focus on three empirically supported and well-established therapeutic psychological interventions for depression: cognitive behavioral therapy (CBT), behavioral activation therapy (BAT), and interpersonal therapy (IPT). These interventions were selected because (1) CBTs are evidence-based treatments and are guided by well-established principles of learning theories, behavioral science and cognitive psychology (19); (2) CBT is one of the most empirically evaluated forms of therapy in relation to emotion regulation and cognitive control; and (3) CBT and IPT are considered to be the gold-standard treatments of depression (20).

Although, nowadays, CBT is considered to be an umbrella term for a wide range of interventions, the common premise is that maladaptive or dysfunctional beliefs and biased information processing contribute to the development and maintenance of depressive symptoms. Based on this model, addressing maladaptive thoughts is a first step toward reducing the risk for relapse (21). The goal of BAT is to help patients engage more in rewarding behaviors while also reducing withdrawal and avoidance (22). BAT has been found to be as effective as CBT to reduce depressive symptoms and prevent relapse (23, 24). IPT is a short, present-oriented, form of psychotherapy that views interpersonal issues as the primary trigger for the development and maintenance of psychological distress (25, 26).

We reviewed existing publications that included both neuroimaging and clinical outcome measures to evaluate the efficacy of psychotherapy. We restricted our search to those studies with adult samples and who described their participants as suffering from depression. We searched PubMed, Scopus, Ovid, and Cochrane for articles containing the terms "depression," "psychotherapy," "cognitive therapy," or "behavioral therapy" combined with terms referring to widely used structural and functional neuroimaging techniques including "MRI," "fMRI," "DTI," "photon emission," "positron emission," or "spectroscopy." We additionally included electroencephalogram (EEG) measures as they provide neural indices of cognitive processes of relevance for psychotherapy (e.g., cognitive control and self-monitoring). We also reviewed studies discussed in Weingarten et al. and Fournier et al.'s systematic and meta-analysis reviews on neuroimaging

and psychotherapy in psychiatry (27, 28). Although this search has no claims of being fully exhaustive, it aimed to provide comprehensive evidence of the state of the science in the field of imaging and psychotherapy.

For ease of reading we present our findings in two different sections. The first section examines the effects of psychotherapy on the brain, and the second section discusses the imaging predictors of psychotherapy response. Table 20.1 summarizes the primary findings of this review.

20.3 Effects of Psychotherapy on the Brain in Depression

To put our findings into context, it is important to provide first a brief overview of the structural and functional brain networks associated with mood disorders. Frontal (orbitofrontal, dorsolateral, and ventromedial), limbic (amygdala, hippocampus, and insula), and anterior cingulate cortex (ACC) are closely connected key emotion-processing regions (29, 30). Fear processing and anhedonia are prevalent in depression, and have been linked to poor functioning and connectivity within and between basal ganglia, striatum, and para/hippocampal regions (28, 31). The well-established evidence of the reduced connectivity between the prefrontal, cingulate, and limbic-striatal structures (32) supports the hypothesis of a fronto-limbic disconnection leading to the mood dysregulation observed in mood disorders (33). This disconnection is hypothesized to disrupt cognitive control or "top-down" processes, and may lead to increased emotional or "bottom-up" activity (34). There is general agreement that psychotherapy may strengthen the cognitive "top-down" network by teaching individuals to implement effective problem-solving and coping skills to manage stressful situations (28).

Overall, the majority of the studies retrieved in our systematic review have focused on CBT, and to a lesser extent on BAT and IPT. To date, most imaging studies of psychotherapy have used fMRI and positron emission tomography (PET), and only few studies adopted sMRI, magnetic resonance spectroscopy (MRS), and EEG techniques. In the following section, we will discuss available imaging findings illustrating the effects of psychotherapy on functional, metabolic, and structural brain measures.

Table 20.1 Summary of the imaging studies of psychotherapy included in the current review

Studies	Design	Age (mean ±SD)	Gender	Diagnosis depression at baseline	Medicated during psychotherapy?	N of CBT sessions	Definition of responder	N of responders	Imaging technique	If fMRI: type of task
Brody et al. (51)	14 IPT 10 paroxetine 16 HC	40.7±11 36.4±12.2 35.6±18.3	57%	HAMD: 20.5±5.3 17.8±5.5 0.8±1.3	No	12 weeks	None	IPT: 38% decrease Paroxetine: 61.4% decrease	PET	
Costafreda et al. (56)	16 CBT	40±9	13	HRSD21±2	No	16	HDRS<8	9	fMRI	Implicit processing of sad faces
Dichter et al. (64)	12 BAT 15 HC	11.4±2	6	HAM-D:30.8±9.7	No	15	HAM-D<6	9	fMRI	Monetary incentive reward
Dichter et al. (43)	12 BAT 15 HC	39±10.4 30.8±9.6	6 9	HAM-D:23.8±2.3	No	8 to 14 sessions	HAM-D≤6	9	fMRI	Cognitive control using sad stimuli
Fu et al. (62)	16 CBT 16 HC	40±9	13	HDRS:21±2	No	8	HDRS<8	8	fMRI	Sad faces recognition
Goldapple et al. (50)	14 CBT 13 paroxetine	41±9 (based on completers and not completers, not reported for paroxetine)	Not reported	HDRS 20±3, 22.8 ±3.6	No	17.7±2 sessions over 26 ±7 weeks	50% HDRS decrease	9	PET	
Kennedy et al. (41)	12 CBT 12 venlafaxine	30±9.8 41.25 ±9.4	7, 8	HAMD:20.6±3.4, 20.3±3	No	16	50% HAMD decrease	5, 3	PET	
Konarski et al. (67)	12 CBT 12 venlafaxine	29.45±18.8 38.95±10.3	7 7	HAMD:20.8±3.35 20.5±3.05	No	16	50% HAMD decrease	7 CBT	PET	
Martin et al. (52)	13 IPT 15 venlafaxine	38±4.9 39.4±8.3	9	HAMD:22.7±2.7 22.4±3.1	No	6 weeks	Not reported	Not reported	SPECT	

Table 20.1 (cont.)

Studies	Design	Age (mean ±SD)	Gender	Diagnosis depression at baseline	Medicated during psychotherapy?	N of CBT sessions	Definition of responder	N of responders	Imaging technique	If fMRI: type of task
Ritchey et al. (37)	15 CBT	36±10	9	BDI:27±7	No	On average 30	BDI decrease by at least 8 points & final BDI score ≤ 14	12	fMRI	Evaluation of emotional pictures
Siegle et al. (35)	14 CBT 21 HC	45±9	7	BDI:25±12	No	12	BDI<8	62%	fMRI	Sustained attention to emotional words
Yoshimura et al. (36)	23 CBT 15 HC	37.3±7.2 36.7±8.2	7 7	HAMD:14.7±4.4	Yes	12	Not reported	Not reported	fMRI	Self-referential to emotional stimuli

20.3.1 fMRI

Most fMRI studies of psychotherapy employed task-based protocols requiring the explicit or implicit processing of emotional stimuli. The primary outcome measures of these studies are typically the pre- to post-psychotherapy changes in either brain activation or functional connectivity. It is noteworthy mentioning that, unless otherwise specified, the findings here below refer to treatment-related changes in brain functioning in patients with depression. When compared to their pretreatment imaging measures, CBT-treated patients showed reduced activation in the medial prefrontal cortex and ventral ACC during the evaluation of negative stimuli (35) and increased activation in these regions in response to positive stimuli (stimuli included self-referential and non-self-referential cues)(36, 37). CBT was also associated with increased activation in the amygdala, caudate nucleus, and hippocampus, which are regions involved in emotion, reward processing, and emotional memory, respectively (38). Interestingly, prior to CBT, depressed patients were found to have stronger fronto-cingulate connectivity compared to healthy controls (39). The CBT-related improvement in depressive symptoms correlated positively with the reduction in fronto-cingulate connectivity (39). This finding suggests that these brain regions might underlie some of the dysfunctional thoughts targeted as part of CBT. This is also partially in line with findings showing that a decrease in connectivity between the dorsal anterior and subgenual ACC regions is linked to lower levels of self-reported worry in anxious patients (40). CBT also led to an increase in connectivity between the amygdala and frontoparietal regions during a task evaluating feelings and thoughts triggered by emotionally salient stimuli (37). These findings are consistent with previous evidence that low connectivity in the fronto-limbic network predicts poor response to both psychotherapy and antidepressant medication (41, 42).

One of the few studies examining the neural predictors of BAT outcomes found that having been treated with BAT was associated with decreased activation in the prefrontal, cingulate and paracingulate, caudate nucleus, fusiform, and cerebellar regions in response to sad stimuli (43). The frontal regions have noteworthy a high clinical relevance and play an important role in cognitive control and information processing (44). For example, the orbitofrontal cortex has been implicated in affective processing, decision-making, and suicidal thoughts (45, 46). As Dichter et al. (43) pointed out, this finding stands in contrast with the previous pharmacological literature showing an increase in prefrontal activation alongside symptom remission (47, 48). While differences in task protocols could contribute to such inconsistent results, these findings could also suggest that psychotherapy and medication lead to symptom remission by targeting different brain networks. For instance, in Dichter et al.'s study, psychotherapy induced changes in activation in the pars triangularis, which is important for language and motor control but is not directly involved in emotion regulation or cognitive control.

20.3.2 PET and SPECT

CBT-related serotonin changes were measured with positron emission tomography (PET) using a serotonergic 5-HT_{1B} receptor-selective radioligand (49). CBT was associated with a 33% reduction in serotonergic binding potential in the dorsal brain stem. This finding is not surprising given that this brain region includes the raphe nucleus, a key node in the serotonin pathway (49). The authors argued that a reduction in serotonergic binding may reflect the downregulation of the inhibitory 5-HT_{1B} receptor and the increase in serotonin release to emotion-processing areas such as the prefrontal and limbic regions. It is noteworthy mentioning that all the patients involved in this study responded successfully to CBT, thus suggesting a strong link between CBT outcomes and serotonin production. A (^{18} F)-2-fluoro-2-deoxy-d-glucose–PET study by Goldapple et al. (50) compared CBT to paroxetine, a selective serotonin reuptake inhibitor. CBT-treated patients displayed an increase in glucose metabolism in the prefrontal, cingulate, and hippocampal regions, which are brain areas associated with mood regulation (50).

Few studies have examined the impact of IPT on functional brain measures. IPT was associated with increased glucose metabolism in the left insula compared to paroxetine (51). Further, IPT-treated individuals showed increased brain blood flow (measured with single-photon emission computed tomography or SPECT) in posterior cingulate brain regions when compared to the serotonin-norepinephrine reuptake inhibitor venlafaxine (52). It is noteworthy that this study did not detect the changes in activation in cingulate or frontal regions observed in the fMRI psychotherapy studies discussed in the previous section.

The divergence of results may be due to the selection of regions of interest included in the analyses. It is also important to remember that the fMRI and PET techniques measure different physiological processes. While fMRI findings are task-specific, PET measures are closely related to the brain metabolism at rest.

20.3.3 MRS

Two proton magnetic resonance spectroscopy (^{1}H-MRS) studies measured changes in gamma-aminobutyric acid (GABA) concentrations in the occipital cortex of depressed patients. The selection of this region was based on studies showing that antidepressant treatments such as serotonin reuptake inhibitors and electroconvulsive therapy were associated with an increase in occipital GABA concentrations (53, 54). CBT was not found to alter occipital GABA levels in either of these studies (55, 56). This suggests that, while previous pharmacological treatments targeted the GABAergic pathways, CBT interventions may not affect this brain circuit.

20.4 Imaging as a Predictor of Psychotherapy Response

Functional and structural neuroimaging have, so far, shown that psychotherapy targets fronto-limbic and fronto-cingulate networks. As part of this review, we also examined whether these same regions could predict the likelihood of response to CBT, BAT, and IPT.

20.4.1 fMRI

Hypoactivity in the ACC (35) and sustained hyperactivity in the dorsolateral prefrontal cortex during an emotional task were associated with favorable response to CBT (57). In the latter study, CBT nonresponders showed increased activity in the right amygdala at baseline, which may indicate that an overactive amygdala interferes with CBT. Alternatively, it is possible that some of the patients included in this study suffered from comorbid anxiety. If this were the case, the poor response to CBT may be due to the fact that CBT targeted depression instead of anxiety. Indeed, the amygdala is involved in fear processing and shows increased reactivity in response to stressful events (58).

Increased resting state functional connectivity between subcallosal cingulate regions, the frontal operculum, and ventromedial prefrontal cortex were found to be predictors of a positive response to CBT (59). The same study also found that, before CBT, responders activated a network of brain regions similar to that of healthy volunteers. In another study, baseline hypoactivity in the frontal inferior triangle and right superior frontal gyrus and hyperactivity in the middle frontal and left superior frontal gyrus predicted better CBT outcome (60). Elevated functional activity in the cingulate, paracingulate, temporal, and striatal regions was also found to be a predictor of a better response to CBT (37, 38, 41, 43, 50, 61). More specifically, individuals with high cingulate activation in response to sad stimuli prior to CBT were more likely to respond to CBT (56). Fu et al. argued that ACC hyperactivity, and reduced amygdala-hippocampal hypoconnectivity may be the key predictors for a positive response to CBT (20, 62).

Decreased connectivity between the anterior insula and the middle temporal regions was associated with severe anhedonia and symptom severity prior to CBT treatment. Intriguingly, hypoconnectivity between these regions was also linked to increased likelihood of CBT response (22). ACC activation in response to a reward-processing task was found to be a positive predictor of BAT outcome (63). This finding is not surprising given that BAT encourages patients to engage in activities that give them a sense of purpose. The success of BAT may therefore require high reward responsiveness on a neural level (64).

20.4.2 PET

In line with previously reviewed structural and functional imaging findings, the ACC glucose metabolism was found to be a predictor of positive CBT response (41, 65, 66). High baseline glucose metabolism in subcallosal cingulate (67) and limbic-subcortical areas (65), and reduced metabolism in the insula (68) predicted a better outcome following CBT (65). By comparison, individuals with high glucose metabolism in the insula were more likely to remit in response to medication (70). The findings related to the insula are intriguing since this brain region plays a role in emotional self-awareness and processing of subjective feeling states (69). However, it has yet to be determined whether having low glucose metabolism in the insula means having poor self-awareness and reduced ability to process feelings. An alternative interpretation of this finding may be that the insula contributes to the successful assimilation and implementation of CBT strategies.

20.4.3 Structural MRI and EEG

Structural MRI studies showed a positive correlation between enlarged ACC cortical volumes and reduced depressive symptoms (70). Large cingulate volumes along with strong connectivity between inferior parietal and prefrontal regions were also associated with better CBT outcomes. Specifically, stronger connectivity between these regions prior to CBT was correlated with increased self-reported use of effective "adaptive rumination techniques" (i.e., reflective pondering) (71). Cingulate regions are involved in decision-making, cognitive control, and affective processing (72). One could therefore argue that individuals with enlarged cingulate volumes have better self-monitoring abilities and are more likely to respond to CBT.

In patients with comorbid depression and anxiety, decreased amplitudes in the reward positivity EEG component (which originates from frontal regions and reflects processing of positive feedback vs. breaking even or losing) were found to be associated with a better response to CBT (73). The authors argued that individuals who can resist immediate rewards in favor of long-term rewards may be more likely to benefit from CBT.

20.5 Discussion

This review examined the neural substrates of psychotherapy in patients with depressive disorders. The studies reviewed in this chapter provided consistent evidence that increased activation and glucose in the ACC predicted a positive response to psychosocial interventions,

including CBT, BAT, and IPT. Other regions of clinical relevance included the prefrontal regions and the amygdala (35, 72). These brain regions are key areas for emotion regulation and reward processing and have been previously discussed with regards to the pathophysiology of depression (73). The rostral and subgenual components of the ACC have also been found to predict response to a number of treatments including antidepressant medication (75, 76), transcranial magnetic resonance (77), and sleep deprivation (78). This review showed that the neural effects of psychotherapy extended to regions closely connected to the ACC such as fronto-limbic, cingulate, striatal, and insula regions. These brain regions have clinical relevance as the fronto-cingulate network and the striatum contribute to reward processing (79) and the insula is involved in self-monitoring and emotional awareness (80). Current evidence also shows that individuals who present with hyperactivity in the ACC, decreased frontal activity, and amygdala–hippocampal connectivity comparable to that of healthy volunteers prior to CBT are more likely to respond to treatment (18, 62). This would support the hypothesis suggesting that psychotherapy targets the cognitive control "top-down" pathway (e.g., ACC) to regulate individuals' emotional response (e.g., amygdala) (28).

These findings are in line with previous literature on emotional regulation and resilience. Enlarged ventral medial prefrontal cortex, rostral, and subgenual ACC were found to be key neural markers of resilience to stress (81). Further, reduced cortico-limbic connectivity has been related to increased sensitivity to stress, emotion dysregulation, and increased vulnerability to mood and anxiety disorders (82, 83).

The finding related to the increased fronto-limbic connectivity and activation in reward-processing striatal regions related to cognitive behavioral therapies is not surprising. CBT, IPT, and BAT aim to strengthen the patients' ability to regulate emotions and cope with stressful situations. BAT specifically engages patients in favoring meaningful and uplifting activities over behaviors that exacerbate depression, for example, avoidance or rumination. Given the dearth of findings related to IPT and BAT, additional evidence is, however, needed to build a detailed neural model of action for psychotherapy or perhaps even different psychological approaches or strategies.

When interpreting the presented findings, it seems essential to keep in mind the large number of biological constructs probed by each imaging technique (i.e., structural measures, brain metabolism, cerebral blood oxygenation) and different methods (i.e., activity at rest or during a task). The psychotherapy-related changes in functional and metabolic activity may vary depending on the individuals' resting activity prior to the task, selection of the comparison/control conditions in fMRI tasks, and interindividual differences. The small sample sizes and the lack of correction for interindividual differences at baseline in subsequent analyses may constitute substantial confounding factors. Further, regional brain changes in activation or metabolism may be due to a number of physiological, task-specific, and setting-related factors. For instance, a post-treatment increase in brain activation may suggest functional improvement but may also reflect impaired neural efficiency. This concept refers to the need for additional brain effort to accomplish the same task. It is also important to point out that current studies did not examine whether functional activation and metabolic changes were partly due to practice effects and whether they were maintained over time. Furthermore, studies assessing the predictive power of imaging measures focused either on psychotherapy only or compared psychotherapy to antidepressant medication. These studies could not, therefore, determine if any observed changes in brain metabolisms were specific to CBT, IPT, BAT, or psychotherapy in general. To date, studies have defined "treatment response" based on the reduction of depression severity on mood questionnaires. There are other measures of treatment and remission response such as global functioning, psychosocial adjustment, perceived quality of life or long-term stability of mood after a maintenance period. These measures would provide additional and perhaps more useful information when investigating neural markers of therapeutic success.

20.6 Final Conclusions

The management of depression remains an open challenge as currently treatments are either suboptimal or unsatisfactory. There are several medications and other somatic treatments available to treat depressive disorders, but remission rates are not high, and recurrence remains a challenge for health professionals. Evidence suggests that the combination of psychotherapy and medication can enhance the likelihood of sustained treatment response when compared to monotherapy during the acute phase of the illness (10). However, as highlighted in this review, people's brains differ in how they respond to treatments for depression. Personalized treatments of depression based on individuals' neural signature appear to be a promising way to address this issue. With the advent of sophisticated imaging techniques and methodologies, the goal of identifying predictive neural markers of treatment response is within reach.

As illustrated earlier, response to psychotherapy interventions such as CBT, IPT, and BAT appears to be linked to the fronto-limbic, cingulate, hippocampal, and insula regions. This research field is still in its infancy and additional well-designed randomized clinical trials are obviously needed to distinguish neural processes related to short-term treatment response to those related to long-term treatment effectiveness. It would be important to compare results based on different treatment efficacy measures (e.g., relapse, symptom reduction). Future protocols should also compare therapy interventions (IPT, CBT, BAT, etc.) to treatment-as-usual and/or antidepressant medication. It might also be that the presence or absence of comorbidities (e.g., anxiety disorders) might have been a confounding factor in some of the imaging studies reviewed here. One could also consider integrating multiple imaging modalities to acquire structural, functional, and metabolic measures such as glucose metabolism or blood flow. For fMRI studies, it may be equally helpful to include physiological measures such as heart rate variability or skin conductance to discard potential effects of stress on functional brain activity. The use of functional near-infrared spectroscopy (fNIRS) may provide in vivo information of changes in cerebral flow during therapy. This noninvasive technique involves the use of a skullcap that detects changes in cortical blood flow and could be used to monitor participants' brain response during the course of a CBT session.

In summary, there is limited but promising evidence that psychosocial therapies modulate brain function and metabolism and this may help predict treatment response and clinical outcomes in depressive disorders. Additional research in this field is needed to refine these findings and establish their reproducibility.

References

1. Whiteford HA, et al. Global burden of disease attributable to mental and substance use disorders: Findings from the global burden of disease study 2010. *Lancet*. 2013; **382**(9904): 1575–1586.

2. Park SC, et al. Does age at onset of first major depressive episode indicate the subtype of major depressive disorder?: The clinical research center for depression study. *Yonsei Med J*. 2014; **55**(6): 1712–1720.

3. Kessler RC, et al. Age differences in the prevalence and co-morbidity of DSM-IV major depressive episodes: Results from the WHO world mental health survey initiative. *Depress Anxiety*. 2010; **27**(4): 351–364.

4. Oquendo MA. McGrath P, Weissman MM. Biomarker studies and the future of personalized treatment for depression. *Depression and Anxiety*. 2014; **31**(11): 902–905.

5. Chen C-H, et al. Brain imaging correlates of depressive symptom severity and predictors of symptom improvement after antidepressant treatment. *Biological Psychiatry*. 2007; **62**(5): 407–414.

6. Li C-T, et al. Cognition-modulated frontal activity in prediction and augmentation of antidepressant efficacy: A randomized controlled pilot study. *Cerebral Cortex*. 2014; **26**(1): 202–210.

7. Cuijpers P, et al. The effects of psychotherapies for major depression in adults on remission, recovery and improvement: A meta-analysis. *Journal of Affective Disorders*. 2014; **159**: 118–126.

8. Cuijpers P, et al. Psychological treatment of depression: A meta-analytic database of randomized studies. *BMC Psychiatry*. 2008; **8**(1): 36.

9. Cuijpers P, et al. A meta-analysis of cognitive-behavioural therapy for adult depression, alone and in comparison with other treatments. *The Canadian Journal of Psychiatry*. 2013; **58**(7): 376–385.

10. Karyotaki E, et al. Combining pharmacotherapy and psychotherapy or monotherapy for major depression? A meta-analysis on the long-term effects. *Journal of Affective Disorders*. 2016; **194**: 144–152.

11. Cuijpers P, et al. Adding psychotherapy to antidepressant medication in depression and anxiety disorders: A meta-analysis. *World Psychiatry*. 2014; **13**(1): 56–67.

12. Chakrabarty T, Ogrodniczuk J, Hadjipavlou G. Predictive neuroimaging markers of psychotherapy response: A systematic review. *Harvard Review of Psychiatry*. 2016; **24**(6): 396–405.

13. Linden D. How psychotherapy changes the brain– the contribution of functional neuroimaging. *Molecular Psychiatry*, 2006. **11**(6): 528.

14. Frewen PA, Dozois DJ, Lanius RA. Neuroimaging studies of psychological interventions for mood and anxiety disorders: empirical and methodological review. *Focus*. 2010; **8**(1): 92–109.

15. Beauregard M. Functional neuroimaging studies of the effects of psychotherapy. *Dialogues in Clinical Neuroscience*. 2014; **16**(1): 75.

16. Barsaglini A, et al. The effects of psychotherapy on brain function: A systematic and critical review. *Progress in Neurobiology*. 2014; **114**: 1–14.

17. Roffman JL, et al. Neuroimaging and the functional neuroanatomy of psychotherapy. *Psychological Medicine*. 2005; **35**(10): 1385–1398.

18. Fu C, Steiner H, Costafreda SG. Predictive neural biomarkers of clinical response in depression: a meta-analysis of functional and structural neuroimaging studies of pharmacological and psychological therapies. *Neurobiol Disease*. 2013. **52**: 75–83.

19. Beck JS. *Cognitive Behavior Therapy: Basics and Beyond*. Guilford press; 2011.

20. Parker G, Fletcher K. Treating depression with the evidence-based psychotherapies: A critique of the evidence. *Acta Psychiatrica Scandinavica*. 2007; **115**(5): 352–359.

21. Beck AT. *Cognitive Therapy of Depression*. Guilford press; 1979.

22. Crowther A, et al. Resting-state connectivity predictors of response to psychotherapy in major depressive disorder. *Neuropsychopharmacology*. 2015; **40**(7): 1659–1673.

23. Dimidjian S, et al. Randomized trial of behavioral activation, cognitive therapy, and antidepressant medication in the acute treatment of adults with major depression. *Journal of Consulting and Clinical Psychology*. 2006; **74**(4): 658.

24. Dobson KS, et al. Randomized trial of behavioral activation, cognitive therapy, and antidepressant medication in the prevention of relapse and recurrence in major depression. *Journal of Consulting and Clinical Psychology*. 2008; **76**(3): 468.

25. Klerman GL, et al. *Interpersonal Psychotherapy for Depression*. Lanham, Maryland, USA: Rowman & Littlefield; 1996.

26. Cuijpers P, et al. Interpersonal psychotherapy for depression: A meta-analysis. *American Journal of Psychiatry*. 2011; **168**(6): 581–592.

27. Weingarten CP, Strauman TJ. Neuroimaging for psychotherapy research: current trends. *Psychotherapy Research*. 2015; **25**(2): 185–213.

28. Fournier JC, Price RB. Psychotherapy and neuroimaging. *Focus*. 2014; **12**(3): 290–298.

29. Drevets WC. Neuroimaging and neuropathological studies of depression: Implications for the cognitive-emotional features of mood disorders. *Current opinion in neurobiology*. 2001; **11**(2): 240–249.

30. Hariri AR, Bookheimer SY, Mazziotta JC. Modulating emotional responses: Effects of a neocortical network on the limbic system. *Neuroreport*. 2000; **11**(1): 43–48.

31. Fales CL, et al. Altered emotional interference processing in affective and cognitive-control brain circuitry in major depression. *Biological Psychiatry*. 2008; **63**(4): 377–384.

32. Vargas C, Lopez-Jaramillo C, Vieta E. A systematic literature review of resting state network–functional MRI in bipolar disorder. *J Affect Disord*. 2013; **150**(3): 727–735.

33. Radaelli D, et al. Fronto-limbic disconnection in bipolar disorder. *Eur Psychiatry*. 2015; **30**(1): 82–88.

34. Phillips ML, Swartz HA. A critical appraisal of neuroimaging studies of bipolar disorder: toward a new conceptualization of underlying neural circuitry and a road map for future research. *Am J Psychiatry*. 2014; **171**(8): 829–843.

35. Siegle GJ, Carter CS, Thase ME. Use of fMRI to predict recovery from unipolar depression with cognitive behavior therapy. *American Journal of Psychiatry*. 2006; **163**(4): 735–738.

36. Yoshimura S, et al. Cognitive behavioral therapy for depression changes medial prefrontal and ventral anterior cingulate cortex activity associated with self-referential processing. *Social Cognitive and Affective Neuroscience*. 2014; **9**(4): 487–493.

37. Ritchey M, et al. Neural correlates of emotional processing in depression: Changes with cognitive behavioral therapy and predictors of treatment response. *Journal of Psychiatric Research*. 2011; **45**(5): 577–587.

38. Fu C, et al. Neural responses to sad facial expressions in major depression following cognitive behavioral therapy. *Biological Psychiatry*. 2008; **64**(6): 505–512.

39. Yoshimura S, et al. Cognitive behavioral therapy changes functional connectivity between medial prefrontal and anterior cingulate cortices. *Journal of Affective Disorders* 2017; **208**: 610–614.

40. Assaf M, et al. Neural functional architecture and modulation during decision making under uncertainty in individuals with generalized anxiety disorder. *Brain Behav*. 2018 August; **8**(8): e01015.

41. Kennedy SH, et al. Differences in brain glucose metabolism between responders to CBT and venlafaxine in a 16-week randomized controlled trial. *American Journal of Psychiatry*. 2007; **164**(5): 778–788.

42. Konarski JZ, et al. Relationship between regional brain metabolism, illness severity and age in depressed subjects. *Psychiatry Research: Neuroimaging*. 2007; **155**(3): 203–210.

43. Dichter GS, Felder JN, Smoski MJ. The effects of brief behavioral activation therapy for depression on cognitive control in affective contexts: An fMRI investigation. *Journal of Affective Disorders* 2010; **126**(1): 236–244.

44. Burgess PW, Dumontheil I, Gilbert SI. The gateway hypothesis of rostral prefrontal cortex (area 10) function. *Trends in Cognitive Sciences*. 2007; **11**(7): 290–298.

45. Wright P, et al. Dissociated responses in the amygdala and orbitofrontal cortex to bottom–up and top–down components of emotional evaluation. *Neuroimage*. 2008; **39**(2): 894–902.

46. Jollant F, et al. Decreased activation of lateral orbitofrontal cortex during risky choices under uncertainty is associated with disadvantageous decision-making and suicidal behavior. *Neuroimage* 2010; **51**(3): 1275–1281.

47. Fales CL, et al. Antidepressant treatment normalizes hypoactivity in dorsolateral prefrontal cortex during emotional interference processing in major depression. *Journal of Affective Disorders*. 2009; **112**(1–3): 206–211.

48. Harmer CJ, et al. Antidepressant drug treatment modifies the neural processing of nonconscious threat cues. *Biological Psychiatry*. 2006; **59**(9): 816–820.

49. Tiger M, et al. Reduced 5-HT(1B) receptor binding in the dorsal brain stem after cognitive behavioural therapy of major depressive disorder. *Psychiatry Res*. 2014; **223**(2): 164–170.

50. Goldapple K, et al. Modulation of cortical-limbic pathways in major depression: Treatment-specific effects of cognitive behavior therapy. *Archives of General Psychiatry*. 2004; **61**(1): 34–41.

51. Brody AL, et al. Regional brain metabolic changes in patients with major depression treated with either paroxetine or interpersonal therapy: Preliminary findings. *Archives of General Psychiatry*. 2001; **58**(7): 631–640.

52. Martin SD, et al. Brain blood flow changes in depressed patients treated with interpersonal psychotherapy or venlafaxine hydrochloride: Preliminary findings. *Archives of General Psychiatry*. 2001; **58**(7): 641–648.

53. Sanacora G, et al. Increased cortical GABA concentrations in depressed patients receiving ECT. *American Journal of Psychiatry*. 2003; **160**(3): 577–579.

54. Sanacora G, et al. Cortical γ-aminobutyric acid concentrations in depressed patients receiving cognitive behavioral therapy. *Biological Psychiatry* 2006; **59**(3): 284–286.

55. Abdallah CG, et al. Decreased occipital cortical glutamate levels in response to successful cognitive-behavioral therapy and pharmacotherapy for major depressive disorder. *Psychother Psychosom*. 2014; **83**(5): 298–307.

56. Costafreda SG, et al. Neural correlates of sad faces predict clinical remission to cognitive behavioural therapy in depression. *Neuroreport*. 2009; **20**(7): 637–641.

57. Siegle GJ, et al. Toward clinically useful neuroimaging in depression treatment: Prognostic utility of subgenual cingulate activity for determining depression outcome in cognitive therapy across studies, scanners, and patient characteristics. *Archives of General Psychiatry*. 2012; **69**(9): 913–924.

58. Ressler KJ. Amygdala activity, fear, and anxiety: Modulation by stress. *Biological Psychiatry*. 2010; **67**(12): 1117–1119.

59. Dunlop BW, et al. Functional connectivity of the subcallosal cingulate cortex and differential outcomes to treatment with cognitive-behavioral therapy or antidepressant medication for major depressive disorder. *Am J Psychiatry*. 2017; **174**(6): 533–545.

60. Thompson DG, et al. fMRI activation during executive function predicts response to cognitive behavioral therapy in older, depressed adults. *American Journal of Geriatric Psychiatry* 2015; **23** (1): 13–22.

61. Forbes EE, et al. Reward-related brain function as a predictor of treatment response in adolescents with major depressive disorder. *Cognitive, Affective, & Behavioral Neuroscience*. 2010; **10**(1): 107–118.

62. Fu C, et al. Neural responses to sad facial expressions in major depression following cognitive behavioral therapy *Biol Psychiatry*. 2008; **64**(6): 505–512.

63. Carl H, et al. Sustained anterior cingulate cortex activation during reward processing predicts response to psychotherapy in major depressive disorder. *J Affect Disord*. 2016; **203**: 204–212.

64. Dichter GS, Felder JN, Bodfish JW. Autism is characterized by dorsal anterior cingulate hyperactivation during social target detection. *Social Cognitive and Affective Neuroscience*. 2009; **4** (3): 215–226.

65. McGrath CL, et al. Pretreatment brain states identify likely nonresponse to standard treatments for depression. *Biological Psychiatry*. 2014; **76**(7): 527–535.

66. Yoshimura S, et al. Cognitive behavioral therapy for depression changes medial prefrontal and ventral anterior cingulate cortex activity associated with self-referential processing. *Social Cognitive and Affective Neuroscience*. 2013; **9**(4): 487–493.

67. Konarski JZ, et al. Predictors of nonresponse to cognitive behavioural therapy or venlafaxine using glucose metabolism in major depressive disorder. *Journal of Psychiatry & Neuroscience: JPN*. 2009; **34** (3): 175.

68. Seminowicz D, et al. Limbic–frontal circuitry in major depression: A path modeling metanalysis. *Neuroimage*. 2004; **22**(1): 409–418.

69. Critchley HD, et al. Neural systems supporting interoceptive awareness. *Nature Neuroscience*. 2004; **7**(2): 189.

70. Fujino J, et al. Anterior cingulate volume predicts response to cognitive behavioral therapy in major depressive disorder. *J Affect Disord*. 2015; **174**: 397–399.

71. Sambataro F, et al. Anterior cingulate volume predicts response to psychotherapy and functional connectivity with the inferior parietal cortex in major depressive disorder. *Eur Neuropsychopharmacol*. 2018; **28**(1): 138–148.

72. Pizzagalli DA. Frontocingulate dysfunction in depression: Toward biomarkers of treatment response. *Neuropsychopharmacology*. 2011; **36**(1): 183.

73. Burkhouse KL, et al. Neural reactivity to reward as a predictor of cognitive behavioral therapy response in anxiety and depression. *Depress Anxiety*. 2016; **33**(4): 281–288.

74. DeRubeis RJ, Strunk DR. *The Oxford Handbook of Mood Disorders*. Oxford University Press; 2017.

75. Salvadore G, et al. Anterior cingulate desynchronization and functional connectivity with the amygdala during a working memory task predict rapid antidepressant response to ketamine. *Neuropsychopharmacology*. 2010; **35**(7): 1415.

76. Keedwell P, et al. Neural markers of symptomatic improvement during antidepressant therapy in severe depression: Subgenual cingulate and visual cortical responses to sad, but not happy, facial

stimuli are correlated with changes in symptom score. *Journal of Psychopharmacology* 2009; **23**(7): 775–788.

77. Weigand A, et al. Prospective validation that subgenual connectivity predicts antidepressant efficacy of transcranial magnetic stimulation sites. *Biological Psychiatry*. 2018; **84**(1): 28–37.

78. Wu J, et al. Prediction of antidepressant effects of sleep deprivation by metabolic rates in the ventral anterior cingulate and medial prefrontal cortex. *American Journal of Psychiatry*. 1999; **156**(8): 1149–1158.

79. Kringelbach ML, Rolls ET. The functional neuroanatomy of the human orbitofrontal cortex: Evidence from neuroimaging and neuropsychology. *Progress in Neurobiology*. 2004; 72(5): 341–372.

80. Kurth F, et al. A link between the systems: Functional differentiation and integration within the human insula revealed by meta-analysis. *Brain Structure and Function*. 2010; **214**(5–6): 519–534.

81. van der Werff SJ, et al. Neuroimaging resilience to stress: A review. *Frontiers in Behavioral Neuroscience*. 2013; 7: 39.

82. Drevets WC, Price JL, Furey ML. Brain structural and functional abnormalities in mood disorders: implications for neurocircuitry models of depression. *Brain Structure and Function*. 2008; **213**(1–2): 93–118.

83. Shin LM, Liberzon I. The neurocircuitry of fear, stress, and anxiety disorders. *Neuropsychopharmacology*. 2010; 35(1): 169.

Index